STRONG
MEDICINE

STRONG MEDICINE

How to Save Canada's Health Care System

MICHAEL RACHLIS, M.D.
AND CAROL KUSHNER

HarperPerennial
HarperCollins*Publishers*Ltd

First published in hardcover by HarperCollins Publishers Ltd: 1994
First HarperPerennial edition: 1995

Canadian Cataloguing in Publication Data

Rachlis, Michael
    Strong medicine : how to save Canada's health care system

1st HarperPerennial ed.
Includes index.
ISBN 0-00-638061-1

1. Medical care – Canada.   2. Medical policy – Canada.   3. Public health – Canada.   I. Kushner, Carol.   II. Title.

RA395.C3R33 1995   362.1'0971   C94-932391-8

---

95 96 97 98 99 ❖ HC 10 9 8 7 6 5 4 3 2 1

This book is dedicated to two of Canada's greatest health care system visionaries—Dr. Vince Matthews and Mother Marguerite D'Youville. As Medical Officer of Health for Swift Current in the 1950s, Dr. Matthews was decades ahead of his time in linking public health with a more efficient health care delivery system. Two centuries earlier, Mother Marguerite D'Youville founded the Order of Gray Nuns in Montreal and became the first in Canada to demonstrate the power of primary care nursing to heal the health care system.

Contents

Tables

Figures

Preface

This book is about saving Medicare, Canada's most popular social program. After almost twenty-five years' experience, it's very clear that the principles governing our system for public health insurance work well by enabling Canada to provide the fruits of modern health care to all of our citizens. However, we are convinced that in order to save Medicare for future generations, we must make major changes in the way we organize and pay for health and health-related services.

We know that some readers will be disappointed that we haven't focused more attention on the other more important determinants of health—the social, economic, and environmental conditions that shape the quality of our lives, and hence our health. However, we think it is absolutely crucial for Canada to fix its health care delivery system now, before we lose public health insurance altogether. That said, we hope to redeem ourselves by writing yet another book specifically addressing the development of a broad strategy for health (as opposed to health care) in Canada.

In preparing the text of *Strong Medicine*, we have made every effort to be clear by using common terminology to explain some key medical or scientific concepts. However, we have also relied on endnotes wherever additional detail seemed necessary to fully explain a complex point or to delve into some side issue not immediately relevant to the principal argument. We hope that academic readers will agree that, by and large, technical precision has not been sacrificed as a result.

We have used the following convention when making reference to specific case examples. We give a last name initial whenever an individual has requested anonymity or when the profile is really a composite of typical cases. Our use of full names for patients is reserved for real people who either have given their permission to be identified or have already gone public.

We think Medicare's potential has only begun to be expressed. The problem is that old habits, old ways of doing things, may be blinding us to what's really possible. We want Canadians to develop a more expansive vision of Medicare's future.

This doesn't mean, however, that we think we have all of the answers. In fact, we've barely tapped into the creativity and innovation of Canada's health care policy makers, researchers, and service providers. However, by sharing some of these ideas from around the country, we hope that we can kickstart some needed reform and help Medicare survive—and even thrive— into the twenty-first century and beyond.

After our first book was published (*Second Opinion: What's wrong with Canada's health care system and how to fix it*; HarperCollins, 1989) it was a great pleasure to hear people say we had provoked them to think about health policy in a different way. We hope this book, too, will stimulate debate and invite readers to address their comments to our publisher. Constructive feedback has always been a positive force in our thinking and we look forward to a continued dialogue with our readers.

Of course even *two* authors need considerable assistance to write a book of this scope, so we would like to thank a number of people who helped to make *Strong Medicine* a reality. First, we would like to thank the hundreds of people working in the health care system and in government who agreed to be interviewed. We would particularly like to thank the provincial civil servants who helped us to assemble our material on health costs. Thanks also to Rick Hudson, Jonathan Lomas, Julia Abelson, Greg Stoddart, Stephen Birch, the Polinomics discussion group, and Joel Lexchin who read portions of our text and helped to make it more accurate and intelligible. (Obviously, though, the opinions and conclusions expressed in the text are our own and should not be attributed to anyone else.)

We are very grateful to our editor Catherine Marjoribanks for her patience and her sage advice. Thanks also to the wonderful staff at HarperCollins, and especially to Tom Best who continued to see the potential in our work and offered us endless encouragement. We would like to thank our agent, Dean Cooke, and his predecessor, the late, great Peter Livingston. Michael Rachlis continues to owe a great debt to the faculty and staff of the Department of Clinical Epidemiology and Biostatistics and the Centre for Health Economics and Policy Analysis at McMaster University and wishes to thank the instructors and students involved in the Health Policy Analysis course at McMaster over the past four years. He would also like to sincerely thank his parents for instilling in him the twin values of social justice and efficiency in public services.

Finally, we both want to thank our friends, and especially our families—Danny, Debby, Linus and Leila—for their unflagging love and support.

STRONG MEDICINE

Chapter 1

Medicare:
Miracle or Mistake?

ON HIS WAY TO A MEETING of health and finance ministers in June 1992, Chris Decker, then Newfoundland's health minister, was down in the dumps. "I'm beginning to think," he said, "that maintaining a universal health care system into the next century may not be possible unless we become filthy rich all of a sudden."[1] Many of his provincial counterparts seemed similarly discouraged.

The provinces are having a hard time coping. Declining federal support for health care and falling tax revenues at home continue to curb their capacity to finance government programs. The recession's lasting impact adds a further measure of gloom as thousands of the unemployed join the welfare rolls each month. Today, for the first time since its inception, our health care system—the crowning jewel of Canada's social programs—is directly behind the eight ball as governments search for ways to control deficits.

The threat to Medicare's* future is substantial. Health care— the single largest spending item in provincial budgets—has become an obvious target for restraint initiatives. Suggestions about how to curb government liability for health care abound. For example:

---

* Strictly speaking, the term "Medicare" refers to our system for insuring the costs of physician services. But today it is widely understood to encompass all publicly financed health care services, including those received in hospitals or long-term-care facilities, as well as drug benefit programs, home care, and other services. We use the term in its widest meaning.

- British Columbia economist Michael Walker, from the Fraser Institute, argues that health care services in Canada should become a taxable benefit. This would mean that the sickest among us—those with the highest health care costs—would pay more.[2]
- Private clinics are now doing 40 percent of cataract surgeries in Alberta and are charging patients $1,000 out of their own pockets. Ignored is the fact that waiting times in the publicly funded system for this non-urgent operation could easily drop to weeks instead of months if proper management systems were in place.[3]
- A group of disaffected physicians in British Columbia have completely opted out of the provincial health care plan and are now charging patients directly for their services.[4]
- The Ontario government is working with its medical association to come up with a list of services to delist from the provincial health insurance plan, hoping to decrease costs by $20 million. The proposals include everything from routine annual health exams to sterilization reversals to inserting testicular prostheses in cancer patients. Initially, patients wanting these services will be stuck paying for them alone. But ultimately the decision to delist services could throw patients into the arms of the private insurance industry.
- It's no secret that at least two provinces (Alberta and Quebec) would like to introduce user fees to health care, despite evidence that charging patients does not achieve the policy objectives they claim.

Tax-back schemes, privatization, opted-out doctors, cutbacks on benefits, user fees—all of these so-called solutions make it look as if publicly financed health insurance, Medicare itself, were the real problem. It's not. If our political leaders are determined to pursue these kinds of policy changes, Medicare in Canada will soon be a fond memory. What we'll end up with instead is a two-tiered system where ability to pay rather than need determines who gets care. Overall costs for health care will rise, not fall, as private insurance steps in to fill the void left by retreating government programs. The wealthy and the healthy will do fine. Poor people—and especially those who are sick—will not.

So before we go down this path any further, Canadians need to know that our method for financing health care insurance is fundamentally sound. Public health insurance provides universal coverage and has helped to hold Canada's health care spending in check. But our health care system isn't strapped for cash, either. Both points are key to understanding how to save Medicare.

What really needs fixing is the unplanned, uncoordinated, and unaccountable way we deliver health care. Making these repairs will involve fundamental changes in how we plan, organize, and pay for health care delivery. As far as we're concerned, the target we should all be aiming at is a better system for all Canadians.

Symptoms of Dysfunction

In September 1993, Judy L., age fifty-two, discovered a small knot of tissue in her left breast. It was cancer. Because the tumour was small and appeared localized, Judy's doctor recommended removing the lump alone (lumpectomy) instead of removing the entire breast (mastectomy).

Following the lumpectomy, Judy needed to have post-operative radiation therapy to forestall the recurrence of cancer in that breast. But when Judy left the hospital after her surgery, she found she'd have to wait twelve weeks to get radiation treatment in Toronto, where she lived. That was too long to wait, according to Judy's doctor, and he offered an alternative. She could get treatment right away if she agreed to travel to Sudbury or Thunder Bay. Ontario's ministry of health would pay for her accommodation and meals during her stay, but she'd have to pay the transportation costs herself.

Feeling both scared and angry, Judy got in touch with a local breast cancer support group and found she wasn't alone—in the previous six weeks, eight other cancer patients from Toronto had travelled north for radiation treatment. In fact, between June 1992 and January 1993, 228 breast cancer patients—mainly from Toronto—were referred out of town for treatment.[5] "Apart from giving birth to my children, this was the first time I ever felt totally dependent on Medicare," Judy said. "I always thought it would be there for me when I really needed it. Now I feel let down, betrayed, and frightened."

What Judy's case reveals is a serious problem of mismanagement in health care delivery. To pinpoint how the health care system failed this patient we can look to a number of factors: a lack of planning, a lack of standards governing medical treatment, and an appalling lack of coordination. In combination, these failings lower the quality of care and the quality of service that should be available in our system.

To begin with, the Ontario Cancer Treatment and Research Foundation has been warning the Ontario government of an impending problem with access to radiation treatment since 1985. The incidence of all types of cancer between 1981 and 1988 grew at about 0.7 percent a year.[6] This modest growth is partly due to the aging of our population but also to the increase in screening tests for certain cancers.* Referrals to radiation treatment are growing at 8 percent a year, primarily because of changing physician practice behaviours. For example, more and more surgeons are treating breast cancer with lumpectomy (removal of the cancer alone), which requires post-operative radiation. According to Dr. Meakin, the Ontario Cancer Treatment and Research Foundation's senior policy adviser, about half of all cancer patients could benefit from radiation treatment, but in Ontario only 35 percent are getting access to the service.**

Furthermore, there are currently no standards to guide the delivery of breast cancer treatment and, as a result, the approaches to treatment vary widely from doctor to doctor. A recent Ontario study found forty-eight different approaches to how long patients should receive radiation treatments, ranging from three to five weeks. Doctors apparently also disagree about the dosage of

---

* Some breast cancer screening is worthwhile, but some is of dubious value, as is most screening for prostate and colon cancer. We discuss screening further in Chapter 4.

** Radiation is also an excellent way to relieve pain caused by certain advanced cancers like breast and prostate, but too few patients are presently getting it for palliation.

radiation breast cancer patients need, since this varied too, by over 50 percent.[7] While all centres radiate the entire breast, some also give a "booster" shot of radiation targeted directly at the tumour site. In general, it appears that doctors are tending to favour longer and longer treatment schedules, even though there is no clinical evidence showing that it actually improves survival,[8] and despite the fact that it adds to professional workloads and increases the cost of care.

Another key factor also varies from centre to centre—the productivity of the doctors. The radiation oncologists in Toronto see 50 percent fewer new patients than those in Hamilton. And those in Hamilton see 50 percent fewer new patients than those in Halifax. The oncologists in Toronto do more research than those in Hamilton or Halifax, and clinical research is obviously very important to determine better management of cancer patients. But less than half the difference in the number of patients being seen is due to research activities. Dr. Meakin points out that radiation oncologists in the United States stick to the technical part of the job and leave the responsibility for overall patient care to the internists. By contrast, radiation oncologists in Canada, like those in Britain, typically assume responsibility for all the patient's care needs. In other words, members of this high-demand specialty have developed a practice style in Canada that severely limits their ability to take on new patients—an important factor in waiting lists.[9]

And it isn't as if the non-human resources are used much more efficiently. Radiation machines operate fourteen hours a day in British Columbia, ten hours a day in Ottawa and London, Ontario, but only eight hours a day in Toronto.[10]

The media play a role in the general confusion as well. News reports in 1993 described a "breast cancer radiation crisis" but hardly ever mentioned that radiation therapy does not improve survival.*[11] This point doesn't trivialize the therapy—it is clearly necessary. But, on the other hand, the spectre of women being forced to travel *to save their lives* fuelled the panic. In fact, many cancer patients don't properly understand their true

---

*Radiation therapy *does* prevent recurrence of cancer in the same breast, but it does not appear to stop the cancer from spreading to other sites of the body.

situation, even when their doctors feel they have effectively communicated with them.[12]

Put all of this together and a rather frightening scenario emerges—one characterized by poor planning, a lack of standards, an inefficient use of existing resources, and poor communications. Nor can we comfort ourselves that these kinds of problems are confined to cancer treatment alone. On the contrary, similar examples can be found throughout our health care delivery system.

The challenge facing us now—and the major focus of this book—is to come up with a plan to address these kinds of shortcomings systematically. We can reduce the enormous amount of waste in our system. We can improve the appropriateness of care, and by doing so, boost quality and efficiency. We can protect the people who work in the system, too, by involving them directly in operational decisions and by implementing labour adjustment programs that offer employment security as a starting point. But readers should take heed: stop-gap measures won't work. Nothing short of a fundamental restructuring in how we plan, organize, and pay for health care services will do the job.

How Canadians Value Health and Health Care

A scan of our Constitution, the Canada Health Act, and various provincial commissions reviewing health care in Canada over the past decade reveals a core of values that we think ought to guide the development of any comprehensive, system-wide reform.[13] Table 1.1 offers a list of Canadian values for health and health care derived from these sources.

Ethicists often subdivide values into two categories: "essential" and "instrumental." Essential values are those that should be maximized as long as doing so doesn't threaten other essential values. Instrumental values are those that help achieve essential values.[14]

Equity is arguably the most important value held by Canadians with regard to health and health care. Over the years, most of the arguments about public health insurance have centred on the issue of equality of access to health care services. Furthermore, equality of opportunity for well-being is set out as an objective of Canadian confederation in Section 36 of our Constitution:

Table 1.1

CANADIAN VALUES FOR HEALTH AND HEALTH CARE

Essential Values

1. EQUITY

- Canadians should have equal opportunity to achieve health and well-being.
- Canadians should have equal opportunity to receive health services according to their needs.

2. QUALITY

- Canadian should enjoy as high a quality of life as possible.
- Canadians deserve high-quality health care.

3. INFORMED CHOICE

- Canadians should be encouraged to make informed choices about their health care.

Instrumental Values

1. HEALTHY ENVIRONMENTS

- Public policy should focus on ensuring that all Canadians live in social, economic, human-built, and natural environments that enhance health and encourage healthy choices.

2. ACCOUNTABILITY

- Health care providers should be accountable for the public money they receive—including being accountable for the quality of care patients receive.
- Citizens should be accountable for their choice of primary care provider.

3. EFFICIENCY

- Because resources are finite, it is important that health care services are delivered in the most efficient fashion possible.

4. CITIZEN PARTICIPATION

- Canadians should be encouraged to participate fully in their own care and the care of their families.
- Canadians should be able to participate meaningfully in decisions about their health care system.

> 36. (1) Without altering the legislative authority of Parlia-
> ment or of the provincial legislatures, or the rights of
> any of them with respect to the exercise of legislative
> authority, Parliament and the legislatures, together
> with the government of Canada and the provincial
> governments, are committed to
> (a) promoting equal opportunities for the well-being
>   of Canadians;
> (b) furthering economic development to reduce dispar-
>   ity in opportunities; and
> (c) providing essential public services of reasonable
>   quality to all Canadians.
>
> (2) Parliament and the government of Canada are
> committed to the principle of making equalization
> payments to ensure that provincial governments have
> sufficient revenues to provide reasonably comparable
> levels of public services at reasonably comparable lev-
> els of taxation. [15]

This section holds Ottawa responsible for making sure that
every province has the means to deliver comparable levels of
health care services. In other words, equity appears to be the
underlying value.

In 1984, Parliament unanimously passed the Canada Health
Act. The following five key policy directions for health and for
health care are derived from its preamble and from Section 3.[16]

1. Health policy is much more than health care services.
2. Achieving any health status objective requires a multi-
   sectoral approach.
3. The purpose of health care is to improve the health
   status of all Canadians.
4. Health care services should be available without
   undue barriers.
5. The federal government should continue to help the
   provinces fund their health care systems.

But our health care system doesn't properly reflect these values.
We spend almost all our money for health on treating illness.

And there seems to be little accountability in the delivery system. In fact, the health care system seems to be built on the assumption that all you have to do is make sure there's a doctor and a hospital bed available when a Canadian thinks she needs one.

The Evolution of Public Support for Medicare

When Canadians are asked to name the biggest difference between Canada and the United States, the short answer is often "Medicare." We'd be hard pressed to name a more popular publicly funded program. Poll after poll confirms how much we value the principle of universal access to health services, and how proud we are of having constructed such an equitable system. A September 1993 Gallup poll, found 96 percent of Canadians preferred Canada's system to the one in the United States.[17] The same survey also showed that public confidence in the quality of care our system delivers is also on the rise—89 percent rated it as good or excellent, up from 71 percent in 1991.[18]

But Canadians didn't always attach so much importance to what doctors and hospitals do. In fact, when Canada's first constitution, the British North America Act, was passed in 1867, all of the areas judged to be really important or expensive came under federal jurisdiction—defence, maritime shipping, the regulation of trade and commerce. Responsibility for health care, on the other hand, fell to the provinces.[19] In all probability, this was because health care was something of a flop in the nineteenth century. With little effective treatment to offer, what physicians did was only of minor social and economic importance. The few hospitals in operation in 1867 served marginal populations—for the most part, those who were destitute and dying.

The regulatory environment for health care was equally underdeveloped. Ontario didn't even have a licensing body for doctors until 1869.[20] Surgery was a rare and very painful event in the pre-anaesthesia era, and those brave or desperate enough to risk it often succumbed to massive post-operative infections. These kinds of drawbacks were well understood by the public. Everyone knew that the doctors' pills, purgatives, and leeches were just as likely to harm as to heal them.

However, while curative health care was largely dismissed as ineffective during the nineteenth century, public health, and its forte, prevention, were enjoying the limelight. There were no effective medical treatments for the major health threats of the day—cholera, typhoid, whooping cough, diphtheria, tuberculosis, and other, often deadly, infectious diseases. Antibiotics weren't widely available until after the Second World War. Prevention aimed at stopping the spread of infectious disease was the only viable option. And it worked remarkably well. Death rates from infectious diseases continued their decline as the public health movement gained influence and as living conditions improved. Soon, people came to think of safe water and food, adequate housing, and better working conditions as health issues.

Over the first half of the twentieth century, major advances in biology, chemistry, and human anatomy gradually improved the scientific basis for medical care. As new, more successful treatments were discovered, people began to switch allegiance, attaching less and less importance to public health as the reputation of modern medicine grew. During the Second World War, new surgical techniques came on stream. Doctors rescued soldiers from certain death. The public, understandably impressed by these successes, was even more dazzled when drugs like penicillin became widely available after the war. These "magic bullets" worked so well against infection that they seemed almost miraculous.

It wasn't long before people began seeing the treatment of disease as the single greatest contributor to health. Some people thought that medical science would eventually be able to conquer all human illness. It was just a matter of time.

At the turn of the century, Canadian life expectancy at birth was a mere forty-nine years.[21] By 1950, it had risen to sixty-nine years, largely due to a sharp decline in death rates from infectious disease and tremendous advances in infant survival. Most people thought doctors and hospitals deserved the credit. It took the work of Dr. Thomas McKeown and other epidemiologists to show that these improvements in longevity had little to do with medical treatment.[22] The reason was a simple matter of timing. The bulk of the improvement had already occurred, thanks to better housing, clean water, safe food, and sewers. By the time medicine had something that really worked against these diseases, all that remained was a mop-up job.

The health care system does have some spectacular successes. For example, vaccines for polio and smallpox have virtually eliminated these diseases. But nowadays, among experts, there's little disagreement: how we live, how we love, and what we do for a living—these are the things that really count when it comes to being healthy.

Unfortunately, public perception hasn't fully caught up with this new understanding. Many people still believe that health care is the most important health determinant. It was this conviction, of course, that helped garner public support for publicly funded health insurance. But the downside to overemphasizing the role played by formal health care services is that it has led to a top-heavy system, too reliant on hospitals and doctors and too neglectful of the kinds of social policies and public health programs that could have prevented much of the illness we see today.

Changing Times, Changing Attitudes

Canadian health economists Robert Evans and Greg Stoddart have developed a useful series of models to describe how our understanding of the relationship between health care and health status has evolved over time.[23] Figure 1.1 reproduces the first of these models and represents the kind of thinking prevalent in the 1940s and 1950s, when Canada and other nations were debating whether to set up national health programs.

In Figure 1.1, all the various external factors that might make people sick or keep them healthy are completely ignored. There's an assumption here that as long as people can get access to health care, we don't need to understand what causes illness at all. The model can be compared to the thermostat in your house—the more illness there is, the more health care is provided to treat it. Theoretically, the "temperature" setting on health care's thermostat could be turned down when all health needs are met. Lord Beveridge, who was one of the key individuals behind Britain's National Health Service (the "grandfather" of national health programs), predicted in the 1940s that when everyone had access to health care, the demand for care would decrease over time as their needs were met.[24] But of course he was overly optimistic. Health care systems everywhere in the

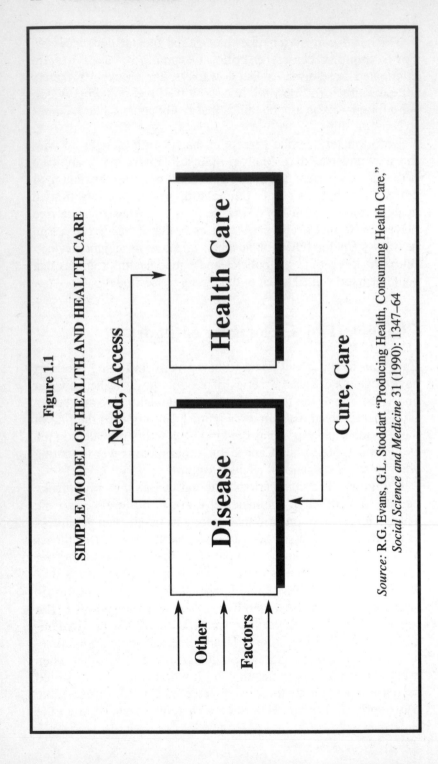

Figure 1.1

SIMPLE MODEL OF HEALTH AND HEALTH CARE

Source: R.G. Evans, G.L. Stoddart "Producing Health, Consuming Health Care," *Social Science and Medicine* 31 (1990): 1347–64

western world have developed a rather astonishing capacity for expansion. Not only are new treatments and therapies entering the field all the time, but new needs get defined as well. All sorts of life's passages have been medicalized—childbirth, adolescence, menopause, dying. And all kinds of problems have been redefined as health care needs—baldness, infertility, anxiety, stress, and so forth.

Even today, a number of misconceptions underlying this conceptual model of health are still alive and well. For example, the public generally believes that:

- experts don't know very much about what causes illness or what keeps people healthy;
- as long as people have access to health care, there's no need to understand what causes health and illness;
- medicine is a precise science—almost devoid of discretion;
- it's easy to define the necessity for medical care.[25]

Let's take a look at each of these beliefs in turn.

Experts don't know what causes illness or what keeps people healthy

In the 1940s and 1950s, this may have been true to some extent, but today, we actually know quite a bit about how health is determined. The World Health Organization's *Ottawa Charter for Health Promotion* is deservedly confident in asserting that "the fundamental conditions and resources for health are peace, shelter, education, food, income, a stable eco-system, sustainable resources, social justice and equity; improvement in health requires a secure foundation in these basic prerequisites."[26]

A recent report by the Ontario Premier's Council on Health Strategy outlines the evidence that these broad influences really are the major determinants of health.*[27] This work singles out the strong correlation between social and economic well-being and health status, noting that, as the gaps between rich and poor narrow, the health status of a population improves.

_____

*The Ontario Premier's Council on Health Strategy was renamed the Premier's Council on Health, Well-being, and Social Justice in 1990.

Quebec's Commission d'Enquête sur les services de santé et les services sociaux (the Rochon Commission of 1988) came to similar conclusions in its review: "Over the last twenty years, we have made considerable progress in developing knowledge in this area: the influence of risk factors and the synergistic effects which may exist between them are all the more clearly defined. In the light of such knowledge, prevention takes on new strategic importance: it is now possible to influence directly certain determinants which are a condition to the appearance of health problems."[28]

However, Canada has had some difficulty translating this knowledge into policy and practice. In this respect, there's a lot we could learn from other jurisdictions. Consider, for example, the approach France took to reducing its infant mortality rates. As in North America, France experienced a dramatic drop in newborn death rates during the 1970s. Most of the improvement here and in Europe had to do with new and better treatments. The rate of premature births, however—a major predictor of infant mortality—had barely budged. The scope for prevention was still enormous.

In the early 1980s, the French government put in place a set of social and economic policies aimed directly at reducing the risk of premature birth. For example, the French government began paying women to attend prenatal sessions and provided them with food supplements during pregnancy. Maternal leave before delivery was expanded to nine weeks. Pregnant women in Paris were given thirty minutes off at the beginning and end of each working day so they wouldn't have to cope with the most hectic part of rush-hour traffic.

The results of these policies were impressive—rates of prematurity fell by 30 percent, and the rate of very-low-birthweight babies dropped by half![29] Today, French infant mortality rates are, along with Canada's, among the lowest in the world, but the French purchased their health improvement with healthy public policies, not treatment.

There's an added bonus to the approach France took. Being born too small often means a lifetime of disability and the need for ongoing and costly medical interventions. But if prematurity is prevented in the first place, so that more and more babies are born full-term, infants have a better chance of reaching a normal birthweight and going on to live a normal life.[30]

As long as people have access to health care, there's no need to understand what causes health and illness

If health care were able to cure most illnesses, and were very inexpensive, this might be true. However, real cures are very rare and treatments are often costly. Even spectacular treatment successes like heart surgery and dialysis usually don't cure the problem. As the late physician-philosopher Dr. Lewis Thomas explained, most medical treatments are *halfway* technologies.

New approaches to most common ailments, like breast and lung cancers, have hardly improved survival at all.[31] It's usually far more efficient to prevent than to treat. Also, while medical and hospital treatment can be very important for some people at some times, they play a relatively small part in determining the overall health status of a population.

In general, *health care cannot compensate for the ill effects imposed by adverse social, economic, and environmental conditions.* When Canadians fall ill they often find themselves like poor Humpty Dumpty, with a problem that cannot be cured, even by "all the king's horses and all the king's men." As startling evidence of treatment's inability to produce health, poor Canadians die at twice the rate of wealthy Canadians, despite reasonable access to the world's most expensive publicly funded health care system.[32]

Medicine is a precise science, virtually devoid of discretion

This assumption is equally misleading. Many people assume that for every set of symptoms there is only one possible cause, an equally straightforward, commonly accepted way to diagnose the illness, and an agreed-upon best way to treat it. Nothing could be further from the truth. Medicine is rife with alternative ways to diagnose and treat illness. A given condition—like heart disease, for example—might be suitable for therapy with drugs, surgery, diet, exercise, stress management, or a combination of the above. Many alternative approaches to treating the same disease have never been evaluated, making it impossible for practitioners to know which ones really work best. To say that medicine is still very much an art, as well as a science, is far more accurate. In fact, real artistry in medicine is necessary precisely because there is so much uncertainty in medical decision-making. But uncertainty isn't the only problem. Sometimes patients don't get the right care at the right time in the right place because the system itself gets in the way. The lack of evidence-based standards, the prevalence of badly designed systems and processes for delivering care, the influence of perverse financial and professional incentives—all of these problems interfere with the quality of care available in our system.

The amount of inappropriate care that has been documented would probably come as a shock to the many people who assume our health care system has a sophisticated approach to quality assurance. At least one-third of services given are either unlikely to help patients or cost more than an equally effective alternative. Patients are often denied the chance to express their own preferences about treatment options and report feeling ill-informed about risks and benefits of various alternatives. The problem of inappropriate care isn't trivial—it kills thousands of Canadians every year and costs the system billions of dollars.

It's easy to define the need for medical care

This is the final faulty assumption tied to the thermostat model for health care. Culture plays a major role in defining the need for health care. For example, the French, Germans, British, and Americans approach certain health practices and illness treatments very differently.[33] As well as modifying personal and professional behaviour, culture also influences the allocation of health care resources. In Europe, for instance, it's quite common for public health insurance to cover visits to health spas for "rest cures," virtually unheard of as an insured benefit in North America. Here in Canada, public health insurance won't pay for relaxation programs or exercise classes, even though both have been shown to delay the onset of coronary heart disease and some other illnesses.[34]

What gets covered is a ticklish issue. Should we consider infertility treatment medically necessary? There's no clear-cut answer. The Canadian Medical Association says that infertility treatment should be considered a health service, but not necessarily one eligible for public insurance coverage.[35] Meanwhile, Canada's Royal Commission on Reproductive Technology recommends that only women whose fallopian tubes are blocked should be eligible for in vitro fertilization (IVF) as an insured service, since other causes of infertility are not as likely to be helped by this technology.[36] To complicate the confusion, Ontario pays for all IVF services while other provinces don't. Sorting it all out is far from easy.

It may not always be practical to try. For example, in 1993, the Ontario Medical Association and the provincial government began searching for $20 million worth of medical services to delist to reduce health care costs. Early on in the process, the repair of torn earlobes was identified as a promising candidate for the chop, but when women's groups pointed out that torn earlobes were a common injury among victims of wife abuse, a compromise was recommended: continuing coverage for assault victims, but dropping it for those whose earlobes were torn from wearing heavy earrings. This illustrates the danger of instituting sweeping policies about who and what gets covered. Many times what constitutes appropriate care depends on cultural acceptability, individual circumstances, and patient preferences. In our view, these exercises to define "medical necessity" are a waste of time.

The question of who needs care is also closely related to the question of which health care provider they should see and what type of service they really need. The term *medical* necessity actually implies the need for a *doctor*, but many services that could benefit patients don't require a physician's extensive training. In fact, some community nursing programs can reduce death rates by 25 percent or more—a record any doctor would envy.[37]

Guardians and Traders: Improving Health versus Improving Health Care

An important step in making our health care system more efficient and effective is to examine the respective roles of governments and service providers. Medicare is often called a government-run system, but of course only the insurance side is publicly administered. Most doctors are in private practice and most hospitals are non-profit, private corporations.* Is this the right public/private mix? What role, if any, should governments play in health care delivery?

---

*Some hospitals are owned by governments—psychiatric hospitals, for example.

Toronto author Jane Jacobs is highly regarded as an original thinker. Her critical insights about how urban design affects city life have revolutionized modern planning principles.[38] In her most recent book, *Systems of Survival: A Dialogue on the Moral Foundations of Commerce and Politics*, Jacobs looks at working life and deduces two completely different moral systems—one for government and one for business. Doing the right thing, according to Jacobs's analysis, very much depends on being clear about what it is you're doing and which moral system applies.

Jacobs explains that in human civilizations, some people maintain order and stability, while others create wealth. Over thousands of years, these two distinct realms of activity have relied on separate, but complementary, value systems: one dictating how politicians and government officials should behave, the other laying down the rules and conventions for commercial enterprises.

One set she labels "Guardian values," since the *raison d'être* for those who govern is to guard territory and protect the population. Guardian values include (among others) fortitude, loyalty, adherence to tradition, respect for hierarchy, and a prohibition against engaging in trade. By contrast, the chief objective of Traders is to make deals and earn money by meeting, and profiting from, the needs of individuals. Trader values include (among others) efficiency, innovation, dissent for the sake of the task, initiative, and a prohibition against the use of force. A complete list of Guardian and Trader values from Ms. Jacobs' book is offered in Table 1.2. Notice how the values in each syndrome are internally consistent but at odds with those in the other syndrome. Guardians value obedience; Traders value dissent for the sake of the task. Traders value innovation, while Guardians adhere to tradition.

Some might think this framework is merely an artificial construct, but in fact, there's strong evidence of its *organic* nature. The Guardian and Trader value syndromes are very consistent in explaining the behaviour of both individual humans and their institutions. For example, according to medieval law in Europe a man couldn't train to become a knight if even one of his eight great-grandparents had engaged in commercial activities. Japanese samurai faced a similar prohibition. Two completely different societies and cultures held a common view that deal-making experience—of the type common in normal, everyday

Table 1.2

THE GUARDIAN AND TRADER VALUE SYSTEMS

The Guardian Value System

Shun trading
Exert prowess
Be obedient and disciplined
Adhere to tradition
Respect hierarchy
Be loyal
Take vengeance
Deceive for the sake of the task
Make rich use of leisure
Be ostentatious
Dispense largesse
Be exclusive
Show fortitude
Be fatalistic
Treasure honour

The Trader Value System

Shun force
Come to voluntary agreements
Be honest
Collaborate easily with strangers and aliens
Compete
Respect contracts
Use initiative and enterprise
Be open to inventiveness and novelty
Be efficient
Promote comfort and convenience
Dissent for the sake of task
Invest for productive purposes
Be industrious
Be thrifty
Be optimistic

Source: Jane Jacobs, *Systems of Survival: A Dialogue on the Moral Foundations of Commerce and Politics* (Toronto: Random House, 1993).

business operations—could make the military vulnerable to bribery and other kinds of corruption. To avoid this possibility, Guardians throughout history, and in many different cultures and societies, have tended to shun trading.

As in the past, modern-day governments value loyalty, observe traditions, enjoy dispensing largesse, and institute policies to protect the interests of the collectivity. So Guardian values are very much alive and well today. Similarly, our current crop of entrepreneurs, whether engaged in for-profit or not-for-profit activities, all tend to esteem efficiency, innovation, and the primacy of the individual, as good Traders should.

Jacobs's framework also helps to explain why governments have so much difficulty with innovation. A public official faces severe consequences for taking the kind of risks involved in new ventures. A civil servant foolhardy enough to take ten risks could easily lose her job, even if only one of the risks turns out badly and the rest succeed. A 90 percent success rate couldn't protect her (or her minister) from the fallout produced by a single major disaster. On the other hand, a commercial trader might be quite happy to score only one win in ten tries—provided the success was a big one, and the losses from the failures were limited.

One potential criticism is that Ms. Jacobs's analysis is somewhat coloured by a nineteenth-century, liberal view of government. Historically, Canadians have been more comfortable with a more significant and interventionist role for government than Americans ever have.[39] Our system of universal public health insurance is a good example of this difference.

Also, a quick read-through of the values for each syndrome might leave you with the impression that Guardian values are somehow less admirable than the Trader values. In fact, Jacobs herself stresses the interdependency of Guardians and Traders, pointing out that Traders really need Guardians to enforce the basic societal rules governing honest dealings and respect for contractual obligations. "Each syndrome," she points out, "is good for its functions, and if you mix them up—if you try to run a government as if it were a business—it is a disaster. Or if you try to run a business as if it were a government it is equally a disaster. You must have both syndromes. Each is bad in the wrong place, but each is necessary and good for its suitable function."[40] Without Guardians minding the shop, Traders would be constantly tempted to cheat. Good Guardians are essential to keep criminal activity in check, allowing businesses to prosper in a regulated, yet relatively free, environment. By the same token, Guardians must rely on successful and innovative Traders to create wealth and provide the tax base.

Now, what relevance does all this have to saving Medicare and reforming our health care system? In a word, plenty. Protecting the public's health and ensuring access to necessary health care are essential Guardian activities. Only the state can set limits on individual freedoms to protect the public's well-being. An overall strategy to improve the health of Canadians may involve other players, but government action to set broad policy goals, pass laws, and enforce regulations is absolutely central.

By contrast, delivering health care is more of a Trader activity, one that could benefit enormously from individuals who are committed to the comfort and convenience of patients and who value innovation, industriousness, and thrift. Guardians do not share these values, a factor that helps explain why governments have generally failed to introduce new delivery structures to prevent and treat illness. Innovations like these, so natural to the culture of Traders, are alien to Guardian capacities.

The new delivery system for health care proposed in this book has made extensive use of Jacobs's analysis. In our proposed system, governments will be able to concentrate on their main job—setting the overall goals for the system and creating the right environment for achieving them. Health care providers, meanwhile, will have much more freedom to exercise their Trader instincts.

Revenge of the "Zombies"

Any offer to radically change Canada's health care system along these lines must first deal with longstanding beliefs about what is really wrong and how to fix it. Some of these beliefs are supported by good evidence; others are not. Most curious of all are those ideas that ought to have been killed off completely because the evidence against them is overwhelming.

Economist Robert Evans calls them "Zombies," ideas "that are really dead intellectually, but keep returning from the grave, bumping into things, doing damage." And the idea that user fees would somehow help our health care system is his favourite example.

User fees

User fees for health care are primarily a mechanism for redistributing wealth: the wealthy and the healthy gain; the sick and the poor lose.[41] In reviewing the evidence, it is clear that user fees do not achieve the policy objectives most often put forward by their proponents:

* user fees do not control health care costs;
* nor do they improve appropriateness of care;
* nor do they improve access by injecting more resources into the system.

Some political leaders think people who can afford it should pay at least some of their health care costs directly. Despite evidence to the contrary, they think user fees would fix our health care system. Both Quebec premier Daniel Johnson and Alberta premier Ralph Klein have seemed determined to introduce them.[42] During her leadership campaign, former prime minister Kim Campbell seemed willing to go along and let provinces that wanted to "experiment with user fees." This blooper, and the Reform Party's adamant insistence that provinces should be free to finance health care any way they wish, helped make Medicare a federal election issue in 1993.

The idea that user fees make good economic sense remains stubbornly persistent, a topic we explore in more detail in Chapter 6.

Private insurance for health care

The arguments for private health care insurance, like those for user fees, are seductive but intellectually dead. A rigorous economic analysis shows clearly that private health insurance is a market failure.[43]

There are three key reasons this is so. The first is that private health insurance cannot take advantage of the inherent *economies of scale* available when the insurance function is consolidated within a single public utility. In the United States—where private insurance predominates—administrative costs are six times higher than in Canada.[44] Then, too, a private system has to spend resources on marketing, and is supposed to make a profit, neither of which apply to a public system. Furthermore, a single, large public insurer is in a much better position to leverage better prices from health care providers than a large number of private insurers.

A second factor causing market failure in private health insurance is the tricky problem of *knowing how much to charge*. We simply don't have enough information to figure out a fair premium rate that factors in the eventual future health costs related to current hazardous risks or exposures. This is a particular problem for occupational diseases with a long time delay between the original exposure to the hazard and the development of an illness in response to it.

A third factor is the problem of *adverse selection*. Consumers have one advantage over insurers: they know their own risk status better than insurers do. And naturally people who expect to need health care will be more likely to purchase health insurance than those who judge that their risk of illness is slight. However, people who know their health status is good aren't going to be happy paying premiums that, in effect, subsidize the costs of those at greater risk.

Private insurers in the United States have tried to deal with this problem by switching from community-wide rate setting to experience-based rate setting. Under the former, all individuals in the community pay the same premium; under the latter, health care costs for a given group of subscribers are monitored and premium rates are adjusted according to their actual use of health care. Of course, this means that people with poorer health will face much higher premiums. Private insurers in the United States have responded to adverse selection rather ruthlessly, by focusing on groups to share the risk and increasingly refusing to provide coverage to individuals. There are many Americans who are truly at low risk for claims who cannot buy a policy at any price. Public insurance avoids this problem altogether. Everyone pays for coverage through their taxes, and in those provinces where health insurance premiums are in effect, there is no adjustment of the cost to reflect individual or group risks. As a result, everyone is covered and no one is penalized because of poor health status.

Taken together, these factors make an excellent case for choosing public over private health insurance,[45] a decision Canada made in stages over a period of twenty-five years.[46] Indeed, for any country that values equity and efficiency, there is only one reasonable way to finance the bulk of health care services—and that is through the public purse.

The belief that Canada's social spending is too high

Over the past five years or so, Canada's social safety net has been under attack from a number of business leaders, economists, and editorial writers. While we agree that our social programs desperately need reform, there is a last zombie that fuels the political demand for change—that Canada's social spending is way out of line, especially considering the extent of our public debt and the persistence of government deficits.

It may surprise you to know that in Canada, government spending as a proportion of our national income (GDP) actually fell during the 1980s. According to Statistics Canada, government program spending contributed only about 6 percent to the growth in our national debt during the 1980s, while tax breaks for high-income families and corporations contributed 50 percent, and high interest-rate policies 44 percent.[47]

We have no desire to minimize the problem of debts and deficits. In fact, we understand that Canada's current situation is serious. We appear to be in a debt trap, which one economist and senior public servant, Michael Mendelson, traces back to 1974 when changes in taxation policy inadvertently weakened the relationship between economic growth and tax revenues.[48]

However, we want to emphasize that Canada's social spending compares well with what other countries spend. We may look like profligates next to Mexico or the United States, but not when you compare our level of social spending to what's spent in European countries.

Even though Canada's *public* spending on health care is near the top of the twenty-four countries belonging to the Organisation for Economic Cooperation and Development, Canada's total social spending in 1990 ranked seventeenth (out of twenty)*

---

*Only ahead of Japan, the United States, and Portugal.

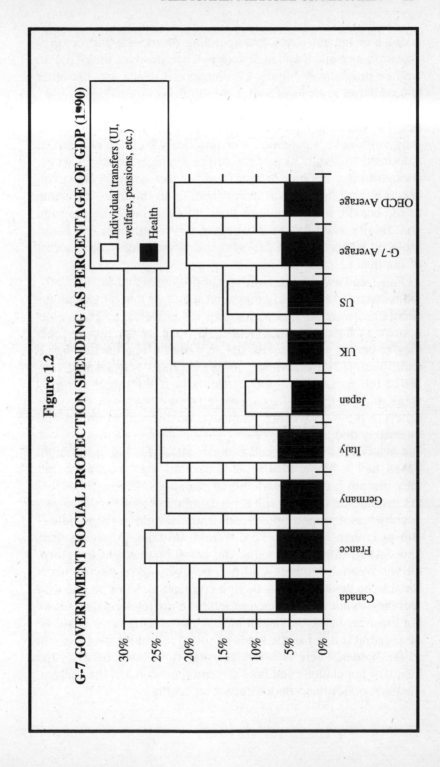

Figure 1.2

G-7 GOVERNMENT SOCIAL PROTECTION SPENDING AS PERCENTAGE OF GDP (1990)

because of our relatively low spending on income support programs. France and Sweden devote twice as much of their GDP to welfare programs.[49] Figure 1.2 compares Canada and the other G-7 countries in terms of social spending.

A lot has changed since we first developed our social safety net. For example, back in 1945, Canada's family allowance program was very generous. For families with three children, it amounted to about 20 percent of the average industrial wage, enough to pay the rent or buy food for the month![50] However, because this program was never indexed to inflation, the value of the benefit was allowed to dwindle over time. The program was finally axed by the Mulroney government in 1993 and replaced with a targeted program that benefits only the poorest of families.

This trend away from entitlement programs and towards programs targeted at special groups has a danger that all Canadians should be aware of. When programs are universal, everyone has a stake in how well they work. As long as the public feels they're getting some benefit, it's very difficult politically to discard them. However, when a program serves only a small subset of the population—and particularly if the target group is weak and poorly organized—there is enormous risk that over time the program will lose support, be allowed to erode, and ultimately disappear altogether.

Canada's tax levels are also under attack for being too high. Taxes may be higher than some Canadians want them to be, but they are not high by international standards. Comparing 1992 tax revenues in Canada with those from other modern developed countries as a proportion of GDP finds us right in the middle.[51] But of course, people have different attitudes to paying their taxes when they really value the services they get in return. Oliver Wendell Holmes said he positively liked paying taxes because he thought he was buying civilization.[52] For people who feel they're not getting much in return, a tax revolt makes sense. On the other hand, the health impact of reducing taxes could be devastating if it led to the kinds of social inequities we see south of the border. There is a fundamental connection between the health of populations and how governments conduct themselves. Taxation policy has a major impact on health.

The Federal Role for Health Care

Much is made of the fact that under Canada's Constitution, health care is a provincial responsibility. However, according to Mr. Justice Estey, health policy may be considered the responsibility of either the federal or provincial governments.[53]

> Health is not a subject specifically dealt with in the *Constitution Act* either in 1867 or by way of subsequent amendment. It is by the Constitution not assigned either to the federal or provincial legislative authority. Legislation dealing with health matters has been found within the provincial power where the approach in the legislation is to an aspect of health, local in nature ... on the other hand, federal legislation in relation to "health" can be supported where the dimension of the problem is national rather than local in nature ... or where the health concern arises in the context of a public wrong and the response is criminal prohibition.... In sum, "health" is not a matter which is subject to a specific constitutional assignment but instead is an amorphous topic which can be addressed by valid federal or provincial legislation, depending in the circumstances of each case upon the nature of scope of the health problem in question.[54]

At a time when Ottawa is considering off-loading even more responsibility for health care onto provincial shoulders, this legal opinion establishes a basis for continued federal involvement. Just as Jane Jacobs's analysis of Guardians and Traders clarifies distinct roles for government and the private sector, we need sensible criteria for assigning roles for the federal and provincial governments in health and health care.

Only the federal government can ensure that health care coverage is portable across the country. Only the federal government is in a position to conduct national health surveys. In fact, it makes economic sense for the bulk of basic health research to be funded federally. But it makes sense for health care services to be planned and managed at the provincial level, or even closer to home. In fact, some provincial governments are already devolving the day-to-day administration of health care to regions and communities.

Ottawa must sustain its cash contributions to the provinces if we are to maintain a truly national system. Unfortunately the federal finance minister, Paul Martin, Jr., is looking to the provinces to solve his financial problems, while the provincial ministers are looking to Mr. Martin for the same quick fix. If Canada's treasurers can work together, and if Ottawa keeps cash flowing to the provinces, health ministers, caregivers, and consumers could revamp Medicare for the twenty-first century and beyond. If we maintain our system of public insurance but make fundamental changes in our delivery system, Canadians will have a double win: we'll save Medicare and have better health care for all Canadians.

Chapter 2

Is Medicare Affordable?

JUST LIKE CLOCKWORK, every fall and spring, newspapers and television reports are full of stories about "the crisis in Medicare." But the "crisis" described depends very much on the messenger. People who work in health care often argue that the system needs more money because it is underfunded. Meanwhile, those who pay the bills—government officials and politicians—claim that health care costs are going through the roof and cannot be sustained. Where does the truth lie?

The claim that the system needs more money has been soundly refuted by a series of authoritative analyses. Almost every province in Canada has conducted a major review of health care in the past decade.[1] None of the reports published in the last five years supports the claim that the system is generally underfunded.

But the idea that skyrocketing costs are making Medicare unaffordable has gripped some of Canada's most prestigious political leaders. Their solution? To shift more costs to the private sector.

Quebec and Alberta are flirting with user fees. Even NDP governments—traditionally strong supporters of social programs like Medicare—are moving quickly to dump certain services and cut eligibility for programs.*

---

* Bob Rae's Ontario government, for example, has delisted a number of drug products from the provincial benefit formulary. Saskatchewan has also decreased eligibility for its public drug program.

Are they right? Is Medicare now unaffordable? Will more private spending help? Let's look at the facts.

The Price Tag

This year, Canadians will spend over $70 billion on health care.[2] If you're like most people, a figure as large as this is utterly incomprehensible, so let's put it into understandable terms. Assuming you have a stack of thousand-dollar bills, with about one hundred to the inch, the average person could reach in and grab a couple of handfuls totalling more than a million dollars without any trouble at all. But $70 billion stacked this way translates into a pile of money over ten miles high! Put another way, it represents over $2,500 for every man, woman, and child in the country—enough to feed a family of four for a year, or to purchase a new colour TV and VCR every three months. Get the picture?

About $50 billion, or 72 percent of total health spending, is publicly funded, mainly through general tax revenues. Some provinces (British Columbia, Alberta, and the Yukon Territory) also charge health insurance premiums, and some (Ontario, Manitoba, and Quebec) levy payroll taxes that are ostensibly for health care.

The remaining $20 billion (28 percent) represents private spending on health care. This includes products and services not covered by provincial insurance plans—including, for example, what you pay for additional dental or extended-care insurance, or what you spend on drugs, eyeglasses, or visits to alternative medical practitioners.[3]

More relevant to the question of affordability than how much money is spent or where the money comes from is the question of whether the current level of funding is appropriate. Are we paying too little, too much, or the just the right amount? Is spending out of control, or is the system starved for lack of funding? Before addressing these questions, let's examine how Canada's much-praised health care system came into being. Table 2.1 presents a chart outlining key dates and events in the development of the Canadian system.

Table 2.1

A THUMBNAIL HISTORY OF MEDICARE

1947   Saskatchewan's CCF government implements public health insurance for hospitals.

1948   Mackenzie King's Liberal government passes the **National Health Grants Program**—mainly used to build hospitals.

1957   St. Laurent's Liberal government passes the **Hospital Insurance and Diagnostic Services Act.**

1962   Saskatchewan's CCF/NDP government implements the **Medical Care Insurance Act** on July 1, and 90 percent of the province's doctors stage a three-week strike.

1966   Pearson's Liberal government passes the **National Medical Care Insurance Act (Medicare)**, implemented in 1968.

1971   All provinces in Canada are fully participating in Medicare.

1977   Trudeau's Liberal government and the provinces negotiate the **Established Programs Financing Act (EPF)**, replacing fifty-fifty cost-sharing for health care with per capita "block grants" to the provinces. Federal funding under EPF is supposed to grow at the same rate as the Gross National Product.

1983   Trudeau's Liberal government imposes anti-inflation measures on the post-secondary education portion of the EPF grant. This lowers the overall base on which future EPF growth is calculated.

1984   Trudeau's Liberal government passes the **Canada Health Act**, which sets out penalties for provinces that allow hospital user fees and physician extra-billing.

1986   Mulroney's Conservative government changes the growth formula for EPF—now it is tied to GNP growth minus 2 percent.

1990   Mulroney's Conservative government passes **Bill C-69,** freezing EPF for three years, after which future EPF growth will be based on GNP minus 3 percent.

1991   Mulroney's Conservative government passes **Bill C-20**, which freezes EPF growth for an additional two years—making a five-year freeze in total—before the new growth formula (GNP minus 3 percent) comes into effect. Also, C-20 makes it possible for Ottawa to withhold *any* federal transfer payments from provinces in breach of the **Canada Health Act.**

The Rocky Road to National Health Insurance

Access to medical care became a major public policy issue as early as 1919, when Mackenzie King convinced the Liberal Party to adopt national health insurance as part of its platform. Various provincial parties took up the issue over the next decade.[4] In 1933, the Regina Manifesto made national health insurance a key plank in the platform of the Cooperative Commonwealth Federation (CCF).

In 1945, a federal-provincial conference was convened to develop plans for a variety of social programs, including a draft bill for national health care, with federal-provincial cost sharing.[5] But the plan faltered because the provinces objected to federal intrusion into this area of provincial jurisdiction.

Instead, North America's very first universal public health insurance program got its start in Saskatchewan, when Tommy Douglas's CCF government implemented hospital coverage in 1947.

Douglas's commitment to public health insurance can be traced back to a key early experience. As a boy in Winnipeg, he'd developed a bone infection in his leg (osteomyelitis). The attending doctors recommended amputation, but, fortunately for Douglas, an orthopaedic surgeon, Dr. R.J. Smith, offered to try to save the leg if Tommy's parents agreed for the boy to be a teaching case. The treatment was successful and Douglas went on to become, among other things, an amateur boxer, a powerful orator, and a very successful politician. Douglas believed that he would have lost his leg if Dr. Smith hadn't kindly offered his services for free.[6]

Former Saskatchewan Premier Allan Blakeney, who served in the Douglas government, recalls how this incident affected his colleague's political views:

> He regarded the recovery that enabled him to do these things as something that had come to him by pure accident, sheer luck. I suppose he would say it was by divine grace, and he was going to see that he spread around the divine grace as much as he could. He had that passion when he became premier, and he was a very strong-willed man, very able and bright. Charismatic. Stubborn.[7]

Those qualities helped Douglas "sell" his plan for publicly funded health insurance, a plan predicated on the idea that "health services ought not to have a price tag on them, and that people would be able to get whatever health services they required irrespective of individual capacity to pay."[8]

The federal government entered the health care arena in 1948 with a National Health Grants Program, fulfilling a small part of its wartime commitment to introduce cost-shared social programs. This program made grants available to provinces for a variety of initiatives, but most of the funds were used to build or improve hospitals, which, at the time, were considered to be inadequate in number and outdated. The federal program set off a boom in hospital construction across the country that was to continue for more than three decades.

British Columbia introduced a hospital insurance program in 1948. Then Newfoundland entered Confederation in 1949, bringing its cottage hospital system. Cottage hospitals served people in the outports and provided care to almost half the province's population through provincially owned facilities in which doctors were paid salaries.[9] In 1950, Alberta also developed a hospital insurance plan, but it only covered the poor.

By 1955, five provinces (Saskatchewan, Newfoundland, British Columbia, Alberta, and Ontario) had hospital insurance plans, but they were finding them very expensive to finance with provincial revenues alone. One of Canada's perennial problems is the fit between federal and provincial governments in terms of their revenues and responsibilities: Ottawa had most of the tax money, but the provinces had to pay for health care, and they wanted Ottawa's help.

Hospital Insurance and Diagnostic Services Act

Pressure from an unlikely source—Ontario's Conservative Premier Leslie Frost—was instrumental in convincing the federal government to respond.[10] In 1957, Parliament unanimously passed the Hospital Insurance and Diagnostic Services Act. With this legislation, Ottawa agreed to pay half the costs to provinces that set up hospital insurance plans. To qualify for funding, however, the provincial programs had to meet certain conditions:

1. Comprehensiveness.
2. Accessibility

3. Universality of Coverage.
4. Public Administration.
5. Portability of Benefits.

The program proved very popular, and in short order every province in Canada was participating. However, the new law meant that only hospital costs were covered; costs for treating patients in the doctor's office were not. As a result, many people were hospitalized for tests or procedures they could have received outside an institution. Because coverage depended not on *what* was done but on *where* it was done, over-reliance on hospitals became entrenched.

In the words of Evelyn Shapiro, former chair of the Manitoba Health Services and professor of medicine at the University of Manitoba, "We had rapid expansion in the institutional sector as a result, because it could be cost-shared, and very little movement in health promotion, home care support, and other terribly important health areas because, for the most part, they were not eligible for federal funding."[11]

Meanwhile, hospital construction continued. Between 1961 and 1971, the number of hospital beds increased twice as rapidly as the population (33 percent versus 18 percent) and occupancy levels remained at about 80 percent.[12]

Doctors come on board

When it came to providing public insurance for physician care, once again Saskatchewan led the way by passing the Saskatchewan Medical Care Insurance Act in 1961. The Canadian Medical Association had supported public insurance during the Second World War,[13] but by this time organized medicine was strongly opposed to government-sponsored insurance. Half of Canadians were now covered by private medical insurance, and the major insurers were doctor-sponsored, non-profit companies.[14] When the act came into force on July 1 of the following year, 90 percent of Saskatchewan's doctors went on strike for three weeks. Eventually, the strike was settled with the assistance of Lord Taylor, a British Labour member of the House of Lords.*

---

* Lord Taylor was also a practising physician who helped to launch Britain's National Health Service after the Second World War.

Four years later, Ottawa once again played catch-up with Saskatchewan by passing its own legislation, the Medical Care Act (1966), implemented in 1968. And again the carrot for participation was the federal government's offer to pay half the costs to any province that set up public insurance plans, this time for doctors' services. This act imposed the same conditions on provinces as the Hospital Insurance and Diagnostic Services Act but strengthened them:

1. Comprehensiveness—the provinces had to cover all "medically necessary" services inside or outside of hospitals.
2. Accessibility—the provinces had to ensure that services were "reasonably" accessible and provided on "uniform terms and conditions." This criterion also required reasonable compensation for health professionals.
3. Universality of Coverage—the act stipulated that 95 percent of the population had to be covered within two years.
4. Public Administration—the provinces had to administer their plans either directly or through a non-profit public agency fully accountable to the provincial government.
5. Portability—the provinces had to ensure that the benefits were portable from province to province.

Cracking the whip: the Canada Health Act

By the late 1970s, there were growing concerns that access to care was being threatened. Some doctors and hospitals were billing patients directly—charges that were over and above what they received from government. Ottawa responded by passing the Canada Health Act in 1984.

The act reaffirmed the program criteria for public health insurance and specified that the federal government could withhold some of its contribution from any province that breached them. But it was only specific about the penalties for user fees and extra-billing: the act stipulated that federal transfers to the provinces would be reduced, dollar for dollar, by the amount collected through direct charges to patients.

Despite strong opposition from organized medicine—including a brief doctors' strike in Ontario—all the provinces quickly complied with the new legislation.[15] User fees and extra-billing ceased within two years.*

The move to block funding

As the economic boom of the 1960s gave way to the "stagflation"** of the 1970s, the federal government grew concerned about its open-ended liability for health costs. Ottawa wanted a more predictable basis for budgeting. Besides, some provinces were unhappy with some of the restrictions inherent in the cost-sharing arrangements; they wanted more freedom to experiment with their delivery systems. For example, health policy analysts pointed to the folly of stimulating the construction and use of hospitals (the most expensive part of the system) while leaving out coverage for home care and nursing homes.

So in 1977, Ottawa and the provinces agreed on a new way to fund health care. The Established Programs Financing Act (EPF) abolished fifty-fifty cost sharing and replaced it with "block funding." This change completely uncoupled the link between provincial health spending and federal liability. No longer would it matter what the provinces spent on health care—the federal contribution was determined separately.

EPF consolidated the existing federal grants to the provinces for both health and post-secondary education. On the health side, in addition to funding for insured hospital and physician care, the grant also included cash transfers for extended health care (long-term care).

Total EPF grants grew in size along with the population and were also designed to increase at the same rate as the economy.

---

* Some physicians do charge patients, however, for services that are not insured. For example, some charge a $50 annual administrative fee to cover the costs of filling out forms for insurance companies, workers' compensation boards, and for providing "sick notes" for employers.

** The term "stagflation" was used to describe a new phenomenon—high inflation and high unemployment. Until then, most economists believed that high levels of unemployment would bring down inflation.

This meant, for example, that if health costs rose faster than the economy, the provinces had to make up the difference on their own. But, by the same token, if costs were contained, the provinces alone reaped the benefits.

The inner workings of EPF are very complicated. The total federal EPF grant comes in two forms: a tax portion and a cash transfer. The tax portion works like this: when EPF came into effect, the federal government decreased its personal tax rate by 13.5 percent and its corporate tax rate by 1 percent. This left the provinces free to increase their taxes without their citizens facing any new tax burden. The difference between the calculated value of the tax portion and the total EPF payment due from the federal government was made up in cash (the cash transfer).

In general, the larger and wealthier provinces were able to collect more of their EPF entitlement through taxes, while poorer provinces were more dependent on cash transfers. Also, Quebec negotiated a slightly different deal, arranging from the outset for a larger tax-point transfer from the federal government. Thus the cash portion of EPF in Quebec has always been smaller than in other provinces.[16]

Shaving the carrot and whittling away at the stick: changes to the EPF

The amounts represented by cash and tax transfers for insured health services under EPF were almost equal when the new block funding was implemented in 1977. But of course it was expected that, over time, cash transfers would drop as inflation and economic growth brought in larger and larger tax revenues, which would then make up an increasing proportion of the overall EPF grant. However, during the 1980s, the federal government took steps that speeded up the erosion of the cash portion.

The first blow came in 1983 when the Trudeau government applied anti-inflation guidelines to the post-secondary education portion of the total EPF contribution. This ratcheted down the base for future EPF calculations.

There was further erosion in 1986 when the Mulroney government changed the formula for increasing EPF. No longer would EPF grow at the same rate as the economy. The new formula linked EPF growth to GNP growth *minus 2 percent*. The most recent changes, introduced in the 1990 and 1991 federal budgets, froze the total EPF contribution for five years; after 1995, it will only grow by GNP growth minus 3 percent.

Although the per-capita EPF payment is still frozen, and will remain frozen until 1995, the value of the transferred tax points will continue to grow because of inflation and real economic growth. As a result, less and less cash is being transferred from the federal government year by year. Because of its special arrangement under EPF for a larger tax-point transfer, Quebec will run out of federal cash for insured health care services first, probably within the next five years. But under the current arrangements, within ten to fifteen years* no province in the country will be getting any cash under EPF at all.[17]

According to a recent paper by the C.D. Howe Institute, the rate of off-loading in health care has actually outpaced other federal spending reductions: "Despite the rhetoric from Ottawa, the health care system is one of the main areas that will bear the burden of federal deficit reduction. The future of Canadian health care may be determined as much by the decisions regarding a new sharing of taxation as by changes in the way health care is actually delivered."[18]

It's important at this point to remember that, constitutionally, the federal government cannot regulate health care or health insurance. Health care is a provincial responsibility. Of course, Ottawa did find a way around this limitation. The power of the federal purse—the enticement of hard cash—was key to creating a nationwide approach to Medicare. Without this kind of active fiscal federalism, Canada's poorest provinces would likely never have been able to establish public health insurance.** But cash from Ottawa also represents the only federal lever available to enforce Medicare's program criteria. So the

---

* The exact timing depends on economic growth and population increases.

** Even with this help from Ottawa, the so-called have-not provinces devote a larger share of their income to health care than wealthier ones. For example, in 1987, Prince Edward Island spent 12.2 percent of its Gross Domestic Product on health care while Alberta spent only 7.7 percent. (Source: Health and Welfare Canada)

carrot is also a stick. Provinces that contravene the Canada Health Act stand to lose part of their EPF cash transfers.

So what happens when the federal cash dries up? How will Ottawa enforce Medicare then?

In its 1991 budget bill, the federal government specified that it could withhold other types of transfers from provinces that breach the Canada Health Act. In theory, this means that federal cash transferred under equalization, or for other cost-shared programs like social assistance or job training, can now be held back as a penalty. But this is only a technical solution.

Will Ottawa Enforce Medicare?

With the Liberals now in power, the question remains: is there real political will to save Canada's public health insurance plan? Recent cutbacks under the Tories betrayed waning federal support for all sorts of social programs:

- In 1990, the Progressive Conservative government imposed a 5 percent growth limit on cost-shared programs (including social welfare programs) under the Canada Assistance Plan for British Columbia, Alberta, and Ontario—the "wealthy" provinces.
- In 1992, Ottawa dropped its plans to introduce a national day-care program.
- In 1993, Ottawa reduced eligibility for unemployment insurance and shortened the benefit period. This meant that unemployed people who were unable to find work ended up on welfare rolls even sooner.

Will the Liberals follow a similar path in their promise to revamp social programs? When EPF was implemented in 1977, some critics worried that without direct federal cost sharing, Ottawa's commitment to enforce Medicare's program criteria would evaporate, and that providers and provinces would pursue their own narrower interests. Neither problem materialized in the short term. But more recent developments suggest that, in the long run, these critics might have been right to worry. The federal and provincial governments are due to renegotiate EPF by 1995. Will the feds pull out altogether to try to solve their fiscal problems?

Limits to enforcing accessibility and comprehensiveness

Figuring out whether provinces are meeting the criteria for accessibility and comprehensiveness really hinges on what's meant by "medical necessity" or "medically required"—the language used in the legislation. Neither the federal government nor any province has ever offered an operational definition of these terms. And frankly we think this may have been wise.

The accessibility criterion also stipulates service delivery on "uniform terms and conditions." In general, this has been interpreted to mean that patients must not face financial barriers to getting the care they need and is widely seen as key to preventing the development of a two-tiered system—one for the well-off and one for the poor. This was the interpretation used to outlaw extra-billing and user fees.

But accessibility as described in the act could also mean—at least theoretically—that similar patients are supposed to receive similar treatment. This would require health professionals to develop standards of practice for insured services, defining explicitly the best-known ways to investigate and treat specific conditions according to currently available scientific evidence. Right now, however, few explicit standards for clinical practice exist. The result? Some services that are useless or even dangerous are provided, while others, known to be effective, are unavailable.

For example, many experimental studies show that monitoring the fetus during labour is useless and probably dangerous for women at low or medium risk for a complication.[19] All the same, this technology is routinely offered in most Canadian hospitals that perform obstetric care. By contrast, high-quality scientific evidence shows that a trained labour attendant can reduce the rate of complications from labour and delivery for women without partners.[20] But, at best, there is scant provision of this type of service across the country.

Without operational definitions for "medically required" and "medical necessity," the federal government cannot meaningfully enforce accessibility or comprehensiveness.

Portability not enforced in Quebec

The portability criterion is meant to ensure that Canadians can receive care under similar conditions in different parts of the country. The province of Quebec has flouted this principle for years.

In 1988, nine provinces signed an agreement promising to pay the prevailing rates when their residents received hospital or medical care in other provinces. Although Quebec follows this practice for hospital services, it still refuses to respect the same policy for physician services. So when doctors in other parts of Canada treat Quebec residents, they receive only the amount that Quebec pays its own physicians for the service—which usually means less than their normal fee.* Despite complaints from provincial medical associations, Ottawa has never taken action to penalize Quebec for this breach.

Universality: provinces that levy premiums may be in breach

Provinces are theoretically free to raise the money for their health programs in any way they see fit, and health insurance premiums are not in any way prohibited by the Canada Health Act. However, the universality criterion is contravened if a resident is denied access to a "medically required" health care service because of failure to pay the premium.

It's a bit like defaulting on your taxes. Revenue Canada can take you to court and sue for the funds, but it can't cut off your mail delivery!

Today, Alberta, British Columbia, and the Yukon Territory all charge premiums for their health insurance plans. The Hall Review of Medicare in 1980 and other more recent reports[21] have documented instances in which residents have been denied access to services because they haven't paid their premiums. The federal government has never investigated this possible breach.

---

* Quebec has, however, signed an agreement with Ontario to pay physicians in the Ottawa area treating Quebec patients at their normal rate of reimbursement.

Except for violations of "accessibility," penalties are not explicitly defined

As mentioned earlier, Ottawa can deduct one dollar from its cash contribution for each dollar of user fees or extra-billing permitted within a province. This penalty proved sufficient to enforce the accessibility criterion—provinces stopped extra-billing and dropped user fees soon after the Canada Health Act was imposed. But when other program criteria are contravened, the act offers no specific penalties.

It's up to the federal government to decide whether to investigate a possible breach. Then it's up to Ottawa to decide whether or not there has been a breach. And finally, even if the federal government finds that a province is in breach, it's still up to Ottawa to determine the amount of the penalty. This highly discretionary process allows the federal government too much leeway. Politics rather than policy could easily determine Ottawa's response. Overall, we conclude that the Canada Health Act is largely unenforceable, with the exception of penalties for user charges.

Armed with some background about Medicare's evolution and current policy status, let's return to our original question concerning health funding: is Medicare affordable?

Too Little? Just Enough? Or Too Much?

According to Professor Robert Evans, a health economist from the University of British Columbia:

> the Canadian health care system has achieved a remarkably good record in both preserving universal access to comprehensive coverage and moderating the growth of health care costs. This performance has been outstanding in comparison with that of the U.S. system, which displays accelerating cost escalation, increasing radical institutional change and deteriorating equity. The Canadian performance also looks good in comparison with that of Western Europe—a more demanding comparison.[22]

Let's look at the facts. By the time all the provinces were fully participating in Medicare back in 1971, health care costs for the country were around $7 billion.[23] Since we're spending $70 billion now, that means costs have gone up 1,000 percent in the past sixteen years!

But using current dollars obscures the fact that the purchasing power of money has declined over time. Think of your own expenditures—you may be spending twice as much on clothes today as you were in 1971, but that doesn't necessarily mean you're buying twice as much clothing. If you use constant dollars to eliminate the effects of inflation, you might discover that spending on your wardrobe has gone up only 25 percent. By using constant dollars to analyse health care costs, we find that health care spending in Canada has more than doubled over the same period.[24]

Economists prefer yet another method for analysing expenditures. They like to express health care costs as a proportion of our national income (Gross Domestic Product, or GDP).* This accomplishes two things: it eliminates the effect of inflation, and it puts spending in the context of affordability.

As income increases, so does the ability to spend. To return to our analogy, expressing your clothing purchases as a percentage of your income might show that you are spending about the same proportion of your wages on clothes today as you did in 1971. Even the effects of spending beyond inflation are softened because your income has gone up as well. If, however, you've become a slave to fashion in the meantime, such an analysis would reveal it by showing that you now spend a greater proportion of your revenues on clothing.

Medicare has kept health care affordable

In 1971, when all provinces had adopted Medicare, Canada was spending 7.4 percent of its GDP on health care. Twenty years later, in 1991, Canada was spending 9.9 percent of its GDP on health care.[25]

---

* The Gross Domestic Product (GDP) measures the value of production within Canada, regardless of who owns the means of production. The Gross National Product (GNP) is the GDP plus the interest, dividends, and income earned by Canadians from work and investment outside the country.

As you can see from Figure 2.1, Canada's health care spending was remarkably stable during the 1970s, with a more or less constant share of national income going to health care. In fact, full public financing for health care seems to have ended the cost escalations we were experiencing during the 1960s. In other words, Medicare in Canada actually kept health care affordable.

Things were not so clear in the 1980s, mainly because the decade was bracketed by two serious economic recessions. During the first one, health care began taking a bigger bite out of our GDP. Professor Robert Evans argues that the intervening recovery wasn't strong enough to make up lost ground before the next recession hit with full force. His analysis shows that if Canada had somehow managed to escape both recessions, we would still be spending the same share of our national income on health care as we did in 1970.[26] In addition, he points out that cost increases actually slowed during the 1980s as compared to the two previous decades.

And even though our per-capita expenditures are the highest in the world (except for the United States), health care spending in Canada also compares well with that of other developed countries. Wealthier nations tend to devote a higher proportion of their income to health care. Figure 2.2, using data from the Organisation for Economic Cooperation and Development (OECD), shows a straight-line relationship between per-capita GDP and per-capita health care spending. As you can see, Canada is just above the trend line. The United States, by contrast, shows the greatest discrepancy. Is it a coincidence that the United States is the only country that doesn't rely primarily on public financing for health care? (In the United States, 58 percent of health spending is private.)[27] We provide more details comparing American and Canadian health spending in Chapter 7.

Where you stand depends on where you sit

Of course, provinces don't take much comfort from this kind of evidence. After all, health spending is the single biggest expenditure in their budgets, ranging today from 24 percent in Newfoundland to 38 percent in Saskatchewan.[28] Health spending eats up so much of the provincial pie these days that there's little left for other public policy priorities.

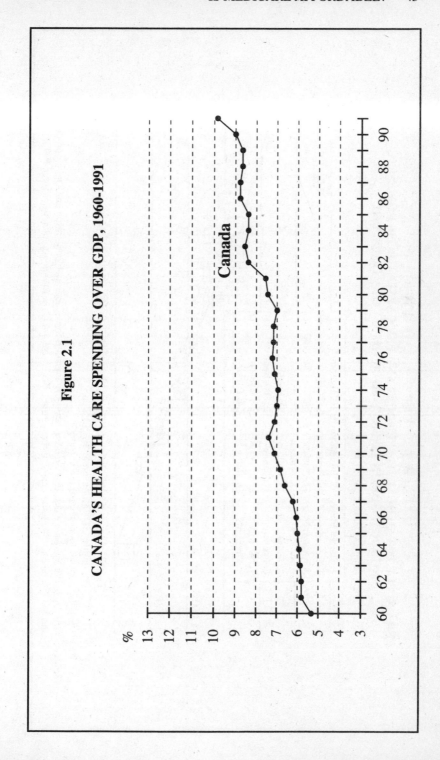

Figure 2.1

CANADA'S HEALTH CARE SPENDING OVER GDP, 1960-1991

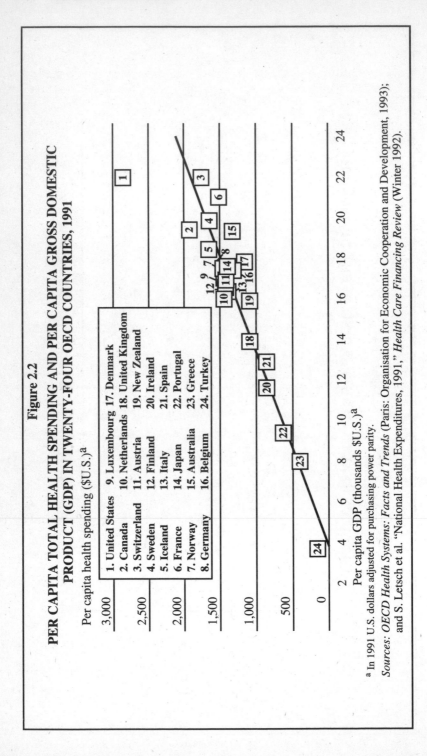

Figure 2.2

PER CAPITA TOTAL HEALTH SPENDING AND PER CAPITA GROSS DOMESTIC PRODUCT (GDP) IN TWENTY-FOUR OECD COUNTRIES, 1991

[a] In 1991 U.S. dollars adjusted for purchasing power parity.

Sources: OECD Health Systems: Facts and Trends (Paris: Organisation for Economic Cooperation and Development, 1993); and S. Letsch et al. "National Health Expenditures, 1991," *Health Care Financing Review* (Winter 1992).

And there are other pressures on the provinces. Progressive declines in federal cash transfers mean that provinces have to come up with more money for health care every year, just to stay even. Ontario, British Columbia, and Alberta have been doubly hit because of the billions lost through cutbacks in federal support for social programs since 1990.[29] High levels of unemployment and a sluggish economic recovery mean declining government revenues and persistent deficits. All of these factors combine to make health care a target of reform on every provincial agenda.

Some provinces have had particular health cost problems. In Ontario, costs exploded during the 1980s, rising at more than twice the rate of inflation during the decade—a period during which most other provinces were more aggressive in moderating health spending through a variety of cost-control mechanisms. But even in Ontario, the runaway train had to be halted. After a decade in which health spending increases averaged 11.2 percent, its 1992-93 health expenditures rose by less than 1 percent.

Where does the money go?

You don't have to be an economist to understand that financial incentives can influence decisions. If something's on sale, we're more likely to buy it. If you had a year's worth of free passes, you'd probably spend a lot more time at the movies. A bargain's a bargain.

When the public first funded hospital and physician services, the cost of the total package was shared fifty-fifty with the federal government. As long as the money went either to hospitals or doctors, every dollar the province spent was matched with another federal dollar. "This policy enticed governments to focus on doctors and hospitals," says Evelyn Shapiro.

Table 2.2 shows a breakdown of provincial government health spending for 1975 compared to 1991.

As you can see, there has been little change in the overall allocation of resources within health care. Admittedly, we've seen a slight decline in the allocation to hospitals, most notably in the amounts spent on capital. But this table shows that doctors have managed to stabilize their share. Home care's piece of the pie has certainly increased, but public health's share has

TABLE 2.2

PROVINCIAL GOVERNMENT HEALTH SPENDING IN CANADA, 1975 AND 1991

	1975	1991
Hospitals, other institutions, and capital expenditures	68.4%	60.0%
Physicians	20.3%	21.6%
Drugs*	1.7%	5.3%
Public health and home care	6.3%	5.7%
Other	3.3%	7.4%

* This category does not include drugs dispensed to patients in hospitals. In-patient drug costs are included with hospital, institution, and capital expenditures.

Sources: Health and Welfare Canada, *National Health Expenditures 1975–87*, and self-reports from all provinces except British Columbia.

actually declined. The most substantial change between 1975 and 1991 is the dramatically increased share going to drugs.

What's more, our spending pattern has barely been affected by a decade's worth of advice from provincial reports reviewing health care. Most of these studies urged less emphasis on acute hospital care and more on a variety of community-based options, such as home care. It hasn't happened, though—at least not on a large scale, not yet. The overall number of hospital beds in the system has declined, but hospitals are actually treating more patients than ever before; the only thing that has really changed is how they do business: many more procedures now are done on a same-day or short-stay basis.[30]

To understand why we haven't seen a dramatic shift towards community care, you need more information about the workings of our system. Let's begin by taking a closer look at hospitals, since they still control the bulk of resources.

Hospitals: The Kings of the Road

The greatest concentration of hospitals in Canada can be found within a stone's throw of the Ontario Legislature. The Toronto General Hospital,* the Hospital for Sick Children, Mount Sinai Hospital, The Queen Elizabeth Hospital, and Women's College Hospital are all within four hundred metres of Queen's Park. And if you expand the radius to about two kilometres you also capture Doctors' Hospital, St. Michael's Hospital, Wellesley Hospital, and many others.

Altogether, within two kilometres of Queen's Park, there are more than 3,300 active acute-care beds, 16,000 full-time and over 5,000 part-time jobs, and a total public expenditure of about $1.3 billion. [31]

It's not as if there's a shortage of beds in the suburbs, either. Extend the radius even further to include all of Metropolitan Toronto and you'll find an additional 6,500 beds. In total, there are just under 9,800 beds for a population of 2.2 million.**

The big hospitals in the downtown core occupy a particularly privileged position, and their proximity to government officials and political decision-makers has paid off handsomely. Former ministry of health and hospital employees freely admit that decisions concerning where to put new programs and how much funding to give them have often been driven by politics rather than need. As one beleaguered bureaucrat put it, "When you know the Premier and the hospital CEO are good buddies, rational planning flies out the window."

---

* The Toronto General Hospital amalgamated with the Toronto Western Hospital to form the Toronto Hospital in 1988.

** It should be noted that Toronto's major teaching hospitals also serve patients who live outside of Metro, especially those referred for highly specialized treatments. Also, Metro's hospital system used to have considerably more beds. Between 1986 and the end of September 1993, 4,800 of Metro's beds, representing just under 30 percent of the total, were permanently or temporarily taken out of service.

Too many hospitals

Of course Toronto isn't the only city with too many hospitals; it's a problem for the entire country. Take Saskatchewan, which has more hospital beds per capita than any other province, many of them in rural facilities too small to deliver cost-effective, high-quality acute care. "Saskatchewan is a Cree word meaning 'too many hospitals,'" jokes Steven Lewis, CEO of the province's Health Services Utilization and Research Commission.

But Saskatchewan's leaders understand the political risks involved in doing anything about the surplus. Back in 1971, Ross Thatcher's Liberal government was ousted, at least in part because they had announced their intention to close nine rural hospitals. Ever since, politicians have been wary of touching the issue. In the spring of 1993, however, the province's dismal economic outlook forced action, and the NDP announced that fifty-two small rural hospitals would lose their acute-care funding. Some will continue to provide long-term care while others will be reconfigured as ambulatory care centres.

Duplication

Another factor in hospital spending is that many small communities are served by more than one hospital. There's too much duplication. As the late Duncan Gordon, former chair of Toronto's Hospital for Sick Children, was fond of pointing out: "Look at the number of communities we have in Canada that have a Catholic hospital on one block and a Protestant one on the next. Each trying to outdo the other, to keep its grip on the community. No one ever questions whether a town of 50,000 really needs two hospitals."

And, of course, when more than one hospital serves a community, the tendency is for them to compete with each other on the basis of resources, staff, and equipment. Each tries to be the best. There's little motivation for rationalization since that means someone has to give something up.

Take, for example, Lethbridge, Alberta. The Lethbridge Regional Hospital, which opened in November 1988, has thirty-five surgical beds, nine ICU beds, and three operating rooms that have never been opened for use. Another three operating rooms are equipped but have no funding for staff. Two hundred metres away sits St. Michael's Hospital, built forty years ago. The provincial government planned to completely rebuild St. Michael's at a cost of $75 million.[32] The new hospital would have focused on long-term care, but the renovations would also have included at least sixty-five acute-care beds and three operating rooms. And, although the community needs long-term care beds now, the acute-care beds were to be built first. Representatives of the Regional Hospital and others in the community asked Alberta's premier and health minister to reconsider their decision, but provincial officials refused.[33] Finally, in the fall of 1993, the Klein government announced major health care cuts and shelved St. Michael's redevelopment plans.

Winnipeg has two open-heart surgery units. Consolidating the two would lower costs and likely improve quality by gathering expertise at a single site, but it has been next to impossible for Manitoba's government to arbitrate the ongoing conflict between the Winnipeg Health Sciences Centre and the St. Boniface Hospital. The latter probably should never have become a major teaching centre in the first place, and it likely never would have if Larry Desjardins, St. Boniface's MLA for many years, had not also been the health minister.

Until very recently, Saskatoon faced the same kind of chaotic competition among its three general hospitals. Each was duplicating most of the services delivered by the others. There was no willingness to rationalize at all. The hospitals even refused to share a common laundry!

Government leadership wasn't getting anywhere until they commissioned a study by Dr. John Atkinson, an Ottawa health consultant. "I've never seen such a scathing indictment of the behaviour that was going on," says Lawrie McFarlane, who is now deputy minister of health in British Columbia. "This report gave government exactly the kind of ammunition it needed." In February 1992, the minister of health abolished Saskatoon's separate hospital boards and appointed a new regional health board to oversee the system. Lawrie McFarlane became its president.*

---

* In fact, the regional board replaced the boards at University Hospital, City Hospital, and the Partridge long-term care facility. St. Paul's Hospital (a Catholic facility) managed to retain its own board, but it is nevertheless subject to the rulings of the Saskatoon Health Board. The regional health board also governs public health, the home care program, and mental health services.

At first, the board concentrated on consolidating the administration and support programs at the three hospitals—laundry services, liability insurance, purchasing, and so on. It didn't touch issues related to patient care at all. The results were phenomenal. "On an annual basis we've already found ways this year of saving $10 million on a combined hospital budget of $190 million," says McFarlane. There was a yearly saving in insurance costs alone of $160,000!

Bearing down on the board

The vast majority of hospitals in Canada are non-profit, private institutions. Some are incorporated and some are not, but all are ostensibly governed by a board of directors.

Being asked to join a hospital board is usually considered something of an honour; the position both confers and reflects social status. The job of the board is governance—which involves policy setting and overall responsibility for the quality of care and the financial health of the organization.

How well are board members equipped to handle these jobs? Well, one study suggests they need more help than they're getting now. In this survey, only half the trustees felt they had enough information to understand and make decisions on complex issues of hospital governance. And only half felt adequately prepared to judge the quality of care provided in their hospitals, or to make policy changes to improve it.[34]

Perhaps you're thinking that this is only natural. After all, the work of hospitals is very specialized—it's hard for people who aren't health professionals to make such assessments. But financial responsibility is another matter. Most hospital boards have gone out of their way to recruit members with extensive backgrounds in finance—accountants, investment managers, corporate lawyers, and so forth.

Toronto's St. Michael's Hospital was no exception. All the same, in the fall of 1990 it became clear that the hospital was in serious financial difficulty, with an accumulated debt of $63 million and a projected deficit for 1990-91 of $16.6 million on an overall budget of $175 million.[35]

An investigation launched by the ministry of health found that a $25 million loss associated with the highly speculative purchase of a downtown office building in 1987 was a major contributor to this financial disaster. Revenues anticipated from this purchase never materialized, and the building was not financially self-supporting. Meanwhile, a number of questionable accounting practices kept St. Michael's burgeoning debt problem from coming to light. For example, the renovation costs associated with the office building were entered in St. Michael's books as an account receivable. The hospital routinely started programs or bought equipment without first determining whether the government was willing to pay and fell into the habit of reporting the funding it hoped to receive as revenue.

The investigators' report highlighted considerable confusion surrounding the role of the board. Board members seemed to have been kept in the dark and were never presented with financial statements regarding the purchase and renovation of the office building. Also, because the hospital was owned by the Sisters of St. Joseph and was not separately incorporated, some board members saw themselves mainly as advisers to the Sisters rather than as the hospital's governing body with overall responsibility.*

Since hospitals use public money to run their operations, it is logical to conclude that hospitals are accountable to the government. But the public may have less right to know the details of hospital operations than we think. In 1991, the Ontario provincial auditor's report noted that the Toronto Hospital refused to let him inspect the details of nine purchases totalling $3.2 million. This included a $1.2 million purchase of a controversial computer system.

Doctors: Gatekeepers to the System

You can't be admitted to a hospital, see a specialist, have a test done, or get a prescription without first seeing a physician. Doctors alone make most of the decisions about what services their patients receive. Canada's doctors have virtually complete clinical

---

* By the fall of 1993, St. Michael's Hospital had cut its debt by more than half by merging programs, performing more day surgery, and laying off some staff. The hospital expects to be debt-free by 1998—two years ahead of schedule.

autonomy. There is little monitoring of their practices by anyone, even other doctors. This contrasts starkly with the situation in the United States, where clinical freedom is evaporating. For many patients, American physicians have to phone and get clearance from a nurse (or sometimes even a clerk) employed by the insurance company in order to arrange hospital admissions, specialist referrals, and increasingly, diagnostic testing.

An Oregon doctor who used to practise in Canada tells a horror story about an elderly patient he admitted to hospital with severe congestive heart failure. After the patient's successful treatment and discharge, the private review agency working for the American Medicare program refused to pay for the hospitalization.* The reviewer, who had never seen the patient, had decided that she wasn't sick enough to be hospitalized. Only after months of filling in forms and making phone calls did the doctor finally manage to get approval for reimbursement.

Most doctors in Canada are paid by government on a fee-for-service basis. In other words, the payment is piecework. The more a doctor does, the more he or she makes. All this would be fine if it were really clear-cut which patients needed which services and doctors made the right decision 100 percent of the time. But, as we discussed in Chapter 1 (and will cover in more detail in Chapter 4), these assumptions are incorrect. The truth is that doctors have a significant amount of discretion in deciding which patients to see, what tests and drugs to order, and which patients to refer to specialists or hospitals.

Over the past twenty years a mountain of research has indicated that fee-for-service as a method for paying doctors increases overall costs by 20 to 40 percent with no clear benefits to patients.[36]

Consider Winnipeg, for example. Between 1971 and 1981, the number of general practitioners rose by two-thirds while the population increased by less than 10 percent.[37] In any normal market, a drastic increase in the number of providers without any similar increase in the number of consumers would produce fierce competition for market share and consequently lower prices. In such a

---

* The American Medicare program is a public health insurance program for those over sixty-five years of age.

situation, some providers would be edged out of the market altogether. At the very least, one would expect physicians' overall incomes to drop. But this didn't happen in Winnipeg. It appears that fee-for-service payment means there are almost no limits to the number of doctors who can gain employment from Medicare.

Fee-for-service also seems to encourage doctors to become workaholics. The financial rewards to those who see more patients and work longer hours are there for the taking and provide a strong temptation to go overboard, even to the detriment of the physician's own mental and physical health. If an Ontario physician who normally works five days a week decides to go into the office on Saturdays, too, that additional eight hours per week can generate an extra $50,000 per year in net income!* Even though this means doctors have less personal time, economic gains of this magnitude are hard to pass up. To this extent, fee-for-service medicine could be just as unhealthy for doctors as it is expensive for the health care system.

Turf Wars

Doctors may exert the most influence over our health care system and the costs it generates, but they are by no means the only players in the field. A host of other providers from as many as forty different occupational groups—nurses, dentists, pharmacists, social workers—are constantly jockeying for position. Relationships within and among these groups are often strained and even acrimonious.

Specialist doctors tend to dominate medical associations and are often accused by general and family practitioners of doing things in their own interests. But that's only one example of struggle within the hierarchy.

Nurses, through their professional associations, are demanding wider recognition of their particular skills and are busy trying to convince doctors and government that nursing is a profession

---

*This calculation assumes that the doctor receives an average per-visit billing of $22 and sees six patients an hour. Both are low rather than high estimates of actual earning potential.

"separate and distinct from medicine, but equally important."
The Canadian Nurses Association and its provincial counterparts
have been lobbying to have all new nurses trained in universities
by the year 2000. In 1986, only 12 percent of nurses held a university degree in nursing; instead, most had diplomas from community colleges.[38] Already, governments in Prince Edward Island
and Manitoba have agreed to insist on a university degree for
entry to nursing practice.

What will this mean for the vast majority of nurses who are
not university-educated? The immediate result is that nurses
have been returning to upgrade their education in droves—
often at great personal and financial sacrifice. But the question remains—is a degree really necessary for the experienced
nurse?

The answer, according to the British Columbia Royal Commission on Health Care and Costs, is no. The commission's final
report, *Closer to Home*, released in 1991, noted that diploma
RNs had already proven themselves to be "competent, valuable
nurses." Besides, requiring a BScN as a minimum requirement
for entry to practice was not consistent "with the principle that
employees within the health care system should not be required
to have a higher level of education, training, or accreditation
than is necessary to perform the required tasks." Adopting such
a policy would only add unnecessarily to the costs of the system.

Another battleground concerns registered practical nurses
(RPNs).* These are the nurses who provide most of the hands-
on, basic bedside care to patients, and they want the importance
of their role acknowledged by the RNs. It's ironic that as RNs
battle for more recognition from doctors they have acted to
constrict and downplay the role performed by the RPNs. Job
competition between RNs and RPNs is fierce, and one way to
protect RN positions is to limit what RPNs are permitted to do
on the job, with no regard for what their training, experience, or
skill level suggests they are qualified to do. From hospital to
hospital, and even from ward to ward, policies about who can

---

* Depending on the province, these health care workers are also known as
licensed practical nurses (LPNs), certified nursing assistants (CNAs), or registered nursing assistants (RNAs).

do what vary widely—policies usually set by the head of the nursing department, who is invariably an RN.

Meanwhile, nurse-practitioners, who have the potential to provide many services traditionally performed by doctors, have few job opportunities in our system. Doctors view their scope of practice as a direct threat to physicians' own territory.

Another example of professions in conflict arises in the field of physical therapy. In Ontario, physicians are allowed to bill for this type of service, even though it may be provided by someone who has no formal training, even a secretary. Doctors' billings in 1991-92 for this type of service were estimated at some $24 million—a 33 percent increase over the previous year.[39] Meanwhile, in the same year, registered physiotherapists were being threatened with severe funding cutbacks.

We could document similar turf battles for many other provider groups, like audiologists, speech therapists, midwives, chiropodists, chiropractors, naturopaths, and homeopaths. Each wants a bigger piece of the action—more autonomy and more money. Clearly, professional egos are getting in the way of rationalizing service delivery so that the health care consumer gets the best care for his dollar.

It's Time to Tune Up Medicare for the '90s

Questioning whether Medicare is affordable is a bit like asking whether you can afford to pay rent. If you need a place to live, you have to pay for it. If you need health care, there's a bill for that, too. It just so happens that the most efficient way to pay the bill for health care is through public financing. It's no coincidence that most modern industrial countries have all arrived at the same conclusion. The only major exceptions are South Africa, Turkey, and the United States.

What's more, Medicare's costs have never been under better control than they are today. Granted, that's partly due to the fiscal crisis experienced at the provincial level. But Canada's health care spending still compares well with the rest of the world. Costs are not out of control here, nor have they been since Medicare was introduced.

Seventy billion dollars is more than enough money to provide all Canadians with good quality health care. Indeed, with a better managed system, we could afford to add public insurance for a whole range of services we pay for privately now, like basic dental care, comprehensive community services, and drug coverage. We'd even have enough left over to take a whack at the conditions that breed illness and injury, like poverty, sexism, and racism.

Of course, none of these options has a chance unless we succeed in tackling the real problems plaguing Canada's health care system. It is only by reorganizing the delivery system that Canadians will be able to get the care they need at a price they can afford.

Chapter 3

The Health
of Nations

WHEN THIRTY-YEAR-OLD Wendy Meijaard needed a bone marrow transplant to treat her leukemia, her Hamilton hospital said it couldn't help her. It had already reached its self-imposed annual limit for the number of procedures.* Although other Ontario hospitals had the resources to do Ms. Meijaard's transplant, the Hamilton Academy of Medicine argued that people shouldn't have to leave their own communities to get the treatment they need. The Academy went to the media and succeeded in embarrassing the government and the hospital into providing the procedure.[1] Implicit in the Academy's arguments was the idea that society shouldn't ever put a dollar value on human life.

In the predictable rhetoric used to wrest more resources for health care, this line of reasoning frequently crops up and effectively ends the debate. Of course (we are supposed to think) society shouldn't scrimp when a life is at stake; the value of human life is beyond price. But it seems to us that society puts a price on human life all the time. Consider the following examples.

Steelworker Joseph Beaulieu was just thirty years old when he died at Hamilton's Stelco foundry. A crane block weighing more than 200 kilograms fell on top of him and crushed him to

---

* At the time only three Toronto hospitals had specific funding from the Ontario Ministry of Health for bone marrow transplants. The other hospitals performing the procedure had to find the funds in their global budgets. The Ministry has subsequently funded Hamilton's program.

death on June 30, 1988. Subsequently, the company was found guilty of failing to take reasonable precautions to ensure the safety of its workers and was fined $20,000.[2]

On February 15, 1991, nine-year-old Jennifer Jarchow went for an afternoon drive with her parents. Robyn, her four-year-old sister, was left behind with neighbours. Robyn never saw her sister again. The family's car was broadsided by a Canadian Pacific freight train at a level crossing in Brampton, Ontario. Jennifer died that day at the Hospital for Sick Children, and her parents sustained critical injuries. The crossing was well known to be hazardous according to police at the scene. As OPP Constable Greg Poulis pointed out, there were no markings at the crossing—no lights, no barriers.[3] Later, a coroner's jury recommended immediate action to warn motorists approaching level crossings. Every year about eighty people in Canada lose their lives at level rail crossings, and several hundred more are injured. The ultimate solution is to completely eliminate level crossings right across the country by building overpasses or underpasses. But this would cost billions of dollars.[4]

On December 7, 1987, Victor Luis, age forty-two, killed his wife, Presciosa, by repeatedly smashing her chest with a pickaxe.[5] Judge Eugene Ewaschuk, who sentenced Luis to twelve years in jail, criticized Toronto police for not arresting Mr. Luis when he continued to threaten Presciosa, contrary to the terms of his probation. Almost exactly two years later, Marc Lepine murdered fourteen female engineering students, shouting "You are all feminists." Women throughout the world responded with horror to this senseless violence and a major debate ensued about what Lepine's crime really meant. Was it the isolated act of a madman? Or was it part of a pattern of growing and widespread violence against women in our society?

When we don't spend what's needed to make roads and workplaces safe, people get hurt in accidents—some die. When we protect people's right to buy and use guns, we are also risking lives. In choosing not to limit the "rights" of men to stalk and threaten women, we trade off women's rights to safety and security, and sometimes their right to life itself.

There's no public debate about whether we should have safer workplaces and rail crossings or more family doctors. There's no rational process for weighing these kinds of trade-offs. The decisions about where to spend public resources, however, do get made, and usually in accordance with powerful interests and prevailing social values.

In this chapter, we'll take a look at the most important factors determining our health and how our values and institutions decide which aspects get attention and resources and which don't.

Changing Attitudes about Health

Our way of looking at the relationship between health and health care has evolved significantly since we first established public health insurance.

In Chapter 1, while discussing the attitudes about health and health care that prevailed during the period leading up to the creation of public health insurance, we referred to a thermostat model that completely overstates the role of health care as a determinant of health and makes no reference to the underlying causes of illness, or to other factors that contribute to or detract from our well-being.

Today, however, a much more sophisticated framework is needed to reflect our growing understanding that a myriad of factors interact in a complex way to determine our health. This more comprehensive model acknowledges that health care services are not nearly as important as social, economic, and environmental factors. In a seminal paper titled "Producing health, consuming health care," Canadian economists Robert Evans and Greg Stoddart traced the evolution of this understanding in a series of models, culminating in the one presented in Figure 3.1.[6]

As you can see, this model is highly sophisticated in its attempt to account for the multidimensional nature of health and illness and the interplay of various causal factors. Indeed, in this model, health itself is not viewed as the ultimate goal, but only as one of several determinants of well-being.

But of course our concept of health is rooted in our culture and values. These are the factors that shape our understanding of how the world works. Unlike other animals, human beings strive for meaning in their lives, ways to explain and cope with their environment. It should come as no surprise, then, that from one

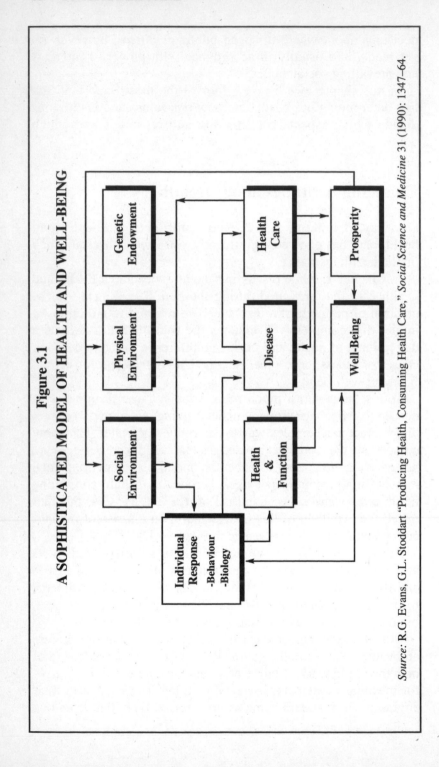

Figure 3.1

A SOPHISTICATED MODEL OF HEALTH AND WELL-BEING

Source: R.G. Evans, G.L. Stoddart "Producing Health, Consuming Health Care," *Social Science and Medicine* 31 (1990): 1347–64.

society to another, from one culture to another, we find enormous differences in the way health is defined, how illnesses are labelled, and in the health status of the population itself.[7]

If, as seems likely, a society's pattern of health and illness reflects its values, culture, and institutions, then several important corollaries inevitably emerge:

1. Fundamental change in a society's pattern of health and illness will require major structural change in the society's values and institutions.
2. Some powerful interests will be threatened by structural changes and will use their positions of privilege to oppose them.
3. Proponents favouring the economic and political status quo will emphasize the treatment of individuals who already have an illness or disease and downplay opportunities to promote the overall health of the population.

These points are well illustrated by the story of tobacco control.

Smoking out the culprits

When tobacco was first introduced into England four hundred years ago, most people thought the product was truly disgusting. King James I deplored the smoking habit as "a custom loatheful to the eye, hateful to the nose, harmful to the brain, dangerous to the lungs."[8]

Despite this early opposition, the use of tobacco spread and, thanks to nicotine's highly addictive properties, large numbers of people got hooked on the habit. Soon smoking became normal and quite acceptable. The growing awareness that tobacco was dangerous to health had little effect on public policy: there were few supports for those who wanted to quit, and little thought was given to the rights of non-smokers to breathe clean air. By the 1950s, half of Canada's adults were smokers, and the social norms of the day meant that they could indulge their habit almost without restriction—in movie theatres, restaurants, grocery stores, even on airplanes.

And, by the 1940s, it was clear that there was a new plague to replace tuberculosis and smallpox—tobacco-related illness. By

1989, Health and Welfare Canada estimated that nearly 40,000 Canadians per year die of smoking-related illnesses, in particular lung cancer and heart disease.[9] Tobacco was estimated to be a $3.3 to $7.7 billion drain on the Canadian economy.[10]

Beginning in the 1970s, public attitudes towards smoking began to change and a coalition of groups opposed to the tobacco industry's unfettered rights to promote a deadly and addictive product picked up steam. The Non-Smokers Rights Association (NSRA)—widely acknowledged to be one of the most effective political lobby groups in the world—has been in the thick of this debate since 1974. Under the leadership of Garfield Mahood and David Sweanor, and operating from tiny, cluttered offices in downtown Toronto and Ottawa, the NSRA has demonstrated just how effective social action can be.

The airline industry was one of its early targets. Passengers often complained about the presence of smoke in cabins. Air Canada began by offering separate seating for non-smokers on 747s in 1971, but this was only a half-way measure, since the smoke really had nowhere to go. Following a major lobby effort by the NSRA, the airline conducted a smoke-free trial on half of its Toronto-Ottawa-Montreal flights for a three-month period in 1986. This was so popular with passengers and crew that the airline banned smoking permanently on all North American flights in 1988. Two years later, the federal government jumped in—again under pressure from the NSRA—and passed legislation banning smoking on all national flights under six hours. The same legislation brought a complete ban on airline smoking in 1993.[11]

You might have expected to find mainstream health organizations front and centre in these debates, given that tobacco causes one-third of all cancer and heart disease deaths and three-quarters of all lung disease fatalities. But in truth, these groups entered the fray rather late and offered less financial support than you might expect.

Among them, the Canadian Cancer Society, the Canadian Heart and Stroke Foundation, and the Canadian Lung Association provide $200 million in grants each year for laboratory research and investigating new treatments. True, all support anti-tobacco legislation and have in recent years been more active in lobbying on the issue. The Canadian Cancer Society, for example, has a public issues office in Ottawa, with a major focus on tobacco policies. All three of these groups regularly support initiatives of the NSRA. All the same, the primary focus of health groups is on finding ways to help individuals rather than on promoting social change. And their spending patterns reflect this orientation—less than 1 percent of their revenues is invested in advocacy activities.

The men and women sitting on the boards of these health groups are part of the elite—leaders in Canadian business, the arts, and academe. If well-educated sophisticates like these view cancer, heart, and lung disease as mainly individual tragedies to be combatted by better medical therapy and fail to see the bigger picture of prevention, it's hardly surprising that average Canadians and the media see things that way too.

For example, in August 1993, Dr. Stephen Lam and biophysicist Branco Palcic of the British Columbia Cancer Agency made headlines in the national press for developing the LIFE imaging system, which allows early diagnosis of lung cancer. Their research, justly regarded as technically brilliant, captured a lot of media attention.[12] No one brought up the fact, however, that by the time lung cancer is detectable, it has almost always spread to other parts of the body. Other trials of early diagnosis of lung cancer have shown that it makes no difference to survival.[13] Nor did the news reports of this story even mention that 85 percent of lung cancers are caused by tobacco.

The print media give almost no space to discussing the health dangers of tobacco, partly because they are dependent on revenues from cigarette ads and promotions.*[14] *Cosmopolitan*'s Helen Gurley Brown candidly admitted, "Having come from the advertising world myself, I think, 'Who needs somebody you're paying millions of dollars a year to come back and bite you on the ankle?' "[15]

Sometimes the only way to protect the health of the population is through tough government action—when vested interests

---

* Sporting events and arts groups have a similar dependance on tobacco sponsorship. In Canada, print advertising for cigarettes is illegal, but there have been increases in advertising for sporting and cultural activities *sponsored* by tobacco companies.

are determined to protect the status quo, only governments have the authority to step in. Research has shown that 90 percent of people who smoke started when they were teenagers. In November 1993, Ontario health minister Ruth Grier introduced some of the toughest measures ever seen to discourage young people from starting to smoke. Now, the maximum penalty for selling tobacco to minors has risen from $25,000 to $75,000, cigarette vending machines are outlawed, and pharmacies are no longer permitted to stock or sell tobacco products.

Unfortunately, in early 1994, progress against tobacco-induced illness suffered a major setback. During the 1980s, the Conservatives massively increased tobacco taxes, so that by 1991, cigarettes in Canada cost at least twice as much as in the United States. These tax hikes were partly based on strong evidence that higher prices discourage cigarette consumption, and are particularly effective in preventing teenagers from taking up the habit.[16]

But the tobacco industry needs a continuous supply of new smokers in order to replace the 3,000 customers who die every month from smoking-related illnesses. They know full well that targeting teens is crucial to their business; it's well established that the older people are, the less likely they are to ever take up smoking.

In fact, the industry's public posture of concern over children using tobacco contrasts sharply with evidence from a Quebec court case, which showed that tobacco companies have been doing extensive research on children's smoking habits, and have even conducted focus groups with teenagers![17] According to one California study, by the time children reached the age of six the cartoon character Old Joe Camel was as recognizable as Mickey Mouse.[18] In fact, in the United States, Old Joe helped make Camels number one in the illegal, under-age market.[19]

Here at home, high taxes were at first quite successful in keeping youth smoking rates under control. However, by 1992, tobacco smuggling in Canada had become a very serious problem. Canadian tobacco exports had ballooned from 1.2 billion cigarettes in 1989 to 19.5 billion in 1993, and it certainly wasn't because Americans suddenly developed a taste for Canadian cigarettes.[20]

The Mulroney government's initial reaction was encouraging. It imposed an export tax of $8 per carton and within a month exports fell by 60 percent. The tobacco industry responded with a warning that Canadian jobs were at stake and hinted that the industry could always relocate south of the border and manufacture for the smugglers directly. Following a massive lobby effort, the industry got its way and seven weeks after being imposed, the export tax was abolished. In return, the tobacco companies promised to limit exports, to help government track the flow of contraband cigarettes, and to design packaging that would clearly distinguish between cigarettes destined for export and those intended for domestic consumption. It appears as though none of these promises was honoured. In fact, Imperial Tobacco set up its own distribution firm and warehouse in upper New York State—an arrangement that made things very convenient for the smugglers. Packages were redesigned, but the effect was to make it even more difficult to distinguish domestic and export products.[21] Quebec journalist Lysiane Gagnon asked, "Why do the cigarette packets shipped to the U.S. bear bilingual labels? Are French inscriptions needed for the American market?"[22]

By the winter of 1993–94, smuggling had reached crisis proportions and demanded government action. Three out of every four cigarettes being smoked in Quebec were contraband. Violence associated with smuggling was on the rise—American junior hockey teams were afraid to come to Cornwall, Ontario, and civic leaders there and in other border communities were reporting threats and other efforts to intimidate their attempts to intervene.

Meanwhile, Quebec Premier Daniel Johnson, facing a tough bid for re-election, saw a chance to restore law and order and remove the profit from tobacco smuggling by lowering the taxes on it. He convinced the Chrétien government to help out by doing the same. Were the tobacco companies counting on powerful allies in Ottawa? Finance Minister Paul Martin, Jr., was a former board member of Imasco, the parent company of Imperial Tobacco. Torrence Wylie, one of Chrétien's closest personal and political friends, had just left his job as executive vice-president of Imasco to become a private lobbyist on Parliament Hill.

As health groups mobilized, reading danger in all these "smoke" signals, Canadians witnessed a heated public debate that seemed close to an undeclared war. But ultimately the tobacco industry prevailed and the federal government and

Quebec slashed tobacco taxes.* The price of cigarettes fell by fifty percent. New Brunswick quickly followed suit by cutting its provincial tobacco taxes. Then, shortly after, Ontario was forced to do the same when confronted with a massive influx of cheaper cigarettes from Quebec. As we go to press, the remaining provinces are holding firm against tobacco tax cuts. If they manage to hold out, perhaps the trend can be reversed.

In fact, health groups might find a spark of hope in the ashes of defeat. Ontario coupled its tax cut with previously unheard of measures to reduce the demand for tobacco products. On February 22, 1994, Ontario Health Minister Ruth Grier announced she would spend an additional $2.5 million on enforcement to ensure that retailers do not sell cigarettes to minors and said she would work with other provinces to move quickly on introducing requirements for plain packaging. Because packaging is key to product recognition and is central to promotion and all forms of marketing, this measure has been bitterly opposed by the industry. This could be the trade-off: lower taxes, but also tough governmental action to reduce the toll of tobacco-related illness. Health groups are seizing this opportunity; they want Ottawa to ban all tobacco sponsorship and promotion, to introduce generic packaging legislation, and to subject tobacco to the same strenuous controls as other products regulated under the *Hazardous Products Act*. Who knows? They may even win.

The story of tobacco control perfectly illustrates that the interests that produce disease are often very powerful. To counter them requires strong Guardian action: legislation, regulation, and strict enforcement.

What Determines Health?

At two in the afternoon, Jane Smith (not her real name) rolls to the side of the bed and lights a cigarette, drawing the smoke deep into her lungs. As the nicotine hits her brain, she slowly gets up to

---

* Ottawa also re-established the $8 per carton export tax and promised to ban "kiddy packs," spend more on health promotion activities against tobacco use, and consider generic packaging.

dress. Her night shift at the factory ended at 7:30 that morning, and she just made it home in time to walk her kids to school. When she returned, she made their dinner and put their plates in the fridge before collapsing in bed to catch five hours of sleep. Now, she's running through the list of all the things she has to do today—grocery shopping, new batteries for the TV's remote control, and, oh yes, call her son's math teacher about the test he failed last week. Since this is swing shift day, everything has to be done before 4:00 p.m. when she's due back at the plant. She groans when she realizes that she missed calling her lawyer that morning about her husband's lagging support payments. Now she'll have to wait another day.

Later, at work, she feels her old back injury act up. But things are so busy, she has little chance to notice the pain. On her break, she rushes to get her package of Cancer Society materials so she can canvass on the weekend. Because both her mother and aunt died of lung cancer, she always tries to do her bit for cancer research.

Back on the line, her back really starts to hurt and she begs off work early. On the way home, she stops in at McDonald's for a Big Mac and fries, but because she's worried about that "extra ten pounds," when she gets home she forces herself to throw up. Her kids are already fast asleep. She kisses each of them on the cheek, downs a double vodka to wash down her blood pressure pill, and collapses into bed. As she drifts off to sleep, she thinks how much easier life seemed to be for her mother and grandmother when she was growing up.

Jane has a point. Her life is amazingly different from life in her mother's or her grandmother's day. In fact, the lives we live, our routines and habits, our diet and social conventions are far removed from the natural environment in which we evolved. All of these factors take their toll on our health.

Food for thought

Each animal species has unique food requirements that developed over millions of years of evolution. It's been about four million years since humanoids first appeared. All of our closest evolutionary relations—the gorillas, orangutans, and chimpanzees—get most of their calories from fruit and other vegetable material.[23] Early humans did, too. Even though we've always had a taste for meat, up until the last fifty to one hundred thousand years our ancestors weren't very successful hunters. As a result, compared to today's typical North American diet, our "natural" diet was very low in fat, protein, and salt, and very high in fibre and water-soluble vitamins, especially vitamin C. It was a very healthy diet, too. Studies show that modern-day hunter-gatherer societies, like our primitive ancestors, have less than one-tenth our rate of heart disease and equally low rates of cancer. Jane Smith's high blood pressure is virtually unheard of among hunter-gatherers.[24]

Jane also suffers from bulimia; she often eats too much, or too much of the wrong thing, and then forces herself to vomit. Sometimes she takes large doses of laxatives, too, in a frantic attempt to keep her body from gaining more weight. Eating disorders like bulimia and anorexia are reaching epidemic levels in North America, as young girls risk their health trying to satisfy modern standards for beauty. Although there are documented cases of these conditions from the last century, they were very rare in an era when women's natural curves attracted admiration. In this century, however, a shapeless slenderness emerged as a new ideal, first in the 1920s with the hipless, breastless flapper, and later—with a vengeance—in the 1960s, '70s and '80s, when film stars and high-fashion models began promoting a painfully thin, unarticulated body shape.

Recently, a new and even more unrealistic demand for beauty has emerged—women must still be very thin, but also strong with large breasts. The result? The typical film star today weighs at least twenty pounds less than Marilyn Monroe or Jane Russell. High-fashion models and ballerinas are expected to be even thinner. The pressure on grown women to emulate these boyish waifs is unrelenting. Donatella Girombelli, who heads up an Italian fashion corporation, laments, "It's weird that very tall, lanky women and anorexics can become symbols of female beauty."[25]

The true confessions of high-fashion models and ballet dancers reveal a constant and painful struggle to measure up. For them, having a healthy woman's body could lead to unemployment. Former cover girl Kim Alexis claims that she was pressured to lose so much weight that she didn't have a menstrual period for two years.[26] Ovulation depends on having enough body fat to support the metabolism of estrogen.[27] Imagine a society whose "ideal woman" can't reproduce!

Substance misuse and abuse

Jane Smith smokes heavily, and although she knows that tobacco causes nearly forty thousand premature deaths in Canada every year, she has never quite managed to quit.

Smoking rates for men have declined greatly over the past thirty years, but women—and particularly young women—have resisted this social trend. One reason may be the fact that tobacco use helps to control weight by suppressing the appetite. Most women know that quitting leads to a five-to-ten-pound weight gain. As a result, almost all high-fashion models say they smoke to stay thin.

Jane also drinks alcohol every day, sometimes heavily on her day off. We aren't the only members of the animal kingdom to use various substances to alter our consciousness, but the practice is much more widespread among humans. Human beings have used wine, beer, and spirits for thousands of years. The Code of Hammurabi, a compendium of ancient Babylonian laws, sets out regulations governing drinking establishments.[28] There's even a theory that beer was what motivated early humans to sow crops.

Alcohol abuse is an important cause of ill health, resulting in a variety of diseases such as cirrhosis of the liver and oesophageal cancer, and a major cause of traffic accidents and family disruption. But alcohol is also a lucrative business in western nations. Today, drinking is thoroughly integrated in our society, and alcohol advertising is the backbone of the magazine, sports, and entertainment industries.

To sleep ...

Human beings, like other animals, need sleep. How much and when we need to sleep depends on daily cycles of hormones, which set an individual's natural sleep cycle. Research suggests that we have evolved to sleep roughly eight hours a day—about six hours at night and two hours in the early afternoon.[29] Our daily hormonal cycle, however, accounts for just over twenty-five hours. What this means is that without being cued by sunrise and sunset, humans would live twenty-five-hour days. Although most of us can adapt to a day that is roughly twenty-three to twenty-six hours long, it's easier for us to lengthen our day than shorten it. That's why we handle the time differences involved in flying west much better than we manage them on our return east.

Poor Jane Smith works shifts. Every week her schedule changes and moves backwards: she is working the swing shift this week, the day shift next week, and the midnight shift the week after. Weekends just aren't long enough for her to adjust. That's why her body is in a constant state of hormonal imbalance. As a result, she is sleepy at work and tired at home. This style of rotating shift work is associated with poor work performance and increased accidents at work and at home, and puts the worker at greater risk for heart disease and family disruption.[30]

Ideally, it would be much better if no one had to work in shifts, but even modifying shift work can make it much healthier. For example, some people actually prefer afternoon or midnight shifts and would like to work the same shift permanently. Rotating shifts every month instead of every week would also make it much easier for people to adjust. Rotating all shifts— day, swing, and midnight—forward instead of backward would also improve Jane's work performance and lower her risk of developing heart disease.[31]

Natural supports

University of British Columbia economist Robert Evans says humans, like construction beams, acquire their strength and vigour from three sources: the material we're made with, the hardening process, and the supports provided.

The basic building material for humans is our genetic inheritance, the chromosomal material that determines eye and hair colour, body size and shape, and, to a great extent, our susceptibility to various diseases. Some illnesses, like cystic fibrosis, are totally determined by our genetic make-up. Others, like early-onset heart disease (before age fifty-five) and manic depressive illness, are partly determined by genes and partly by our environment. By and large, however, it is the latter two factors—the hardening process (our early development) and our support systems (friends, family, meaningful work)—that determine health. Research has established that people live longer if they have more social contacts.[32] For example, married people live longer than singles.

A hallmark of human beings is the traditional family grouping. True, some human societies do not organize around the nuclear and/or extended family, but the majority do. Human interactions in the family set the tone for other relationships between the generations and the genders. Irwin Waller, a professor of criminology at the University of Ottawa, told the Commons justice committee that Canada's dismal record in childhood poverty is also linked to a growing problem with crime.[33] The committee was chaired by Robert Horner, then a Tory MP: "Listen, if anybody had told me nine years ago I'd be studying the social causes of crime, I would have said they were nuts. I'm an ex-member of the RCMP and I'm strictly for law and order. But I can tell you that we can't just continue to build more jails and spend more money on police budgets and have crime increasing the way it is."[34]

There is support for Mr. Horner's viewpoint. Child psychiatrist Dr. Dan Offord did research in an Ottawa housing development in the early 1980s. Children with access to recreational programs and the chance to learn and develop skills in sports and other cooperative games were compared to a control housing project that had no special programs of this type. He found a major reduction in antisocial behaviour and youth crime among the children with access to recreation.[35]

Some lessons have to be learned early or they can't be learned at all. Professor Stephen Suomi and his colleagues at the U.S. National Institute of Child Health have studied the impact of poor social support on young monkeys. They have found that lack of support (particularly the lack of a mother) causes short-term changes in behaviour and various hormone levels. In the longer-term, primates deprived in this way are much more prone to depression.[36]

Work and the social hierarchy

Jane Smith has excellent genes, but she hasn't been so lucky in other respects. Her mother had Jane when she was still a teenager. Jane never knew her father, and, like most Canadian children whose mothers are single parents, Jane grew up poor.

There is a vast amount of evidence that shows that the lower your place on the social hierarchy, the poorer your health is likely to be. This proves true whether you define the hierarchy by education, income, or job classification. For example, Dr. Michael Wolfson of Statistics Canada has documented that poor, middle-aged men are twice as prone to premature death as wealthy men.[37] What is it about being at the top of the totem pole that makes you healthier? What is it about being at the bottom that makes you sicker? Can we just put it down to poor health habits?

So-called bad choices are usually exercised without complete information and within a social context that encourages unhealthy behaviours and discourages healthy ones. For example, Jane knows that smoking is unhealthy, but she's addicted to nicotine. She started to smoke when she was thirteen and all her friends were doing it. She used a forged note from her mother to buy her cigarettes at the corner drug store. Could something really be unhealthy if pharmacists sold it? Later on, most of her workmates were hooked on cigarettes, too. As she got older, smoking helped her stay slim enough to wear a size seven. She timed her breaks at work by how long it took to smoke a cigarette while drinking a cup of coffee.

The social environments of the poor encourage smoking while those for the wealthy are increasingly less tolerant of the habit. Bad health habits, however, are only part of the equation explaining poor health. Most of the health gap between rich and poor is still unexplained. For example, Michael Marmot and his colleagues researched the health of British civil servants, looking in particular at risk factors for heart disease in a series of inquiries known as the Whitehall studies (see Figure 3.2).[38]

A key finding from this research was that deaths, from the highest to the lowest occupational levels in the civil service, followed a set pattern—a stepped gradient—in which death rates rose incrementally in each successively lower occupational level. Instead of an absolute threshold, where everyone earning a certain level of income above the cut-off experienced similar levels of risk, this finding demonstrates that relative differences in income and decision-making authority are associated with relative differences in health.

The study also looked at how many of these differences could be explained by the traditional risk factors. But the researchers discovered that high blood pressure, high cholesterol, and smoking accounted for only a small part of the difference in deaths across occupational groups. For example, while smoking did heighten the risk for heart disease among the most senior administrators in the civil service, the risk of heart disease for manual labourers who smoked was much higher. Even high blood pressure affected

Figure 3.2

WHITEHALL STUDY: AGE-ADJUSTED, ALL CAUSE MORTALITY AMONG FOUR GRADES OF THE BRITISH CIVIL SERVICE OVER TEN YEARS OF FOLLOW-UP

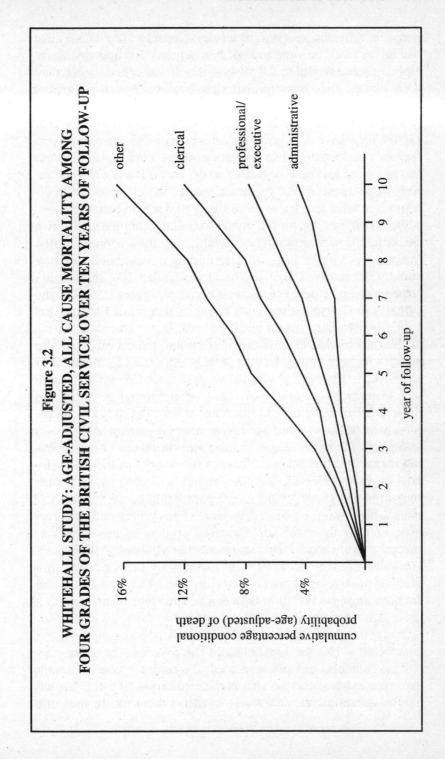

people at different occupational levels differently. All civil servants had higher blood pressure at work than at home. But administrators' blood pressure tended to fall to significantly lower levels once they were home, while blood pressure readings for manual labourers stayed relatively high.

These kind of results complement research showing that highly repetitive and boring jobs—especially where workers feel they lack control over the processes of work—also increase the power of known risk factors to do harm. It's not the executive who's most at risk for heart attack; the clerk in the mailroom is at least four times more likely to develop heart disease.

So where we are on the social and economic hierarchy is a major factor in determining our health, and the steepness of that hierarchy is a major factor in determining the overall health of a society. Recently, a British social researcher has shown that beyond a certain level of income per capita (about $5,000, the same as in Greece), a society's health is determined by the distribution of wealth, not its absolute level.[39]

It could be that income distribution and education are really proxies for something else that is truly important for health. For example, is there a big gap between rich and poor? Is there a steep hierarchy among social and occupational groups? Are there a lot of people in the bottom ranks? Do they feel completely excluded as contributing members in our society?

Societies that answer yes to these questions can't escape having major health problems. Those at the bottom of the hierarchy will be most affected, but the impact will also show poorer overall health status for the entire population compared to societies with a more equal distribution of resources and opportunity. One of the most sophisticated studies in this area was recently published by British researcher Richard Wilkinson.[40] He looked at the changes in life expectancy that occurred in a number of developed countries during the 1970s and 1980s and found a strong correlation between health improvements and a more equitable distribution of income.

It doesn't look like a coincidence that populations with the best health—like the Japanese and the Swedes—have the narrowest gaps between rich and poor. By contrast, countries with the greatest amounts of income inequality—like the United States—demonstrate the worst health indicators. In fact, the

United States, despite its enormous wealth, has the greatest proportion of people in poverty of any wealthy nation[41] and also displays some of the worst health outcomes in the industrialized world. In infant mortality, for example, it ranks twentieth in the world.[42]

More kids live in poverty in the United States than anywhere in the western industrialized world.[43] In 1986, over 20 percent of all American children were growing up in poverty, rising to 54 percent for children living in single-parent families.[44]

But Canada has little to feel smug about. The most recent research shows that:

- our rates of child poverty are twice as high as those in France, the Netherlands, Sweden, and Germany;[45]
- despite Ottawa's 1989 all-party agreement to eradicate child poverty by the year 2000, the number of poor children in Canada swelled by 30 percent between 1989 and 1991, and is continuing to grow;[46]
- in 1991, 1.2 million Canadian children were poor. This means over 18 percent of Canadian children live in poverty.[47]

Humans differ from the rest of the animal kingdom in that only humans seek to explain the universe and their place in it. American sociologist Joseph Campbell and Israeli sociologist Aaron Antonovsky have documented this universal human desire to know who we are, where we come from, and where we are going. For example, virtually every human society has developed explanations to account for the cycle of stars and planets and the mysteries of life, and especially death. This spiritual and intellectual journey towards what Antonovsky calls "a sense of coherence" appears to be yet another requirement for human health, giving people "the feeling that life is comprehensible, manageable and meaningful."[48]

Perhaps for many at the bottom of a steeply sloped hierarchical society there is no meaning to life and no sense of coherence. This factor could well explain yet another dimension of the health impact of social and economic deprivation.

The politics of violence

All human societies have to deal with the issue of aggression, and in particular, male violence against women. The sheer difference in physical size between the genders—on average, men are about 8 percent taller and 20 percent heavier than women— certainly makes it easy for males to dominate females by using force. However, the extent to which they do so very much depends on a given society's tolerance for this kind of behaviour.[49] Culture, values, and institutions can make a dramatic difference in the amount of male violence seen.

Jane Smith suffered considerable psychological abuse while she was still married to her husband, and even some physical abuse. She tried calling the police once, after a particularly bad beating, but on that occasion, her husband promised he'd never do it again. She didn't press charges.

Until quite recently, this scenario was typical. Police in most Canadian cities would not take action themselves unless the woman involved was prepared to lay a charge. And Canadian society has always been more tolerant of male violence directed against a sexual partner than against a stranger.

For example, Ontario provincial court judge Sidney Harris displayed this bias when he asked about wife assault: "Is every such outburst to be made the subject of criminal proceedings? Is this criminal division of the Provincial Court to be involved whenever transitory passion triumphs for a brief instant over reasoned and reasonable solutions to problems?"[50] Although Judge Harris said he didn't condone violence against women, his remarks suggest he doesn't think that our criminal justice system should play a dominant role in dealing with the issue.

But our values and social institutions are changing. We now recognize that 10 percent of women live in abusive relationships, and that up to half of all female trauma patients are the victims of male abuse.[51] In 1994, physicians, nurses, and social workers asked the Ontario Hospital Association to negotiate a policy change that would allow them to breach confidentiality in order to report suspected cases of abuse, even when the women themselves were reluctant to do so.[52] Jane Smith was able to get legal aid to help deal with her husband. And by the time the couple had separated, the police had a new chief who was determined that his constables would enforce court injunctions against men who harassed their wives.

Communities like London, Ontario, are showing the world how to deal with this age-old human problem. Since 1972, the police force in London has had a Family Consultant Service to help officers intervening in violent domestic disputes. Staffed with social workers, clergy, and other professionals, this service is available twenty-four hours a day to provide on-the-spot advice and other kinds of assistance to victims. London police have a strict enforcement policy: they will lay charges against suspected wife-batterers themselves, even when the victims are reluctant to do so. As a result of this program, the number of core families—those with a history of frequent calls for help with domestic violence— has fallen by 20 percent.[53] Other supports in the London community include a shelter for victims and an advocacy clinic to provide abused women with legal advice. In combination, these institutional and structural changes signal a decided shift in a central social value: tolerance for wife abuse is on the decline.

Prevention versus Cure?

Jane Smith is very concerned about her health and the health of her family. She sees her family doctor regularly to keep tabs on her high blood pressure. She makes sure her kids have regular medical check-ups, too. And on top of canvassing every year for the Cancer Society, she helped raise funds in the community for the hospital's CAT scanner.

On the other hand, like many Canadians, Jane doesn't appreciate the importance of diet to health. She knows that cigarettes can cause lung cancer but has no idea that 85 percent of lung cancers are caused by smoking. She's also misinformed about lung cancer treatment. She thinks it's much more effective now than when her mother and aunt died, when in fact it's only marginally better.

Dr. James Hurowitz suggests two factors to explain why people focus on sickness as a problem for individuals rather than looking at the social and economic causes of illness:[54]

- First, governments are often very reluctant to draw attention to the social factors that determine illness—the

issue only calls attention to the structural inadequacies
of other government policies.
- Second, health care providers benefit when more
  resources are devoted to their activities, most of which
  aim at individualized diagnosis and treatment.

Dr. Raynauld Pineault of the University of Montreal notes how
hard it is to "sell" prevention. "Organ transplantation is much
sexier than making sure every kid in poor neighbourhoods gets
a glass of milk every day."[55]

Besides, what motivation do politicians have to address the
social and economic determinants of health? Most social health
researchers would claim that reducing inequality is the most
important step any government could take to improve the population's health. But of course this means more for the poor—a
policy unlikely to hold much attraction for well-heeled political
supporters. "Politicians and taxpayers are more excited by the
opening of a new hospital neonatal ward for underweight and
premature babies than they are by programs to prevent the
problem by feeding pregnant women," according to Kate Dunn,
a former *Montreal Gazette* health reporter.[56]

Over the past decade, various provincial government commissions have stressed the need for a broader approach, in which
health care is only one tactic within an overall strategy aimed
primarily at improving the social and economic conditions
known to affect the health of the population. We're still waiting.

Government as a Guardian of the Public's Health

If it is true that patterns of health and illness reflect a society's
values and institutions, then the only hope for improvement in
health is to change the structure of these values and institutions.
This means fighting against the status quo, and against those
with a vested interest in preserving it.

While non-governmental groups play a role in pushing for
and supporting change, confronting the private interests and
institutions that cause and contribute to ill health is primarily a
job for government. To succeed, it must rely on two key Guardian

values: a willingness to display prowess and a demonstration of fortitude.

The health of Canadians has improved dramatically over the past century. In fact, we now live longer and healthier than at any other time in history. Government action is responsible for much of this improvement. Recent examples include legislation for occupational health, auto safety, seat-belt use, and various anti-tobacco laws and regulations. Not surprisingly, the manufacturers (or private interests) opposed these measures as too costly, but government, in its role as a good Guardian, prevailed.

Victorian victories

Conflict between private interests and the public's health has a long and well-documented history. During the Industrial Revolution, Britain's growing urban industries were hungry for labour and looking for ways to fill their factories. Most of the population, however, lived as tenant farmers in the countryside. Mounting pressure from industry led Parliament to pass various Enclosure Acts, which drove masses of peasants off the land but failed to bring them into the cities.[57] England's Poor Laws—dating back to Elizabethan times—were the obstacle. These laws made it possible for able-bodied poor people to stay in their own communities, subsisting on alms from local poorhouses and workhouses.

To the leading economists and political philosophers of the day, however, this kind of state subsidy was anathema. They argued vehemently that the Poor Laws interfered with the "free" labour market. Their arguments reflected a newly emerging set of values, called "philosophical necessity." Advocates of philosophical necessity thought state intervention in social policy was contrary to nature.* Joseph Priestley claimed, "Individuals when left to themselves are, in general, sufficiently provident and will daily better their circumstances."[58] Like today's neo-conservative movement, supporters of philosophical necessity argued that withdrawal of the state from economic and social policy

---

* Proponents of philosophical necessity based their idea of "what was natural" on Isaac Newton's depiction of an ordered and measurable universe. As far as they were concerned, governments had no more need to intervene in social or economic policy than they had to regulate planetary orbits.

would increase overall wealth and ultimately eliminate poverty and lead to moral improvement—a nineteenth-century version of the trickle-down theory.

On the recommendation of a Parliamentary Royal Commission in 1834, the Poor Laws were soon amended. With the reduction in state support, large numbers of peasants were forced to seek employment in industrial towns. This massive migration had an enormous impact on English life. In 1801, only 17 percent of Britons lived in towns; sixty years later, the proportion had more than doubled.

The industrial cities of England were ill prepared for such rapid expansion. Factories and housing were thrown up wherever the developer owned land, without planning and at the cheapest possible cost. There were no municipal by-laws against overcrowding, so thousands of working families slept more than four to a bed. There were no indoor toilets, which meant communities were quite literally choking on their own filth. In 1841, 70 percent of Liverpool's 223,000 citizens were industrial workers, and almost two out of three workers lived in conditions described as "crowded, dirty and insanitary."[59] One area of Manchester had only two privies for 250 people.

Obviously such neighbourhoods were perfect breeding grounds for infectious disease. Virulent epidemics killed thousands. As the Industrial Revolution spread throughout Europe, the United States, and Canada, the pattern was repeated: vile urban conditions, epidemics, and death.

Cholera posed a particular threat, since it spread rapidly and could kill even a young, healthy person within hours. During one cholera epidemic in London, over ten thousand died within three months.[60] People contracted cholera through contaminated food or drinking water, or by having unsanitary contact with infected individuals.

During the 1840s, various reform groups sprang up as the dreadful consequences of unplanned industrialization became apparent. One of the most vocal of these early lobby groups was the Health of Towns Association, founded by the physician Southwood Smith. Dr. Smith's lobby borrowed strategies developed fifty years earlier by John Howard, the great prison reformer: first, they educated the public; then, using public pressure to get attention, they convinced legislators to pass remedial laws, which the reformers had often drafted themselves!

The reform movement reached a crescendo in 1848. These were revolutionary times: Marx and Engels had just published *The Communist Manifesto*, there were rebellions in Europe, particularly in the German states. Remembering the French Revolution, the most enlightened members of the English ruling class knew that harsh conditions for the poor were as likely to breed revolt as disease. News that a cholera epidemic was sweeping through Europe helped ensure the passage of Britain's Public Health Act that year. This law established a General Board of Health with the power to initiate surveys and investigations and to appoint local health boards. These local boards, in turn, had some authority over water supply, sewage control, and certain aspects of occupational health and safety.

In 1854, another cholera epidemic swept into Britain. Dr. John Snow* was a committed scientist with a passion for tracking cholera epidemics. He traced the outbreak in one part of London to a pump on Broad Street and immediately presented evidence to the local authorities asking them to remove the pump's handle; they complied, and the outbreak was halted.

At the time, water supplies in London were controlled by private sector companies, who were enraged at this interference. In retaliation, they joined forces with local councils (which were often dominated by property developers and their friends) and the College of Physicians (whose members chafed at being less effective against cholera than public health officials) to eliminate the Board of Health. But their impact was only temporary; Parliament eventually re-established the Board.

Lessons from history

The effects of the Industrial Revolution and the history of cholera in Victorian England provide a perfect example of how society's values, institutions, and interests affect health. Regular cholera epidemics were virtually guaranteed by the unsanitary

---

* Dr. Snow is also famous as a pioneer of anaesthesia. Queen Victoria was his most famous patient—he administered chloroform to ease labour pains during the births of two of her children.

living conditions associated with unplanned, rapid growth of industrial cities. Legislation to overturn the Poor Laws was promoted by private industrial interests and reflected an abrupt departure from Britain's traditional social values: laissez-faire favoured by the reformist Whigs was in; paternalistic interference by the more patrician Tories was out. The extreme political philosophy of the day temporarily stripped the government of key Guardian tools to protect the population's health. Ultimately however, values changed again, allowing Guardian institutions—like the General Board of Health—to protect the public from overzealous private interests.

We face a similar dilemma today. Canadians are being repeatedly told we have to get "lean and mean" to compete in an increasingly global marketplace. Reducing government deficits by cutting social spending is seen as essential to creating a more "favourable environment" for business. The ideology driving these policies is called "neo-conservatism" today, although "neo-liberalism" would be a more accurate label. Whatever you choose to call it, this modern economic movement has at least two elements in common with those who advocated philosophical necessity during the Industrial Revolution. Both assert the primacy of the marketplace unfettered by regulation. And both endorse the trickle-down theory by assuming that favours to capital will ultimately increase everyone's wealth.

What worries us, however, is the fact that massive cuts to government spending could do serious harm to the public's health. Many recent government health reports recommend that all major policy changes be reviewed for their impact on health. As far as we know, this is not happening with respect to current plans for tackling government deficits. We want to flag the urgent need to conduct health-impact assessments on these sweeping changes to economic policy. Recently, Lloyd Axworthy, federal minister of human resources, announced a two-year review of Canada's social programs with a view to completely overhauling them. Proposals emerging from this exercise should also be subject to a comprehensive health impact assessment.

The Rich Get Richer ... the Poor Get Sick

Journalist Diane Francis has been a major critic of Ontario's income support system, claiming: "... it's made payments so rich nobody will get off welfare.... Not only will this system create an underclass of parasites on an unimagined scale, but it will drive interest rates higher and, if not legislated out immediately, double property taxes in no time." Of course, most of the people who depend on welfare in Ontario and across Canada are single women and their children. If welfare payments were all that rich, Canada's record on child poverty wouldn't be so dismal.

Some members of Canada's business elite seem more concerned about the excesses of the marketplace. Ontario lieutenant governor and financier Hal Jackman, in an address to the University of Toronto's 1993 convocation, said: "... business leaders during the 1980s began to seek new economic justifications for their role. Free-market or classical economic theory was misinterpreted to justify the pursuit of selfish and short-sighted aims at the expense of long-term growth and industrial stability.... In the 1980s, it became fashionable to justify this activity by equating nineteenth-century utilitarianism with twentieth-century cupidity and greed."[61]

The debates raging now over social and economic policy in the 1990s sound a lot like Britain's nearly two hundred years ago. A federal paper on social policy leaked during the 1993 election criticized Canada's social safety net as "a barrier to people leading active and rewarding lives."[62] This is virtually identical to the critique that proponents of philosophical necessity used to overturn the Poor Laws. Supports to the poor are held out as bad economics and not in the best interests of the poor. We're told we have to cut social benefits in order to liberate the needy from their "dependence."

As already mentioned, substantial evidence from epidemiology, sociology, and immunology supports the conclusion that widening the gap between rich and poor increases illness. These findings, however, are largely ignored in the current economic debates about social policy in this country. Indeed, Canadians are being urged by some quarters to adopt American-style social policies. In fact, we've already started. For example, in early 1993, the Mulroney government changed the rules for unemployment insurance, making it more difficult for people to qualify for it and reducing the amount of the payments from 60 percent of prior earnings to 57 percent. David McLean, chairman of the Canadian Chamber of Commerce, championed these changes: "People who quit work for no good reason or who are unemployed because of their own misconduct do not have the right to expect to be supported by working Canadians."[63] But, of course, without jobs to go to, lower benefits and a shorter period of eligibility will only increase poverty and shift more and more people onto welfare.

Still, advocates of social spending cutbacks would like us to believe that this is necessary to spark economic growth. The resulting economic inequality, they assure us, will only be a short-term problem. Eventually greater overall wealth will be more evenly distributed. It is incumbent on those who make these arguments, however, to offer some demonstration that this, in fact, would occur. We believe these tax and social policy changes would magnify economic inequalities and greatly increase illness and social strife. Just look south.

Economics and health or economics versus health?

Some researchers are suggesting new ways to measure the economic health of a society besides looking at the Gross Domestic Product and unemployment rates. For example, Amartya Sen, a Harvard economist, thinks we should highlight more "human" indicators, such as mortality, illiteracy, crime, and homelessness.[64]

Economists use the term "externalities" to refer to the health consequences of social and economic inequality. Robert Evans offers this colourful definition of externalities or external effects:

> One person or organization's behaviour may affect others, independent of any voluntary transaction. My playing of loud music at night disturbs your sleep; my refusal to be immunized increases your chance of getting polio, my failure to wear seat-belts increases your taxes to pay my hospital bills. Conversely my beautiful garden not only gives you pleasure, but raises your property value. Insofar as my behaviour fails to take account of such effects, because others have no way to induce me to respond to their preferences, I will (from a society-wide perspective) over-indulge

in activities with negative externalities and under-indulge in
those with positive externalities.[65]

Clearly, the adverse health impact of greater social inequality has
major economic consequences. However, these costs are not usually borne by those who benefit financially from inequality.

This is changing in some policy areas, however. For example, new laws and regulations are beginning to require polluting
industries to clean up the sites they have contaminated. These
new demands reflect a substantive change in Canadian values
and beliefs. We no longer think companies have the "right" to
destroy the environment for private gain. This begs a question:
do Canadians really think we should abandon the millions of
poor so the rest of us can live the good life?

Economic efficiency demands that we allow private enterprise to grow or contract according to market forces. But that
doesn't mean workers should be treated like widgets. In effect,
it's a pay now or pay later proposition. If society as a whole
doesn't cover the cost of sane and humane labour adjustment
now, we'll have to pay eventually through our health care and
criminal justice systems.

Healthy Communities

In the early 1980s, Dr. Trevor Hancock, a leading public health
physician and consultant to the World Health Organization, had a
brilliant idea. Like a modern-day Southwood Smith, Dr. Hancock
was advocating that cities consider the health of their citizens in
their planning and urban development processes. He tested out this
idea in a workshop for Toronto planners, where it was greeted with
enthusiasm. Soon, the Healthy Communities movement captured
national and international attention. By 1993, more than one thousand communities were participating from all over the world.

The Canadian Healthy Communities Project got its start in
1988 with support from the Canadian Institute of Planners, the
Canadian Public Health Association, and the Canadian Federation of Municipalities. Its goal is to improve the health of Canadian communities through the participation and empowerment
of community residents and local government officials.[66]

But today the movement is weathering some heavy criticism. For example, the Toronto office came close to being closed when city council inadvertently passed a motion to that effect. The ensuing debate over whether or not to reinstate it revealed the fact that many politicians had doubts about its effectiveness. Councillor Kay Gardner, for example, complained that the Healthy City Office "is not able to create one job, or provide one living unit. It's a waste of $400,000. Nobody knows what it is and they [sic] couldn't care less."[67]

Kingston's former mayor, Helen Cooper, supplies a similar critique. She says the whole idea of healthy communities is tough for most politicians to grasp unless they have a background in the area. For many, she says, it's "an airy-fairy concept," and too many other more immediate issues are taking precedence.[68] The Kingston project's coordinator, Sue Hendler, admits that they have a major problem with how they are perceived: "They just see us going to these meetings and never getting anything done, which is really unfortunate."

Even academe is throwing darts. Michael Stevenson, a professor of political science from York University, says the health promotion movement's relatively "narrow bureaucratic base" is yet another factor limiting its ability to produce concrete results.[69] Contrasting it with the women's movement and the environmental lobby, he says health promotion "is not a social movement but a bureaucratic tendency; not a movement against the state, but one within it."

This may or may not be a fair comment. Improving health requires a political action against the status quo—a direct challenge to society's values and institutions. But if many of the participants are civil servants themselves, how can they be expected to do this effectively? Government officials are supposed to implement policy, not attack it. Sharon Martin, now executive director of the Vancouver health region, thinks the Canadian approach to healthy communities has been too "top-down." She would like to see more of a community development focus. Dr. Hancock notes the criticism but claims that both tactics are needed—"top-down" and "bottom-up"—to effectively mobilize communities to promote their health.

Certainly the Canadian Healthy Communities movement has helped to broaden awareness about the determinants of health and to create new audiences for health status information. The extent to which this awareness gets translated into concrete and effective action, however, remains something of a question.

The central problem is that health really is "politics writ large," to quote nineteenth-century German pathologist Rudolf Virchow. Many health problems involve major conflicts between different groups with different interests. To resolve them, these conflicts have to be confronted openly, not avoided. For the Healthy Communities movement, this may prove to be an insurmountable challenge.

Improving health and improving our health care system require quite different strategies. This book is mainly concerned with the latter issue, especially how to encourage more innovation and more entrepreneurial behaviour among health care providers, and how to create incentives that encourage Trader values. In this chapter, we have examined a broad question: how to improve overall health. Most of the time, major shifts in the overall pattern of health and illness require structural change in society's values and institutions. Powerful interests can be expected to oppose these changes. Active political pressure from "the other side" can help set the stage for reform, but only governments, in their role as good Guardians, have the authority to effectively counter these private interests.

One hundred and fifty years ago, Rudolf Virchow observed that major socio-economic change always brings changes in health.[70] Today, Canada is embroiled in the most extensive period of socio-economic change since the end of the Second World War. We are already beginning to see the impact of these changes on the health of our citizens. But we also have the knowledge to moderate this change to protect the health of Canadians. The question is whether Canadian governments will use this knowledge or whether they will sacrifice our health for somebody else's wealth.

Chapter 4

Quality of Care: Doing the Right Things Right

FORMER ONTARIO HEALTH MINISTER Frances Lankin created a stir when she claimed before a national audience that as much as one-third of medical care delivered in Canada was inappropriate.[1] Her comment triggered loud protests among many members of the medical profession, who were attending a conference on physician resource management. But was Ms. Lankin really off the mark?

This is a scary subject. To suggest that some patients receive services that are unnecessary or dangerous sounds harsh. So is the suggestion that some patients aren't getting the kind of care they require. Nevertheless, there is strong evidence that there's a lot of inappropriate care in our system.

This problem is not confined to Canada alone. Health care systems around the world are grappling with the same issue: how to improve the quality of care by reducing inappropriate servicing.

It's late Friday night in 1989, and Susan G. is in hard labour in the maternity unit of the Oakville Trafalgar Hospital. At first, Susan makes good progress, but after she's given a spinal anaesthetic to freeze the lower part of her body, her labour slows. As the hours pass, Susan becomes more and more tired and her husband more and more anxious. Meanwhile, her doctor is increasingly worried about the pattern of the baby's heart rate showing up on the electronic fetal monitor.

Finally, the doctor rests his hand on Susan's distended abdomen and says reassuringly, "That's all right, Susan. You've given it a good go, but now it's time for us to take over. I'm going to have to perform a Caesarean section to make sure your baby comes out nice and healthy."

While Susan isn't happy about the prospect of surgery, she was prepared for this news. Both her doctor and the leader of her prenatal class had warned her that a C-section might be necessary if her labour didn't progress well enough. And anyway, she's glad the baby's going to come sooner rather than later.

An hour later, with her infant at her breast, Susan is too full of joy to dwell on such unimportant details. Sure, she would have preferred to deliver her baby "normally," but she has accepted what happened and is grateful that modern medicine was there for her when she needed it.

What Susan didn't know is that the Oakville Trafalgar Hospital had one of the highest Caesarean section rates of any Ontario community hospital—28.8 percent of all births.[2] She also didn't know that if she had gone to a different hospital— for example, the Credit Valley Hospital just 25 kilometres to the east—she might not have had a Caesarean at all. In 1988, Credit Valley had a Caesarean section rate of 18.2 percent.

In the 1960s, Caesarean sections were relatively rare—in Canada in 1969, only about 5 percent of births were surgically delivered, and many reputable obstetricians had a C-section rate under 3 percent. But the frequency of surgical deliveries gradually increased over the next twenty years until, by 1989, about 20 percent of all births were delivered by Caesarean section— one birth in five. By 1990-91, Caesarean section was the fifth most common in-patient surgical procedure.[3] In comparison to the rest of the world, our rate of surgical birthing was close to the top.[4]

True, over the last thirty years infant and maternal death rates in Canada have fallen dramatically, but little evidence links this improvement to the increasing frequency of Caesarean sections. In fact, in the Netherlands, where one baby in three is born at home with a midwife in attendance, the Caesarean section rate is only 7 percent, about one-third the Canadian rate. Dutch mothers and babies appear to do just as well as those from countries with much higher rates of surgical intervention. This should not come as a surprise. Perinatal and maternal mortality are not strongly linked to the method of delivery, but rather to prenatal care and to other social and economic factors.

Canada's very high rate for Caesarean sections suggests that many of the surgical deliveries we perform in this country are inappropriate. It is one indication of a major problem in the quality of care our system delivers.

Here's another.

Melanie B. is forty-five and has gone to consult her doctor about her increasingly heavy menstrual periods. After a physical examination and a chat, her physician suggests the problem might be caused by fibroid tumours. The doctor explains that these growths are almost always non-cancerous, but that they can sometimes cause heavy bleeding. Following an ultrasound to confirm the diagnosis, the doctor recommends a hysterectomy as a way of dealing with the problem "once and for all." He tells Melanie that a myomectomy—a more complicated operation to remove the tumours while leaving her uterus intact—is a possible alternative, but points out that in her case it would be much more difficult because of the number of tumours involved. Reluctantly, Melanie agrees to the hysterectomy.

Unfortunately, life after the operation isn't at all what Melanie expected. For one thing, her recovery takes a very long time—she still feels weak even two months after the surgery. She also experiences a decline in sexual desire and no longer has orgasms.[5]

Melanie's experience of sexual dysfunction following her operation is quite common. According to Dr. Kurt Semm, an internationally respected gynecologist from Germany, the iatrogenic (physician-caused) destruction of female sexuality is seldom given a second thought.[6]

One afternoon, three months after the operation, Melanie is talking to some friends. One of them mentions the fact that fibroid tumours usually shrink with menopause. This is earth-shattering news to Melanie. "My goodness," she says, "does that mean if I had just waited for a few more years, I might never have had needed to have a hysterectomy?"

Hysterectomy is the ninth most common surgical operation in Canada, according to the Hospital Medical Records Institute. If you're a woman, whether you have one or not varies a lot depending on where you live. Rough province-to-province rates (per 100,000 men, women, and children) range from 639 in Newfoundland to 426 in Alberta.[7] Dr. Marsha Cohen, an epidemiologist and senior scientist working with the Institute of Clinical

Evaluative Sciences in Toronto, is studying surgical rate variations in Ontario. In the case of hysterectomy, she reports no variation at all when the diagnosis is cancer, for example, a clear-cut case for surgery. But she has found very large county-to-county variation when the surgery was being performed for other reasons.[8] "When heavy bleeding was listed as any of the diagnoses, the variation was enormous," says Cohen. A woman living in the county with the highest rate was *eighteen times* more likely to have a hysterectomy than a woman living in the county with the lowest rate.[9] (Just for comparison, the variation data that triggered intense media interest in breast cancer treatment found an eight-fold difference in the chances a woman would have a lumpectomy with radiation rather than mastectomy.) Asked whether further studies were planned to investigate the reasons for the variation in hysterectomy provision, Dr. Cohen said there were none that she was aware of.[10] (Women's groups take note.)*

Gillian W. was shocked when doctors at the hospital said they had no choice but to amputate her mother's gangrenous foot. Mrs. B., Gillian's mother, has adult onset diabetes, first diagnosed ten years earlier when she was sixty years old. Mrs. B. has always been careful to follow her diet and take her medication as ordered. All the same, she developed a serious foot infection that wouldn't heal. Her daughter can't understand why the problem wasn't caught earlier—especially since her mother is in the habit of seeing her physician regularly. She was annoyed to discover that her mother's doctor did little more than take her blood pressure, check her diabetes control, and renew her prescriptions. In all the years she has had diabetes, her mother never properly understood the dangers from infection, nor did she realize the importance of proper foot care.

Complications from chronic illnesses like diabetes, high blood pressure, and heart disease are a common reason for hospitalization and a major cause of death. Primary care can catch problems early, before they become major threats to health.

---

* These and other data appear in *The Ontario Practice Atlas*, a publication of the Toronto Institute for Clinical Evaluative Sciences. This is a highly useful tool for researchers, health planners, and clinicians.

Poor Quality Care Kills Thousands of Canadians Every Year

In 1984, some of the world's best health service researchers from Harvard University made a thorough study of the incidence and nature of injuries in New York State hospital care.[11] The study involved a random sample of over 30,000 hospital records that were meticulously scanned for evidence of adverse events and negligence. The investigators found that:

- 4 percent of the patients had suffered an adverse event from their hospital care;
- care for 1 percent of patients was clearly negligent;
- one out of every two hundred patients died from the adverse consequences of their care;
- one out of every five hundred patients acquired a permanent disability from their hospitalization.

Altogether in 1984, nearly 7,000 residents of New York State died and an additional 1,700 were permanently disabled because of negligent hospital care.

Robert Pritchard, president of the University of Toronto and chairman of a Canadian task force that looked into medical malpractice, described the Harvard study as "the best single empirical analysis of the frequency of medical injuries caused by negligence ever done. It is a superb study done by excellent people." And yet, Dr. Stuart Lee, secretary-treasurer of the Canadian Medical Protective Association (the major malpractice insurer for Canadian physicians), questioned whether the study's results had any relevance for Canada: "One has to keep in mind that Canadian hospitals are subject to regular review by accreditation boards. I don't believe that is the case for the bulk of New York hospitals."[12] In fact, New York hospitals are routinely reviewed by state and federal regulatory agencies.

According to Paul Weiler, a Canadian professor of law at Harvard and one of the architects of the study, there is little difference between the quality of health care provided in New York State and in Canada. Dr. Alex McPherson, former president of the Canadian Medical Association, says the findings of the Harvard study are very relevant to Canada.

However, since a number of studies have found that Canadian patients are treated less aggressively than American patients, hospitalized Canadians might actually be less likely to experience injuries as the result of treatment. The fact that the Harvard study found more injuries among intensively treated older persons tends to support this possibility.[13] But even if we assume that Canada's injury rate from hospital care is only half the level found in the Harvard study, we still face a serious quality problem:

- 5,000 deaths a year due to negligent hospital care;
- over 1,300 cases of permanent disability, every year;
- and over 20,000 total cases of negligence within hospitals.[14]

We need to remember that the Harvard-New York State study only categorized adverse events as "negligent" or "not negligent." It did not consider other quality problems in health care, such as poor primary care leading to an avoidable hospitalization.

What is Appropriate Care?

Pinpointing the exact proportion of health care that is inappropriate, and estimating accurately how much inappropriate care costs us, are very complicated tasks. However, it isn't difficult to support Ms. Lankin's assertion that one-third of medical care delivered in Canada is inappropriate. Indeed, the proportion could be even higher. According to Dr. John Wennberg, a professor of epidemiology from Dartmouth Medical School and the director of the Centre for Evaluative Clinical Sciences, perhaps as much as half of all elective surgeries are inappropriate because patient preferences are not properly taken into consideration in the decision-making process.

A study done by a joint task force of the Ontario Medical Association and the ministry of health estimated that Ontario spends $200 million annually on physicians' services for the common cold.[15] Several studies have shown that relatively simple education can reduce physicians' services for colds and other minor illnesses by up to one-half.[16]

However, to conclude whether care is appropriate or not requires some consensus about what appropriate care means. One popular definition in current use describes it as: "the *right* service, at the *right* time, delivered by the *right* person, in the *right* place." This definition helps to highlight the complexity of actually delivering appropriate care to an individual patient. Obviously it involves clinical decision-making, management efficiency, and technical skill. But it also requires sound macro policies and careful planning so that resources and coordinated systems are in place to support appropriate care. A system that consistently delivers appropriate care is a responsive system.

Another definition zeroes in on clinical decision-making and costs and takes a decidedly prospective view: "A service is considered appropriate when the best scientific evidence indicates in advance that it would be of some net benefit to the patient and when the service costs no more than an equally effective alternative."

In Table 4.1 we look at some of the dimensions of appropriate care and attempt to classify them according to the first definition offered.

Variable variations

Many people mistakenly believe that for every set of symptoms there is only one correct diagnostic work-up, and for every illness diagnosed there is only one correct treatment. In fact, modern medicine is rife with alternative and competing diagnoses and therapies. One problem is the fact that most of these investigations and therapies (drugs are a major exception) have never been rigorously evaluated to determine whether they work or how well they work compared to alternatives. "Perhaps only 20 to 25 percent of what we do [in health care] has been adequately evaluated," says Dr. David Naylor, an epidemiologist and director of the Institute for Clinical Evaluative Sciences.[17]

As a result, there is enormous uncertainty among doctors about the best ways to treat patients for many common conditions. This high level of uncertainty shows up in large variations in the provision of services among different countries, different provinces, different counties, different cities, and even between individual hospitals and individual doctors.

Dr. John Wennberg spent the early years of his career documenting variations in the provision of specific treatments, particularly

Table 4.1

DIMENSIONS OF APPROPRIATE CARE

1. THE RIGHT SERVICE
   - is likely to provide a net benefit to patients according to the best available scientific evidence;
   - is guided by the preferences of patients who are fully informed about possible risks and benefits;
   - costs no more than an equally effective alternative service.

2. THE RIGHT TIME

   Services are provided according to scientific evidence about timing. For example,

   - childhood immunizations are done according to schedule;
   - risk factors are identified (e.g. hypertension);
   - effective screening programs are implemented;
   - anticipatory care is provided to patients with chronic illnesses to prevent deterioration.

   Effective services are provided without lengthy waiting;

   - urgent cases receive care without delay.

3. THE RIGHT PROVIDER

   Patients have access to experienced and competent providers;

   - providers have sufficient technical skill to deliver their care.

   Patients have access to the most cost-effective provider;

   - Many services are provided by family doctors instead of specialists and others are provided by nurses or other health professionals instead of doctors. Patients are taught, as much as possible, to manage their own health problems.

4. THE RIGHT PLACE
   - Highly specialized services are clustered in regional and teaching hospitals while more routine care is provided in community hospitals. Nursing homes offer palliative care, oxygen, and suctioning to prevent unnecessary transfers to hospitals.
   - Some community care is delivered in home-like alternatives to the acute-care hospital—e.g. hospices for palliative care, birthing centres, adult day-care, etc.
   - Many services are available in the home according to patient preferences.

surgeries. In comparing medical services in Boston and New Haven—two New England communities with reputations for academic excellence in medicine, and remarkably similar populations—Dr. Wennberg reports that:

> Residents of New Haven were about twice as likely to undergo a bypass operation for coronary artery disease as their counterparts in Boston. On the other hand, Bostonians were much more likely to have their hips and knees replaced by a surgical prosthesis than were New Havenites. Bostonians were more than twice as likely to have a carotid endarterectomy—an operation to clear plaque from the large artery in the neck. By contrast, hysterectomies for non-cancerous conditions of the uterus were more commonly performed on New Havenites.[18]

Enormous cost differences arise from these kinds of variations. Dr. Wennberg reports that for patients over the age of sixty-five, 1982 hospital reimbursements in Boston amounted to $1,894 per person, while those in New Haven were $1,078. If Boston patterns of practice were like those in New Haven, the system could have saved $63 million in one year. He notes that the difference between Boston's and New Haven's costs relates mainly to differences in the decisions doctors make about whether to treat three very common conditions—low back pain, pneumonia, and gastroenteritis—in home or in hospital, the higher costs being associated with hospital care.

Canada's health care system displays equally remarkable variability. For example:

- A patient is three times more likely to have a tonsillectomy in Saskatchewan than in Quebec.[19]
- In Ontario, county-to-county rates of coronary artery bypass surgery vary two-and-one-half-fold. [20]
- Depending on the facility, the length of a hospital stay for heart attack patients in Ontario ranges from 6.6 days to 12.9 days—a difference of almost 100 percent. Available information on patient and hospital characteristics only explained a small proportion of this variation.[21]

The presence of high variation in our system calls for more serious study. Which rate is right? Should low-rate areas increase their provision of service to match high-rate areas? Or do these variations mean that high-rate areas are providing too many unnecessary services?

The answer requires more research. Before we can say the high rates are too high or the low rates are too low, we need to know what constitutes appropriate care. In other words, we need standards or practice guidelines based on rigorous scientific evidence about what works.

The right service

When retired professor Frank S., aged seventy-five, first saw the urologist after a referral from his family doctor, he hadn't realized that the problems he was experiencing in emptying his bladder were very common among men his age. After reassuring the patient that his condition was not caused by cancer, the urologist explained that an enlarged prostate gland was the source of his trouble and, after exploring the options, recommended surgery. Frank had the operation, but like 10 to 20 percent of patients who have this type of surgery, he is now impotent as a result.[22] "I hadn't realized my chances of having this kind of complication," he says. In fact, it turns out that some men have even more prostate symptoms *after* the surgery.[23] "If I had only appreciated the risks of the surgery and the real chances that my bladder problem would be cured, I might have decided against the operation."

Even when good evidence is available about the risks and benefits of alternative approaches, often the decision about whether or not a particular elective surgery is appropriate cannot be made without taking the patient's particular point of view into account. Two people with the same severity of symptoms often have completely different reactions. What seems intolerable to one person might be considered only mildly annoying to another. Also, people vary in how they respond to risk. A 3 percent chance of becoming incontinent might deter one person from having an operation, while another might think those odds well worth the risk.

Because of these differences among individuals, there is generally no way to determine appropriateness unless patients are fully informed about risks and benefits and are actually encouraged and assisted to make choices based on their own individual preferences.

To address these issues, Dr. Wennberg developed an interactive video for patients with benign prostate disease. Patients could scan the video material in about an hour and learn about the relative risks and benefits of having surgery as compared to "watchful waiting" (monitoring symptoms). All of the patients in the video were also doctors; some chose to have the surgery; others opted for watchful waiting. Demonstrating that even doctors make different choices helped patients feel free to make decisions based on their own personal preferences.

In a study comparing patients who had access to the video with those who merely talked the options over with their doctors, Wennberg found that the "video patients" were only half as likely to choose the operation, leading him to suggest wryly that "patients appear to be more risk-averse than their surgeons."[24] What's more, he notes that willingness to undertake the risk of the operation did not seem to be related to the severity of symptoms.

Dr. Wennberg helped establish an organization, the Foundation for Informed Medical Decision Making, which has developed interactive videos for a number of conditions, including low back pain, mild hypertension, and breast cancer treatment.[25] For many of these conditions, he says, "an appropriate clinical decision requires the active engagement of the patient in choosing the treatment that is right for him."[26]

The right provider

Gail F. is a nineteen-year-old university student. She was prescribed the birth control pill six months ago by her family doctor just before beginning a sexual relationship with her boyfriend. After gaining ten pounds, however, she stopped taking the pill and she and her boyfriend began using condoms. Unfortunately, her boyfriend had never been schooled in their proper use. Once, after ejaculating, the condom slipped off. It was the wrong time of Gail's menstrual cycle and she became pregnant.

If Gail had been able to see a primary care nurse she might have avoided this unwanted pregnancy. A session with a nurse to discuss her birth control options at greater length might have led her to decide it was worth it to stay on the pill. Even if she'd decided to switch to condoms, the nurse would have provided information about how to use them properly and likely would also have recommended using spermicidal foam as a backup to the barrier method.

A literature review done by the American Nurses' Association has shown that nurses' patients often have better outcomes than physicians' patients—partly because of better communication—and the costs are much lower.[27]

The right place

Elizabeth H. is an eighty-four-year-old woman who broke her pelvis in a fall at home. An ambulance brought her to the emergency department of her local hospital, where it was decided to admit her. After the first day in hospital, Elizabeth became very confused, unable to recognize her daughter or her doctor. After seventy-two hours, she regained her senses, but had become very apathetic and depressed staying in bed. Three weeks later, Elizabeth has deteriorated significantly. She is very weak and can do very little for herself. Her family and doctor are considering a nursing home placement. There doesn't seem to be any other option.

And yet all this might have been avoided if Elizabeth's local hospital had had a "quick response team" in the emergency department. With such a team in place, a social worker could have helped her family mobilize the appropriate community services to keep Elizabeth at home over the crisis period. A broken pelvis needs nursing and personal care, but not necessarily hospital services. A hospital stay can often be disastrous for a previously normal elderly person, leading to rapid deterioration of mental and physical functions. More often than not, home is the right place for many patients who are currently being hospitalized.

Why Is There So Much Inappropriate Care?

What is really causing our high levels of inappropriate care? Is incompetence the main problem? Who's responsible?

Although it may be tempting to think that individual failings are to blame for inappropriate care, the bulk of the problem has little to do with the knowledge and skills of health care professionals and administrators.

"We live in a universe filled with flaws," says Dr. Donald Berwick, who heads the Institute for Healthcare Improvement in Boston. When problems with quality arise, he says, most of the time the cause has nothing to do with the talents or motivation of the people doing the work. Instead, the problems are embedded within the systems and processes that govern how care is delivered. While it is possible to design processes and systems that are error-resistant, in most health care organizations, how the work is done has evolved willy-nilly. Things go wrong all the time. Files get lost, patients arrive late for their x-rays, orders get misread.

Any number of structural conditions can make errors more likely. For example, if two pills look exactly the same, they are more easily confused than if they have different shapes and colours.

A great deal of inappropriate care in Canada is linked to the structure of our health care system, with its over-reliance on hospitals and nursing homes, underdeveloped home care and supportive housing options, and a poorly coordinated and fragmented primary care system. To ensure the quality of care Canadians deserve at a price they can afford, our health care delivery system needs a complete overhaul.

There is little quality assurance in Canada's health care system

Most Canadians would be shocked to find out how inadequate our programs for quality assurance really are. Most hospitals, for example, pay more attention to the quality of floor cleaning than to the quality of medical care they provide. If the grain or auto industries displayed the same lack of attention to quality, we wouldn't export a single kernel or car door.

And yet there is a generic process for quality assurance that is as applicable to medicine or nursing as it is to manufacturing. (See Figure 4.1.) Health care is only beginning to employ it.

The first requirement is to set a standard for performance and make sure that it is up to date. It is possible for standards to relate to structural issues—for example, how many and what kind of staff are needed in a given intensive care ward. It is also possible for standards to relate to process issues—for example, the steps to be followed in an emergency room in examining

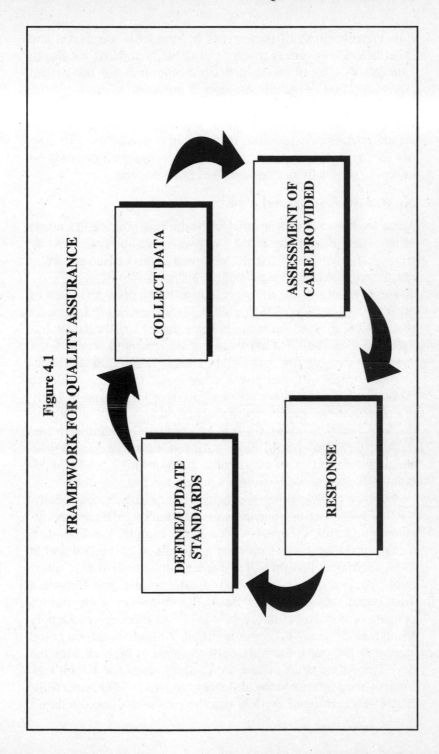

Figure 4.1
FRAMEWORK FOR QUALITY ASSURANCE

rape victims. Both of these types of standards are useful and necessary. However, as much as possible, standards for health care quality should relate to desired outcomes for the patient (survival, relief of pain, restoration of functioning, etc.).

Next, you must monitor performance and see if it falls short, matches, or exceeds the standard. When performance is below standard, action is required to make improvements. Figuring out the "right" action or actions to take very much depends on understanding why the standard was not achieved.

No standard for standards

There are few explicit standards for health care practice in Canada or anywhere else in the world. And when we compare our system's performance to those in the United States or Europe, we're not always sure how to explain the differences we find.

For example, Canadians are more likely than residents of other countries to have their gallbladders removed.[28] It appears that most Canadian surgeons believe that if a gallbladder has gallstones, it should almost always be removed, even if the stones are causing few if any symptoms.[29] Some Canadian doctors take issue with this position and point to strong evidence that surgery for people without significant symptoms is likely to cause more problems in the short run than will be allayed in the long run.[30] Even so, there is no explicit Canadian standard describing who should have gallbladder surgery and who should not. The lack of standards is a major drawback in developing effective quality assurance programming.

So is the proliferation of competing standards. Occasionally, we find two or more standards promulgated by different organizations, offering different advice. For example, the Canadian Cholesterol Consensus Conference, an ad-hoc group that met in 1988, recommended that all Canadian adults have their cholesterol checked on a regular basis.[31] Meanwhile, the Canadian Task Force on the Periodic Health Examination, a prestigious permanent task force that reports to the Conference of Deputy Ministers of Health, recommended a much more targeted screening program, focusing only on those at high risk for the development of heart disease.[32] A survey done for a joint task force of the Ontario Medical Association and the Ontario Ministry of Health found in 1990 that the province's doctors didn't seem to follow anybody's guidelines.[33] Conflicting standards are almost worse than no standards at all. They just add to the general confusion.

Also adding to the muddle is the question of who has the authority to set standards for health care practice. The Royal College of Physicians and Surgeons of Canada is chartered by Parliament to certify specialists, but it doesn't set standards for practice. In some provinces, the legislation that regulates health professionals and establishes licensing agencies also refers to establishing and maintaining standards of practice, but in others, this objective isn't even mentioned. With respect to medicine, the provincial Colleges of Physicians and Surgeons have the statutory authority to discipline doctors. But in Ontario, for example, the professional association—the Ontario Medical Association (OMA)—disputes the right of the college to set standards of practice. The OMA wants to do it, and it prefers to call standards "guidelines."[34]

In truth, neither the provincial colleges nor the provincial medical associations really have the expertise to elaborate standards unilaterally. The real expertise lies within national specialty and sub-specialty medical societies. When the Ontario College of Physicians and Surgeons initiated a process to develop standards (which they now call "parameters") for in vitro fertilization clinics, they relied heavily upon the Society of Obstetricians and Gynecologists of Canada and the Canadian Fertility and Andrology Society. However, these specialty societies are voluntary, non-statutory bodies.

To have legitimacy, standards of practice should be based on the best available scientific evidence, properly gathered and reviewed by acknowledged experts according to an accepted process. Some standards have been developed without recourse to the most basic groundwork—a methodical literature review.[35] On many occasions, however, the needed scientific evidence is sadly lacking, and instead standards are based almost entirely on expert opinion.

Patients or guinea pigs?

James S. was a fifty-four-year-old auto worker when he had his first heart attack in 1987. After James recovered, his cardiologist performed tests showing that James was prone to developing an abnormal heart rhythm (arrythmia). Even though James was feeling no symptoms at all, his doctor prescribed the drug encainide, which was touted to suppress these abnormal rhythms.

The doctor based his decision on a decade of medical consensus that drugs should be used routinely for patients like James. It was conclusively known that patients prone to arrhythmias, like James, were at increased risk for sudden death. It was also known that these arrhythmias could be suppressed with drugs like encainide. Bingo! If the drug could suppress the arrhythmias then it would save lives. One of the early advocates of this approach was Dr. Bernard Lown of Harvard University, who was to become internationally known as a co-founder of Physicians for Social Responsibility and recipient of the Nobel Peace Prize in 1985.[36]

Nine months after his heart attack, James suddenly keeled over at work. Co-workers started cardiopulmonary resuscitation right away and paramedics took over when the ambulance arrived. But all to no avail. James was dead by the time he got to the hospital. His wife and family were greatly saddened but took comfort in knowing that everything had been done to prevent his death. They never even suspected that, maybe, too much was done.

It wasn't until 1989 that a full evaluation of the use of antiarrhythmic drugs for people like James became available. The Cardiac Arrythmia Suppression Trial (CAST), which issued its initial report in that year, showed that encainide was more likely to kill patients than save them—two and one-half times more likely.[37]

Almost overnight, cardiologists stopped prescribing encainide and other similar drugs. But it was too late for James and thousands of others. Dr. Joel Morganroth of Philadelphia estimates that 1,500 to 2,000 Americans died annually from use of these antiarrhythmic drugs in the 1980s.[38] No comparable survey has ever been performed in Canada, but these drugs were also in wide use here. It's safe to conclude they killed hundreds of Canadians as well.

How could dangerous therapies like these antiarrhythmic drugs become so widespread without a proper evaluation? Are there other dangerous and improperly evaluated diagnostic tests and therapies presently being used?

The answer is yes. Typically, a new diagnostic test or therapy is performed on a few patients who appear to be good candidates for success. Then their condition is compared to what it was prior to the procedure, or their condition might be compared to other, similar patients who were treated in the past.

The problem is that these kinds of studies are likely to greatly overstate the usefulness of the new procedure. They are popular, however—particularly if there is money to be made. A clever public relations firm will take these early "promising results" and try for maximum media play. Professionals will adopt the innovation and insurers will pay for it. Finally, years later, if there's enough scepticism, a proper randomized controlled trial will be conducted. Professors John and Sonja McKinlay, American health researchers, have documented this phenomenon, which they have called "seven stages in the career of a medical innovation":[39]

1. A promising report
2. Professional and organizational adoption
3. Public acceptance and state (third-party) endorsement
4. Standard procedure and observational reports
5. Randomized controlled trial
6. Professional denunciation
7. Erosion and discreditation

Why aren't medical services better evaluated? There are two major reasons. First, rigorous evaluations can be expensive and logistically difficult. Second, some doctors and others resist good evaluations.

Evaluation: you get what you pay for

The simplest evaluation study is a case report. A doctor will write up the results for one patient or a series of patients who have had the new test or treatment. Sometimes, the patients' conditions are compared before and after the procedure—a so-called before-and-after study. This type of study is very simple to conduct but it often provides incorrect results, for three main reasons:

1. Most illness is self-limiting
Most illnesses clear up on their own, given enough time. For example, most respiratory infections are caused by viruses that

are not responsive to antibiotics. Chicken soup, vitamin C, and a couple of days of rest and the cold has run its course. However, if a patient sees a doctor and is prescribed a useless antibiotic, she will still get better in a few days. The only problem is that the patient will likely credit the drug for her recovery.

2. The high variability of chronic illnesses
People with chronic illnesses, like arthritis and heart disease, find that their symptoms wax and wane even though, in the long term, their condition usually gets progressively worse. In general, patients will tend to consult their doctors whenever their symptoms worsen. If they receive treatment and their symptoms improve, patients and doctors might think the treatment worked, even though the improvement might have come about anyway due to the high variability of their condition.

3. The placebo effect
If a patient thinks a new treatment will help his condition, the treatment is more likely to be effective.

While most people are familiar with the placebo effect for headache or insomnia, it can also improve symptoms of heart disease and other serious organic illnesses. For example, in the late 1950s, before the advent of modern coronary artery bypass surgery, doctors experimented with a procedure called internal mammary artery ligation. In an elegant study, the doctors randomly assigned heart patients to have the surgery or a "sham" operation. After the operation, 75 percent of patients in *both groups* reported symptom reduction. Both groups also had comparable reductions in their use of medication and ability to tolerate exercise, and both groups also showed improvement in their electrocardiograms (EKGs) during exercise.[40]

For all of these reasons, good evaluations of medical treatments must include a control group—individuals who are not subject to the intervention being studied. The best evaluation is when the control and experimental groups are established by a random process—the randomized controlled trial (RCT).

Screening tests: the false god of prevention
Screening tests are a special case for evaluation. These tests are used on healthy people either to catch disease in its early stages

or to uncover and modify risk factors that might lead to disease before it occurs. The theory is seductive—if we can identify disease in its early stages, we should be able to treat it before it causes damage. The Pap smear screening test for cancer of the cervix is an example of a worthwhile screening test. It is cheap and can be performed by family doctors or primary care nurses without special equipment. When read by competent personnel, it is reliable and valid. Cervical cancer grows quite slowly, so if it can be detected before it has spread it can be cured, and without disfiguring surgery.[41]

However, most screening tests are far less effective than the Pap smear. Some can even kill you.

Margaret B. was forty-two years old when she had her first mammogram x-ray for breast cancer. She was at no particular added risk for breast cancer, but she had heard that the American Cancer Society recommended that all women her age have mammograms. Her doctor agreed to her request. When the x-ray showed a small lump in her left breast, he referred her to a surgeon, who arranged a biopsy to check for cancer. Unfortunately, Margaret suffered a rare complication that can occur any time under general anaesthetic—she had a heart attack and died.

Is this just a hard-luck story, or is there a lesson here for others?

The only way to conclusively determine the effectiveness of a screening test is to assess it with a randomized controlled trial in which patients are randomly assigned to have either the test or conventional care. Canadian researchers astounded the world when the results of the Canadian National Breast Screening Study were released in 1992.[42] The study showed no survival improvement for women in their forties who were screened with mammography but a thirty percent reduction in cancer deaths for women 50 to 69 years of age.* American radiologists, perhaps alarmed by the potential loss of a lucrative part of

---

* There is an important difference between a "screening mammogram," performed on a healthy woman with no signs or symptoms of disease, and a "diagnostic mammogram," performed to diagnose specific breast disorders after a sign or symptom has been discovered. Also, most doctors would agree that women who have a strong family history of breast cancer should have mammograms earlier than age fifty.

their business, attacked the Canadian study on methodological grounds.[43] In fact, the American Cancer Society held a conference on the study that allowed only one of the Canadian investigators, Dr. Cornelia Baines of Toronto, a few minutes to respond to the criticism from four American doctors featured in the program.[44] Since then, however, the Canadian results have been vindicated by other studies and commentaries.[45] Finally, in late 1993, the prestigious U.S. National Cancer Institute recommended against initiating routine mammography until women reach age fifty.[46]

The esteemed British epidemiologist Dr. Archie Cochrane said it's more important to prove the benefits of a screening test than to prove the benefits of a treatment.[47] He explains that there is an ethical difference. When patients arrive at a doctor's office with symptoms, they are asking for help. But it's quite a different matter when a doctor, or a cancer society, or a shopping mall offers a screening test, because in doing so they imply that the benefit of testing outweighs the harm. The problem is that we can't reach that conclusion without first subjecting each screening test to evaluation. Careful study is necessary to avoid some statistical traps that can make a test look better than it really is.

For example, suppose we start a screening program for lung cancer and take sputum samples and chest x-rays from all heavy smokers every six months. Undoubtedly this kind of program would turn up a number of lung cancer cases earlier than would normally be discovered, because many of these patients would be diagnosed before they began to experience symptoms. Survival of cancer patients is usually measured from the time of diagnosis until death. Because the screening program moves the date of diagnosis to an earlier point, the statistics from our program could make it appear that we had actually improved the patients' length of survival. But this conclusion is wrong, and here's an example to show why.

Suppose Uncle Gene was fated to be diagnosed with lung cancer in June and to die in December. But instead he enters our screening program and we diagnose his cancer in March, three months earlier. Uncle Gene still dies in December, but it *appears* that we have increased his length of survival after diagnosis by 50 percent.[48] In reality, however, his life span remains exactly the same. Our screening program has only added to his time of dying, not to his time of living. Epidemiologists call this statistical trap "lead time bias."[49]

The best way to assess the effectiveness of a screening test is to perform an RCT, like the Canadian National Breast Screening Study. If an RCT is not available, we have to be very careful not to overestimate the effectiveness of the test.

The following list of questions can help to determine whether a screening program does more good than harm:[50]

1. Are there treatments available that work should the test results be positive?
2. Does the screening test relate to a serious or common illness?
3. Is there a good screening test available or does the test produce false-positive and false-negative results?
4. Can the program reach those who could benefit from it?
5. Does the health care system have the resources to cope with the screening program and its findings?
6. Will those who screen "positive" comply with subsequent advice and interventions?

Technology: what you don't know can hurt you

Technology has become an increasingly important component of modern health care. But is technology being used to provide the highest possible quality of care? What safeguards are in place to protect us from its possible adverse effects?

Technology assessment in Canada is inadequate and uneven. Protections for the public are few. For example, investigative reporter Nicholas Regush documented the inadequate staffing in the Health Protection Branch of Health and Welfare Canada in his book *Safety Last*. He noted that senior positions previously held by respected scientists were increasingly being filled by administrators, who lacked the necessary scientific background to protect Canadians from defective medical devices.

The government, stung by his criticisms, announced in the summer of 1993 that it was going to add thirty to fifty scientists to its staff to bolster the ability of the Health Protection Branch to assess new technologies.

In 1989, the Conference of Deputy Ministers of Health established the Canadian Coordinating Office for Health Technology Assessment (CCOHTA). The CCOHTA has an annual budget of $500,000—half for salaries and half for operating expenses. Despite the dedication of its staff, the CCOHTA has been fairly described as a fax machine in a broom closet. Quebec and British Columbia have established health technology assessment agencies. Ontario has also announced its intention to establish one. Given their budgets and scope, however, all these organizations put together can barely scratch the surface when it comes to conducting evaluations or diffusing their results to decision-makers.

To remain efficient and competitive, most developed countries and progressive corporations spend at least 3 percent of gross revenues on research and development. But Canada spends less than 1 percent of health care expenditures on any form of research.[51] And even then, the vast majority of these funds are used to conduct basic laboratory research or the pharmaceutical trials required before licensing a new drug product. (Most of these drug trials are for "me-too" products—slightly different versions of already existing drugs.)

Only a tiny proportion of Canada's research funding is spent on epidemiology, public health research, technology assessment, quality assurance, health services organization, or management operations research. Most of this funding comes from the National Health Research Development Program (NHRDP). But Ottawa cut this program by 8 percent in 1991-92 and slashed a further 13 percent in 1992-93.[52] The Medical Research Council budget has been increased, but this won't compensate for the other cuts.

Who Monitors Quality of Care?

In the United States, doctors often have to get approval from an insurance company nurse before hospitalizing a patient or conducting an elective surgery. By contrast, Canada does little to monitor the performance of our physicians. Most Canadian doctors aren't even scrutinized by other doctors. A number of Canadian commissions have concluded that there is very little peer review or outcome assessment in hospitals:

> Hospitals *do* keep information on the age of the patients they treat, the number of days they stay in hospital and their condition throughout their stay. But there is no standard recording of the state of patients upon admission and discharge, or of patients' health after they leave hospital unless they are readmitted. This makes it difficult to evaluate the long-term effect of hospital care.[53]

> In New Brunswick there is insufficient attention being given to utilization management. Hospital boards are quite passive on the question and most hospitals do not have an individual assigned to coordinate utilization management activities.[54]

There's even less scrutiny of care provided outside hospitals in clinics and doctors' offices. A Canadian survey of provincial licensing bodies for physicians, nurses, dentists, pharmacists, and optometrists found the organizations were unlikely to have comprehensive quality assurance programs in ambulatory care.[55] In particular, only four of fifty organizations had any explicit standards that related to patient outcomes. Only six had explicit prospective criteria for assessing a practitioner's performance. Only three had formal review processes for updating standards. Of over 350,000 licensed health professionals, only 0.04 percent (approximately 1 in 2,500) had their licences suspended because of concerns about quality during a three-year period. Only 0.01 percent (approximately 1 in 10,000) had their licences revoked because of concerns about quality during this period.

New legislation governing health professions in Ontario was proclaimed at the end of 1993.[56] Now each of twenty-three health professions must develop and implement a quality assurance program to continuously improve quality of care.

The College of Physicians and Surgeons of Ontario (CPSO) has operated a random quality audit since the late 1970s, in a program widely considered one of the most comprehensive in the country. Each year the practices of 400 randomly selected doctors—both GPs and specialists—are reviewed. Of the 1,142 assessments conducted between 1981 and 1988, fewer than half the practitioners got a clean bill of health for their practices, although most of the problems discovered were relatively minor.[57] Even so, the program's former director, Dr. Roy Beckett, says they are still finding "major deficiencies" in the practices of one out of every seven family doctors in Ontario.[58]

Watching is not enough

Even if we carefully monitor the quality of care, what can we do to improve quality when we find problems? Currently, there are very few mechanisms available to amend performance when it turns out to be below standard.

Still, Dr. Beckett says that the majority of doctors found deficient through his program clean up their act within a year. "Many of them tell us, 'All I needed was a push, and you gave it to me.'" For the 20 percent who refuse to correct serious problems when asked to do so, the program makes a referral to the CPSO's education or executive committee for further action.[59]

There is still some question, however, about the best ways to bring about real changes in practice behaviour. Dr. Robert Kinch, a former chair of the Department of Obstetrics and Gynecology at both the University of Western Ontario and McGill University, has practised obstetrics in England, Canada, and the United States. He says that quality assurance and peer review vary from hospital to hospital and even from department to department. A study conducted by the New Brunswick Commission on Selected Health Care Programs also found tremendous variation in how quality assurance programming was implemented.[60]

For example, contrary to popular belief, the vast majority of women who have already had a Caesarean section are able to deliver vaginally, provided they get the chance. This is amply documented in the standards for Caesarean section developed in 1986 by a highly credible body, the Society of Obstetricians and Gynecologists of Canada. These standards have been widely promulgated to all doctors attending births and have never been challenged.

However, in 1989, Dr. Paula Norman, a family doctor at the Toronto General Hospital, found that only 42 percent of the women eligible for a vaginal birth after a Caesarean section (VBAC) were being allowed to try for one.[61] In the article describing her study, there's no mention of any action taken to help physicians change their style of practice, even though their behaviour is contrary to the standards set by their own specialty society. Dr. Norman's article ends with a plea, not a plan: "All physicians who perform obstetrics or provide antenatal care should be advocating VBAC and providing ongoing support."[62]

The Hospital Medical Records Institute and individual hospitals know their overall rate for Caesarean sections and their rate for repeat Caesareans, and provincial governments have access to this information as well. It's very clear, however, that the mere existence of a sensible, scientific standard—even with good monitoring—is insufficient to ensure high-quality obstetrical care.

How Do We Change Clinical Behaviour?

American health services researcher Dr. John Eisenberg outlines six mechanisms to modify clinical performance that is below standard:[63]

1. Education
2. Feedback on performance
3. Participation of practitioners in designing systems
4. Administrative rules that enhance performance
5. Financial incentives to improve performance
6. Financial penalties to discourage poor performance

Education and feedback about practices can sometimes improve the quality of care.[64] For example, the volume of thyroid tests being done in Saskatchewan fell by 31 percent in less than one year after the province issued guidelines about the appropriate way to conduct the testing. More than $1 million was saved as a result, according to Dr. Stewart McMillan, chairman of the Health Services Utilization and Research Commission, which issued the voluntary guidelines.[65] This suggests that when the real source of a problem is an actual lack of knowledge about the best ways to proceed, producing evidence-based guidelines can change behaviour. It tends to support Dr. Berwick's assertion that doctors and other health professionals (and indeed virtually all workers) want to do a good job.

However, most of the time much more effort is necessary to improve quality. Merely establishing and promulgating a standard isn't enough.[66] In fact, researchers have documented that usually the other four strategies work better than education and feedback alone, and that combinations of strategies are usually more effective than any one strategy alone.

The Quality of Mercy

If we want a better quality of health care, we need to explore new models for quality management in our health care institutions.

Dr. Donald Berwick, head of the Institute for Healthcare Improvement, argues that traditional quality assurance programs rely too much on "sticks" and not enough on "carrots."[67] An apostle of Dr. William Demming, an early promoter of industry quality in Japan and in America, Dr. Berwick is convinced that regulatory approaches that rely primarily on inspection and punishment are actually counter-productive. "They create a very negative environment—a climate of fear among employees," he says. "It's a very human reaction—instead of becoming actively involved in supporting a quality assurance program, workers will try to undermine it—by tampering with data, for example."

To illustrate this point, he describes what happened to him when he was in charge of quality assessment at the Harvard Community Health Plan. Waiting times in the ambulatory clinic were too long. After months with no improvement, suddenly the average waiting time fell to exactly two minutes and stayed there. Dr. Berwick went to congratulate the manager of the clinic and to find out what she'd done to solve the problem. That's when the manager admitted lying in her reports. "I just got tired of telling the same bad news month after month. I know people are waiting too long, you know people are waiting too long," she said, "but who can tell me what on earth we can do about it?"

This helped convince Dr. Berwick that instead of looking for scapegoats, health care organizations needed to create environments that enhance their employees' ability to do a good job. The health care system is rife with structures and processes that make it very difficult for doctors, nurses, and other providers to deliver high-quality care. If the x-ray department is twenty minutes away from the emergency department, patient flow will be inefficient. If one medication looks exactly like another, there will be more medication errors. We need to reduce the amount of rework, complexity, and waste in our system, factors that Dr. Berwick says create major quality problems and add to costs. Berwick claims that an organization designed to continually improve quality will produce higher-quality goods and services than an organization that simply eliminates bad apples. "Motivation is not the problem," he argues. "To solve the problems of quality, we have to begin with the assumption that the vast majority of health care workers want to deliver the best possible quality of care."

To this end, many health care institutions, especially hospitals, have adopted programs of Total Quality Management (TQM) and Continuous Quality Improvement (CQI). These programs, already well established in industry, are viable alternatives that can break the regulation-inspection-punishment cycle.

However, TQM requires nothing less than a sea change in the culture of a traditional organization, and a real commitment from boards and managers, involving a significant investment of time, training, money, and leadership. But if the goals are clear and the investment is made, the payoffs can be enormous. Pleasing, even delighting customers becomes the overriding objective. In health care, of course, the main customer is the patient, but there are also internal customers: when a physician orders a lab test, she becomes a customer of the lab department.

Continuous Quality Improvement (CQI) is one very practical element in Total Quality Management, in which workers in teams collect and use data to track their own performance and test solutions. Often the answer lies in changing the way work is done.

Once a quality concern is identified, the organization pulls together a team of six to eight workers who are actually involved in that part of the system experiencing the problem. Typical teams include workers of all ranks, thus breaking down some of the traditional hierarchy among and between professions, other types of workers, and managers. All team members are provided with some basic training in statistical analysis and they have access to an expert facilitator. Then these standard steps are followed as the team addresses the quality problem:

Defining the problem
This involves clarifying the goal of the team in measurable terms. For example, a team's goal might be to reduce average

waiting times by 50 percent. Often this step involves redefining the problem to make it more manageable.

Diagnosing the cause

The tendency when dealing with problems is to look for someone to blame. Doctors blame nurses, nurses blame reception, reception blames doctors. Everyone thinks they know the source of the problem, and it's always someone else. This step in the CQI process tries to enlighten these opinions with facts. The team collects data to verify assumptions. Since workers are often familiar with only a few of the steps involved in any complete process, a key element in diagnosing the cause is to come to an understanding of all the various components involved. Using collected data, brainstorming, and a variety of analytical tools, the team develops an understanding of the root causes of the problem.

Hypothesizing and testing solutions

Having determined the root causes, the team develops specific strategies they believe will lick the difficulty. Even though most problems have many different causes, in general only a few account for the majority of the difficulty. The team therefore focuses on resolving these key issues, often changing how work is done by simplifying the process. Overcoming resistance is a major part of solving problems effectively, and the team must pay attention to creating solutions that can be effectively implemented. As possible solutions are tested, the team continues to collect data. If the problem isn't substantially resolved, it's back to the drawing board to find new solutions to test. This implementation-and-testing loop continues until a breakthrough is achieved and the goal is reached.

Implementing mechanisms to maintain improvements

Once the team can document a breakthrough, their work is done. However, monitoring and other measures—for example, training new workers—need to be implemented to make sure the problem doesn't reoccur.

How well is Canada doing with TQM/CQI?

Even though the principles of TQM/CQI are very sound and have been proven in other industries, a number of factors have hampered their penetration in Canada's health care system.

In particular, TQM/CQI has sometimes been used to justify slashing an organization's workforce, so organized labour is legitimately wary. Health care unions are finding that CQI too often works in one direction only. Simplifying work processes by eliminating unnecessary steps sometimes leads to job losses, but when a CQI process demonstrates the need to enrich staffing to promote quality, too often the necessary hirings don't happen.

For example, in 1993 the Manitoba government spent nearly $4 million to hire American consultant Connie Curran. Her job was to restructure the province's two major teaching hospitals.[68] Curran wanted to form task forces of ward nurses, who were expected to help her identify inefficiencies. But the nurses knew that Curran's mission was to cut hundreds of jobs and they didn't cooperate.

Another factor hampering TQM/CQI is the fact that some organizations simply don't provide the training necessary to familiarize workers with the tools and methods needed for success. Undertrained, badly equipped teams are bound to flounder around in confusion, creating a "total quality muddle." This, in fact, happened when Ontario's Ministry of Health first tried to implement CQI within its own bureaucracy. "People involved in teams at the beginning didn't receive the training they needed to do a good job—and the initial results were, not surprisingly, disappointing," according to one bureaucrat.

When health care organizations are committed to these new approaches and make the necessary investments in training and support, the results are very encouraging. Take, for example, Bruce Harbur, CEO of Peel Memorial, a community hospital in Ontario: "We're at the point now where over 500 of our staff have received TQM training. At first many were sceptical, but now people are anxious to get trained. And the hospital hosts a 'quality fair' every year to publicize the results of CQI efforts. It's created a lot of excitement and optimism about the future."

Another major problem with TQM/CQI is that so far, hospitals have opted to use it to address mainly non-clinical issues. It is a lot easier to deal with turnover times for patients in an x-ray department than the question of who should get x-rays in the first place. For one thing, hospital management can request radiology staff come to meetings, but they don't have the same authority over doctors. However, steps are being taken to implement TQM/CQI for some clinical problems as well.

To see how, let's return again to Susan G., whose birthing experience we described at the beginning of this chapter.

When she was admitted to the hospital, Susan had the traditional shave, prep, and enema, standard procedures at many hospitals. None of these "services" has been shown to reduce infection or other complications. Indeed, they may actually slow the progress of labour.

Then Susan was hooked up to an electronic fetal monitor (EFM). While EFMs do show when the baby's heart rate is dangerously low, there is no evidence that they are more effective overall than having a nurse listen to the abdomen, especially for women at low risk for developing an obstetrical problem.[69] On the other hand, it is now very clear that the routine use of EFMs does increase the number of Caesarean sections, probably because doctors tend to interpret the machine's signals as showing fetal distress even when there is none. EFMs have become standard in most hospitals partly because the machine replaces the need to have a nurse continually at the bedside. Over three-quarters of all Canadian hospitals that perform obstetrics have EFMs, and in nearly three-quarters of these hospitals, all patients are monitored at some point during labour.[70]

Like many of her friends, Susan wanted her husband to be with her during labour. Both had faithfully attended their prenatal classes. Susan learned breathing techniques to help her manage the pain of labour, and her husband learned how to support her. But her husband's growing anxiety wasn't very helpful in the end. His tendency to panic meant he wasn't the most appropriate labour coach.

All the same, it has been established that a trained labour coach can reduce obstetrical complications and the need for Caesarean section.[71] Having such a person on hand leaves the husband free to offer emotional support. In fact, if labouring women had an experienced and supportive coach who could monitor blood pressure and periodically check the fetal heart rate, the use of an EFM could be eliminated in most cases. Very few hospitals in Canada, however, offer these attendants.

The spinal anaesthetic Susan received markedly reduced her pain, but it also acted to slow her labour. The fact that she was lying on her back—the traditional position most convenient for doctors and nurses—also interfered with the progress of labour.

No one factor alone led to Susan's Caesarean—the whole modern obstetrical experience was at fault. But perhaps not for long.

Dr. Bill McLeod now practises in Eden, North Carolina, but he practised obstetrics for nine years in Windsor, Ontario. He remembers how hard it was to get anyone interested in reducing the city's Caesarean-section rate in the early 1980s. It wasn't until late in the decade that obstetrical guidelines at local hospitals recommended allowing a "trial of labour" for women who had previously had C-sections. But having the new guidelines and advertising them didn't change behaviour.[72] Something extra was necessary.

In 1987, Professor Jonathan Lomas led a team from McMaster University in an experiment aimed at reducing the rate of inappropriate Caesarean sections. The researchers began the Windsor segment of their project by asking the physicians there which local doctor was most knowledgeable about the appropriate use of C-sections. Dr. McLeod was the hands-down winner, and the researchers zeroed in on him to become Windsor's opinion leader on surgical deliveries.

Professor Lomas and his staff worked hard with Dr. McLeod, the labour and delivery staff of the Metropolitan Hospital, and the rest of the community's doctors and nurses to develop a program to reduce C-sections in Windsor. They found the problems in Windsor were similar to those across the country. There was, for example, a high rate of repeat Caesareans with no opportunity offered for a vaginal delivery. In addition, very little was being done to actively manage cases in order to prevent first-time Caesareans.

Some issues, however, were unique to Windsor, which lies across the river from Detroit. American TV blared advertisements from lawyers encouraging patients with bad outcomes to sue their doctors and hospitals. Some felt this might be influencing doctors to play it safe by doing C-sections whenever there was the least doubt about safety. To address this, Windsor doctors needed to know that the Canadian guidelines for C-sections, issued by the Society of Obstetricians and Gynecologists of Canada (SOGC), would stand up in court should there be a malpractice claim. They also needed reassurance that American doctors viewed the standards as valid.

Lomas and his staff and Bill McLeod and the group in Windsor sponsored a lecture series on the SOGC guidelines and demonstrated their similarity to the American guidelines.[73] They concentrated their efforts on older obstetricians, who tended to have higher C-section rates.[74] They made presentations to community groups, printed a pamphlet, and even started a prenatal group specially designed for women who had previously had C-sections. In addition, Bill McLeod began to advocate active management of labour to prevent first Caesareans.

After the dust settled, things had changed dramatically in Windsor's Metropolitan Hospital. In three years, the C-section rate plummeted from 25 percent of all births to 15 percent. Bill McLeod and the Metropolitan Hospital in Windsor had been part of a landmark study on how to improve the quality of health care.

In the late 1980s, various surveys showed that most Ontario doctors who practised obstetrics had heard of the SOGC guidelines, agreed with them, and claimed to be practising in accordance with them. The Caesarean section rate, however, remained at around 20 percent, and data from the province's hospitals indicated that most doctors were not letting women who had previously had a C-section try for a vaginal delivery.

While some were quick to criticize individual doctors, Lomas and his colleagues understood that many systemic factors were involved in the high levels of inappropriate Caesarean sections, including the long-accepted wisdom, "Once a Caesarean, always a Caesarean." They hypothesized that marketing tactics and educational programs developed according to adult learning theory might be more effective than simply issuing and reissuing the guidelines.

Lomas's group identified sixteen community hospitals in southern Ontario and then divided them into three groups.

- Doctors in the first group of four hospitals were sent the SOGC guidelines.
- Doctors in the second group of four hospitals were helped to develop an audit and feedback program. The doctors in these hospitals established their own guidelines and, once every three months, they reviewed all the women who had previously had Caesarean sections.
- In the third group of eight hospitals, the investigators identified and involved opinion leaders like Bill McLeod to develop a suitable local action program.

After twenty-four months, the Caesarean-section rate rose slightly in the first two groups but fell by more than 10 percent in those hospitals using opinion leaders.[75]

The results of this study have had a major impact on how people think about quality assurance and standard setting. While various medical groups like the SOGC were elaborating guidelines in the 1980s, hardly anyone was looking at whether they actually changed behaviour.[76]

Harvard quality-of-care leaders Drs. Glenn Laffel and Donald Berwick refer to the McMaster study as an important contribution to CQI success stories. The U.S. Agency for Health Care Policy and Research now asks the groups they fund to develop guidelines to include specific plans for implementing their research.[77]

Health care resources are scarce. When we spend them on inappropriate care we lose the option of spending them on other, more useful services. Canada spends too much on the wrong services, in the wrong places, delivered by the wrong providers, at the wrong time. If we could curb inappropriate servicing, we could afford to pay for more services that people actually need. A dollar spent on an unnecessary drug is a dollar unavailable for home care. A dollar spent on an inappropriate Caesarean section is a dollar unavailable for a breastfeeding support program.

We started this chapter by explaining that Canada's health care system has a very serious problem with quality of care. But we close it with an example of how Canadian doctors and researchers are starting to take action to turn things around. Quality can be improved. We can learn to do the right things right.

Chapter 5

UnhealthyAlliance: Medicine and the Drug Industry

DORA B., LIKE MANY SENIORS, suffers from osteoarthritis, a painful condition caused by years of wear and tear on her joints. For Mrs. B., it's her knees and hands that cause her the most pain. Over the years, she has taken a variety of medications prescribed by her doctor, and she has always been careful to take her drugs exactly as prescribed. Now she's trying out a new anti-arthritic product, Voltaren SR. Her physician suggested that it might control her pain more effectively, even though it was significantly more costly than other, similar products.

After a few days, Mrs. B. develops an upset stomach and phones her doctor for advice. Never a particularly assertive woman, Mrs. B. doesn't protest when she is told that the doctor can't come to the phone, and she doesn't say anything when the receptionist offers her an appointment three days later. She continues to take her drugs as directed. The evening before her appointment, Mrs. B. collapses at home with a stomach perforation and quietly bleeds to death.

Mr. H. is a fifty-year-old man who has been taking a drug (a beta-blocker) to control his high blood pressure for several years. Recently he consulted his physician about pains in his stomach and the doctor prescribed an ulcer medication, Tagamet. Unfortunately, these drugs taken in combination cause a fatal side effect in the patient. Three days after starting to take his new prescription, Mr. H. suffers a major heart attack and dies before he can reach the hospital.

Millicent G. is in very frail health and has to take many different medications to manage a number of serious medical conditions. She suffers from diabetes, congestive heart failure, chronic kidney disease, and ulcers. She also has a lot of pain from arthritis and is very anxious. Every day she takes more than twelve drugs, including pills to help her sleep. Some of these medications affect her balance and cause confusion, but her daughter, who lives with her, makes sure her mother takes her pills as directed. One evening, Mrs. G. falls in the bathroom and breaks her hip.

What's Really Wrong with Drug Prescribing?

According to Dr. Denis Psutka, a former Ontario assistant deputy minister of health and now an associate professor of medicine at McMaster University, the crux of the problem is that doctors don't know enough about drugs and tend to overlook alternatives. He says that patients often get prescriptions for pills they don't need, or are given new, expensive drugs that don't work any better than older, cheaper ones.[1]

It's a growing problem. Every year we dispense more and more pills to patients. In Canada, between June 1991 and July 1992, pharmacists filled 210.9 million prescriptions.[2] Canada's total drug bill for 1991 was $9.2 billion, almost 14 percent of total health spending, up from 8.9 percent in 1980. By 1994, drug spending is expected to take the same share of health spending as physician services—around 15 percent. The prescription marketplace in Canada is worth about $5 billion in sales. About half of this amount represents government spending on provincial drug benefit programs.

High levels of inappropriate prescribing represent hundreds of millions in wasteful spending by consumers, third-party insurers, and provincial governments. For example, the Canadian Society of Hospital Pharmacists claims that 30 to 50 percent of seniors' medication requirements could be reduced if pharmacists were involved in reviewing the drugs being taken and had an incentive to discuss their patients' medication requirements with prescribing physicians.[3] Since the Ontario government provides free prescription coverage for seniors, inappropriate prescribing for this group alone costs Ontario tax-payers at least $300 million a year. And that's just the cost of paying for the drugs and pharmacy services; it doesn't include physicians' fees or the costs of treating adverse side effects from drugs, which often occur among the elderly.

Evidence of Overprescribing

Are Canadians really taking too many drugs? "It's a huge problem with enormous financial and health implications," says Dr. Joel Lexchin, an emergency room physician and expert on pharmaceutical use in Canada. His recent review of prescribing in Ontario found that the rising cost of the Ontario Drug Benefit Plan "is due to two factors: more intensive prescribing—physicians prescribing to the elderly more often and writing more prescriptions each time they see an elderly patient—and physicians writing prescriptions for more expensive drugs."[4]

Take, as an example, the widespread misuse of antibiotics to treat colds, flu, and other viral infections. These products aren't effective against viruses, but that doesn't stop patients from asking for them or physicians from doling them out. Dr. Peter Jewesson is co-director of Vancouver General Hospital's pharmacy, where they are working hard to implement more appropriate antibiotic prescribing. He estimates that one in ten antibiotics now used in the hospital, and as many as one in four prescribed by general practitioners, is unnecessary.[5]

Dr. Larry Bryan of the University of Calgary estimates that between one- and two-thirds of the antibiotics used in Canada are unnecessary or inappropriately used. Even in hospitals, inappropriate use of these products can be as high as 40 percent according to federal guidelines aimed at reducing overuse of medication.[6]

Particularly disturbing is the increasing use of newer, very expensive, wide-spectrum antibiotics when cheaper products would do the trick. A 1990 study noted that one such product, ciprofloxacin (brand name: Cipro), has achieved "astonishing popularity among physicians."[7] In 1989 in the United States, Cipro was the fourth most commonly prescribed antibacterial product, with one prescription for every forty-four Americans. It was introduced in Canada in January 1989 and is popular here, too—between June 1991 and July 1992, the number of Cipro prescriptions rose by 43 percent.[8]

While Cipro is a very useful drug for some patients, the *Medical Letter on Drugs and Therapeutics* says it should not be used for common out-patient infections as a first-line therapy, despite multi-page ads for the product suggesting the contrary.[9] In the first six months of 1988, Cipro was the second most heavily promoted drug product in U.S. medical journals. The campaign included handing out free samples to doctors and the usual pens, office supplies, and other "freebies" standard in the industry's marketing repertoire. The impact of this promotion blitz has yet to be formally evaluated, but it's tempting to conclude that marketing rather than scientific evidence has been responsible for Cipro's amazing popularity.[10]

Victims of overprescribing: the elderly

Older people are particularly at risk in cases of inappropriate prescribing. "Seniors are being drugged silly," Dr. Psutka told a panel of the Senior Citizens' Consumer Alliance for Long-Term Care Reform in March 1992, pointing out that 80 percent of Ontario's billion-dollar drug program is spent on people sixty-five years of age and over. Elderly people are getting twenty-seven or twenty-eight prescriptions a year, and on average each person over sixty-five is taking four different drugs at any one time, says Dr. Lexchin.

Taking too many drugs isn't just an economic burden. There are serious health risks associated with overprescribing. The federal government estimates that thousands of elderly people die each year as a result of drug side effects.[11] According to Dr. Malcolm Champion, a specialist in digestive disorders at the Ottawa Civic Hospital, up to 2,000 Canadians over sixty-five die each year from internal bleeding as well as heart and kidney failure linked to the use of anti-arthritis drugs.[12] At least 200,000 illnesses among people over sixty-five are due to bad reactions to drugs that are often not needed.

At least 3 percent and perhaps up to 10 percent of all hospital admissions among people over fifty years of age are due to adverse drug reactions.[13] Part of the problem is that doctors often don't take into account the fact that normal adult drug dosages may be too high for seniors. Older people are often unable to clear drugs from their systems as quickly as younger adults. A dosage that's safe for a younger person may well represent an overdose for a senior.

Given the higher probability that seniors will have more than one condition requiring drug treatment, their chance of receiving prescriptions for multiple products is also higher than the general population's. The more drugs taken, the higher the risk of an adverse reaction. Drug-induced mental confusion, ulcers, intestinal bleeding, and dizziness resulting in falls are all too common among this vulnerable population and take a major toll on their overall health.

Take just one class of drugs, the non-steroidal anti-inflammatories, or NSAIDs. These drugs are used to control pain and inflammation associated with arthritis. The best known (and least costly) NSAID is Aspirin, but there are dozens of other competing products in the same drug class that are vastly more expensive and much more popular among prescribers. About one person in eight over sixty-five has osteoarthritis, the most prevalent form of arthritis. Osteoarthritis is quite different from the much more serious and less common disease known as rheumatoid arthritis, which tends to strike younger people.

Depending on the severity of osteoarthritis and an individual's response to treatment, a number of non-drug therapies might control pain and reduce stiffness just as well as medication. These alternatives include applying hot packs, exercise, physiotherapy, and using a walking stick or special insoles to reduce the impact of movement on joints. But there's been little research to establish the short- or long-term benefit of any of these therapies. Drugs are the mainstay of treatment. And although studies comparing various NSAIDs are published at the rate of one every two weeks, there's been almost no research comparing the relative effectiveness of simple pain relievers (like acetaminophen/Tylenol) with the more potent and more dangerous NSAIDs for relieving osteoarthritic symptoms.[14]

There are several problems associated with using NSAIDs for osteoarthritis. One is the fact that, unlike rheumatoid arthritis, inflammation does not play a major role in osteoarthritis.[15] This suggests that NSAIDs, which are specifically designed to reduce inflammation, may not be appropriate for osteoarthritis patients, even though they also relieve pain.

The most serious problem with NSAIDs, however, is that they quite commonly cause serious side effects in the digestive tract. An autopsy study of 713 patients found that NSAID users had fourteen times the rate of intestinal ulcers compared to persons who hadn't used the drugs.[16] Stomach and duodenal ulcers were twice as common, and NSAID users were almost three times as likely to have died from gastrointestinal ulceration and perforation.

Dr. Claire Bombardier, a rheumatologist at Toronto's Wellesley Hospital, estimates that NSAIDs account for one-quarter of all adverse drug reactions, the most serious of which are intestinal bleeding, ulcers, and stomach perforation.[17] And the incidence of these problems is on the rise. According to the U.S. Food and Drug Administration, serious side effects from NSAID use are increasing by 2 percent to 4 percent a year—something Dr. Bombardier feels is "an almost epidemic-like increase" in the number of hospitalizations and deaths. Most at risk are elderly females. More selective use of anti-arthritics and using the lowest dosage possible when medication is indicated could help stem some of these problems, Dr. Bombardier says.

Elderly people also suffer enormously from taking psychotropic drugs. Those over the age of sixty-five who use these medications have a 70 to 100 percent greater risk of hip fracture.[18] In an essay on adverse drug reactions and the elderly, it was estimated that 30,000 hip fractures in the United States every year are related to psychotropic drug use.[19] The authors point out that 10 to 15 percent of patients with hip fractures die within a year, 50 percent lose the capacity to walk independently, and up to one-third of those formerly living in the community will require long-term nursing home care. They estimate that the annual direct costs for medical care alone total $1 billion.

Victims of overprescribing: women

The misuse of psychotropic drugs, especially sedatives, is another example of overprescribing that has a long and continuing history. Studies have shown that women are two to three times more likely than men to be prescribed sedatives and antidepressants.[20] Benzodiazepines are still among the most popular drug products. Past industry standards, like Valium, have been overtaken by the newer, faster-acting hypnotics like Ativan, which in 1992 was the eighth-best-selling drug in Canada.[21] Psychotropic drugs, particularly benzodiazepines, are often prescribed initially as a short-term therapy for sleeplessness or for anxiety, although there are effective non-drug alternatives for these conditions, too.

Women in abusive situations often wind up being prescribed mood-altering drugs by sympathetic physicians. Lisa Coy is a Toronto social worker from the Parkdale Community Health Centre's Domestic Violence Program. She believes that anti-depressants and sleeping pills do have a role in helping patients cope in the short term with high anxiety. But she worries about long-term treatment with psychotropic drugs. "The pills can, in some cases, make things worse by blunting a woman's perception of the danger she's in, making it harder for her to decide to leave an abusive partner," she says.

Evidence for Underprescribing

Most of the evidence concerning inappropriate prescribing points to too many prescriptions rather than too few. There are instances, however—proper drug treatment for pain control, for example— which call for a more liberal use of effective medications.

Providing pain medication on an as-needed basis—the traditional policy in most hospitals—means that about half the time people are given too little medication, says Dr. James Mason, former head of the U.S. Public Health Service. Dr. Mason's organization recently released new guidelines for pain control developed by a panel of experts. According to the guidelines, unrelieved pain not only stalls the healing process, but also impairs the immune system, keeps the patient from coughing as needed, raises the likelihood of pneumonia, and delays the return of normal stomach and bowel functions.[22]

Moreover, recent evidence suggests that strong doses of pain medication just *before* surgery can speed healing and reduce pain and the need for painkillers following the operation. In a study of thirty patients having major chest surgery, half were provided with a strong narcotic just before the first incision and a placebo fifteen minutes after the incision; the other half received a placebo first and the narcotic second.[23] After surgery, all patients were hooked up to morphine pumps that allowed them to control the release of pain medication at the push of a button. Twelve to twenty-four hours after surgery, patients who did not receive the pre-incision narcotic were using the pumps twice as often as those who did.

Only a few years ago, most surgical procedures on premature infants were conducted without deep anaesthesia. What lay behind this apparent barbarism was the mistaken belief that babies couldn't really experience pain at such an early stage of development. Also, because many premature infants have respiratory problems, there was legitimate fear that a general anaesthetic might compromise their breathing abilities even further. But a 1992 study from the *New England Journal of Medicine* concluded that intense, long-lasting pain actually makes surgery riskier for newborns, suggesting that physicians might want to use deep rather than light anaesthesia for babies.[24]

Undertreatment is also a problem for patients with high blood pressure. Because the risk of stroke and heart attack is higher among people with elevated blood pressure, appropriate drug therapy is an important preventive strategy. A study in Laval, Quebec, found that only 20 percent of newly diagnosed hypertensives were being treated two years after detection, and only half of these had their hypertension controlled.[25]

Why Are There So Many Prescribing Problems?

"One of the reasons that doctors don't do a good job in prescribing is that they don't know enough about the products they are using to treat patients," says Dr. Joel Lexchin.[26] Although this sounds like a harsh indictment, at least some Ontario physicians appear to agree. In a 1989 survey of 842 doctors conducted by the Ontario Medical Association (OMA), less than one-third said they were satisfied with their knowledge of equivalencies among similar drugs, different brands of drugs, and non-drug alternatives. Fewer than 20 percent said they were satisfied with their knowledge of drug costs. The OMA's survey did not find doctors blaming patient demand or the need to practise defensive medicine for the increasing rate of prescription drug use. Instead, Ontario doctors seemed to be blaming themselves and the difficulty of keeping up to date in a rapidly changing and expanding field.[27]

Some people do think consumers are at least partly to blame for prescribing problems. The widespread belief that there's "a pill for every ill" is symptomatic of society's unrealistic expectations. Between one-third and three-quarters of physician office visits end with a prescription, so it shouldn't be a surprise that patients expect to leave with one.[28] Tearing off a prescription serves a number of purposes. For one thing, it's a handy way to signal the end of the consultation—useful to doctors with busy waiting rooms. Getting a prescription also validates the patient's decision to seek treatment in the first place.

Sometimes patients even ask for a specific brand of drug. According to Scott-Levin Associates, an American pharmaceutical marketing firm, only 18 percent of U.S. patients were asking their doctors about specific medications in 1987, but by 1992, 54 percent were doing so.[29] This might reflect the impact of new marketing strategies. A number of prescription products are now being promoted directly to consumers through television and print advertising in the United States. Even Canada has shown ads advising patients to see their doctors about new "medical" treatments for baldness or for help in quitting smoking.

At least part of the problem of poor prescribing may be traced to medical schools, where training in pharmacology is extremely limited. In his presentation to Ontario's 1988 Pharmaceutical Inquiry (the Lowy Commission), Dr. Stuart MacLeod, himself a clinical pharmacologist and former dean of Health Sciences at McMaster University, pointed out that Ontario medical students receive only about 140 hours of training directly related to drug therapy.[30] And yet prescribing medication is one of the most common physician services. "There is an immense need for impartial information ... to combat the problem of inappropriately prescribed drugs," he says.

Dr. Jerry Avorn, a professor at Harvard Medical School, says that providing doctors with better information on the best and most cost-effective drugs is the most "do-able" way to control rising drug costs. "It's got to be someone's responsibility to make this information available," he says. "If we as a society leave it up to the manufacturers of drugs to be the only purveyors of information about drugs, then we shouldn't expect them to do anything but to try to increase sales."[31]

Marketing Magic

The drug industry spends about 20 percent of its total sales revenues on marketing. In 1992, over $750 million went to drug promotions and lobbying for the industry—more than twice what the companies invested in research.[32]

Drug companies have a major advantage over manufacturers of most other consumer goods. In order to sell some $5 billion worth of product, the industry only has to reach a small, identifiable group of consumers, the 60,000 doctors practising in Canada today.

Most of the industry's promotion budget goes to pay for its sales force. The Canadian industry employs about four thousand sales representatives—or drug detailers. Each earns on average about $50,000 per year.[33] And the sales reps come in with a well-rehearsed pitch and a clear mission. The objective is to sell as much drug product as possible and help the company make a profit.

Even though most detailers have degrees in science, they are trained to present "the up-side of the drug, much more than the down-side," says Dr. Lexchin. Is the information provided to physicians by detailers always balanced and accurate? Not according to Jody Perez, a former salesperson in Texas with McNeil Pharmaceuticals, a division of Johnson and Johnson. Mr. Perez was featured in a drug industry exposé produced by "Frontline" for the U.S. Public Broadcasting Service. During the program he recalled how he and fellow detailers had been briefed in the early 1980s to sell Zomax, a pain reliever that turned out to be so dangerous it was eventually removed from the market. He claimed that even after the company had discovered that anaphylactic shock was a potential side effect of the drug, it was still telling detailers to downplay the problems.

The typical Canadian physician receives about twenty-five visits a year from detailers. It's a relationship that begins in medical school and continues throughout the doctor's prescribing career.

The industry uses its salesforce strategically by concentrating its efforts on the heaviest prescribers. Low-volume prescribers say they see detailers less than fifteen times a year; those who write a lot of prescriptions report about fifty visits annually. To identify those high-volume prescribers, the drug industry uses regular surveys. One such survey, circulated in January 1993 by the Centre for Medical Communications, a marketing company, asked doctors how many patients they were seeing, how many prescriptions they wrote in an average week, and whether they preferred to see sales reps on a drop-in basis or by appointment only. This particular survey came with a letter offering respondents the chance to win a one-week trip for two to Club Med. Another was accompanied by a five-dollar cheque—just a token thanks for filling out the survey.

More costly offerings from the industry are also common— free lunches and even all-expense-paid junkets to "conferences" at exotic resort locations. The latter are considered "continuing education" by the industry, but in most cases they're really a form of marketing.

For example, in February 1993, about sixty doctors and their spouses attended a weekend conference at a four-star hotel at St. Adèle in the Laurentians.[34] The liquor was plentiful, the $110-a-night rooms were elegantly appointed, and the food was simply sublime. The conference schedule left plenty of time for skiing—only a few morning lectures to attend and the rest was free time. Best of all, the entire weekend's tab was picked up by Searle Inc. of Canada.

Of course, printed materials also play a big role in drug promotion, and again the information is tailored to sell drugs, not to educate doctors. Most medical journals are peppered with ads featuring full-colour artwork and clever slogans. But the scientific information about contraindications and side effects often shows up pages and pages away, and usually in a squint-inducing type size.

Physicians hate to admit that all this hype influences their prescribing behaviour. In a recent Decima survey, 72 percent of doctors claimed to use medical journals and other scientific publications for their information about medications; half the doctors surveyed said drug ads were "unbalanced in their presentation of products' risks and benefits."[35]

External assessments of physician drug knowledge suggest that information from drug advertising can mislead doctors into thinking certain products are more useful than they really are. In 1982, Harvard researcher Dr. Jerry Avorn surveyed eighty-five doctors about their drug knowledge.[36] Of those surveyed, 49 percent thought Darvon, a popular analgesic at the time, was a better pain reliever than Aspirin, an idea nowhere to be found in the scientific literature but definitely suggested by the full-colour ads for Darvon. One-third of the doctors surveyed also thought that blocked blood vessels in the elderly caused mental confusion. Once again, this notion is unsupported by scientific evidence but was common in the ads for drugs that dilate cerebral arteries.

According to a survey of 221 medical journal editors, only 37 percent review ads prior to publishing them, and only 13 percent use a peer-review process for doing so.[37] In 1990, the U.S. Department of Health and Human Services conducted a review of drug advertising in scientific publications.[38] Conducting the reviews were physicians, who themselves were peer-reviewers for scientific journals, and pharmacists involved in educating doctors about drug use. Working in teams of three, the reviewers found "many deficiencies" in the 109 ads taken from leading medical journals during the early part of 1990. Half had little or no educational value, and 59 percent would lead to improper prescribing if the physician had no other information. On average, the reviewers cited 4.3 examples of misleading or inappropriate information per ad; the faulty information was often found in the headlines and frequently involved side effects, referencing, and comparative claims. The reviewers also concluded that the Food and Drug Administration rarely took formal action against those who violated its regulations regarding false or misleading advertising.

What's Hot, What's Not

There are 20,000 drugs currently available for sale in Canada, representing over-the-counter and prescription medications, brand-name products and generics, patented drugs, and those for which the patent has expired. Each year about five hundred new medications come onto the marketplace. Only a handful—perhaps six or seven a year—represent real improvements over products already available. The vast majority are "me-too" drugs—slightly different versions of popular products already on the market.

How can an industry capture an ever-increasing share of the health care market without a lot of breakthrough discoveries? The answer is pretty straightforward.

First, they concentrate on products that have a large number of potential users. No orphan drugs for rare illnesses need apply; there aren't enough customers to warrant the investment. Instead, the industry focuses on the biggest therapeutic markets: drugs for arthritis, drugs for high blood pressure, drugs for ulcers. There are plenty of consumers for these kinds of products, and plenty of profit if the campaign to capture market share is successful.

Then, the challenge is to find a catchy name for the new drug, one that will inspire confidence in doctors. A careful promotional campaign is also key—eye-catching ads for the journals that manage to suggest that this new drug is somehow better than its competitors. "In the final analysis, what stays with you is an arresting photo or graphic, or some figures trumpeted in large print," says Dr. David Naylor, a clinical epidemiologist and director of Ontario's Institute for Clinical Evaluative Sciences.[39] Dr. Naylor has long been irritated by the claims and images used to promote drugs: "It's a real concern and a little bit alarming when you consider that drugs that are heavily promoted tend to find themselves in the top-ten-selling drugs in very short order." Often older but equally effective products get lost in all the glamour surrounding the new product.

Finally, new drug products usually enter the marketplace at higher prices. Drug companies know that if they can manage to convince doctors to opt for the latest formulation, the cost will not likely be an obstacle.

For example, there are about fifteen NSAIDs competing in the arthritic marketplace. Today, in Canada, Voltaren SR is the most popular, but five years ago it was Naprosyn. Is there any scientific basis to the claim that one is better than the other? According to the *Medical Letter*, even though newer arthritis drugs often claim they cause less stomach irritation than older products, there is no clinical evidence that any one NSAID, new or old, is better than another when used in equally effective doses. In fact, one recent study showed that rheumatoid arthritis patients who took aspirin actually had fewer side effects than patients who took other NSAIDs.[40]

Syntex introduced a new NSAID, ketorolac (brand name: Toradol), into the Canadian market in April 1991. University of Manitoba pharmacy professors Robert Ariano and Sheryl Zelenitsky were scathing in their criticism of the company's advertising campaign for the drug: "The advertising and promotion of ketorolac as an NSAID has been subtle and potentially misleading. Statements that refer to the drug as being 'unlike conventional NSAIDs' imply that it is pharmacologically unique.... Ketorolac is not a 'wonder drug' with a mysterious mechanism of action: it is simply another NSAID." Ketorolac is also *thirty times* more expensive than the least expensive alternative—coated aspirin![41] And because of its poor risk/benefit ratio, a number of European countries, including France and Germany, have suspended its use.[42]

Focusing on lots of "me-too" products and promoting them heavily to capture market share have helped make pharmaceuticals the most profitable manufacturing industry in the world. In Canada, multinational producers have achieved more than 25 percent annual after-tax profits on their capital.[43] In the United States, the return on shareholders' equity is more than 50 percent higher than the median of the top Fortune 500 companies.[44] Even at the height of the recession, drug profits in the United States rose by 17 percent.[45]

For those drugs that do represent therapeutic breakthroughs, real improvements over conventional medications, the marketplace is even more receptive.

Consider the short-acting hypnotics like Ativan, used to treat insomnia. These products are commonly prescribed to seniors, who often report problems sleeping, and they can be very effective in the short term. But there are also serious side effects, including dizziness, confusion, rage reactions, and memory lapses. These problems are particularly prevalent among older people.

Investigations showing even more serious side effects have been linked to another drug in this class, Halcion, manufactured by Upjohn and introduced to Canada in 1978. Through the 1980s, Halcion became the most widely prescribed sleeping pill in the world, but reports of serious psychiatric side effects eventually resulted in Great Britain's decision to ban the product in 1991. Shortly afterwards, Canada's Health Protection Branch assembled a team of Canadian experts to review the drug's status in Canada. The team decided that Halcion should stay on the market, but it recommended that doctors prescribe a much lower dosage—one that may be too low to be effective for insomnia but still high enough to induce serious side effects.[46]

Competition in the drug industry rarely means price competition. For the most part, one or two brand-name producers dominate each therapeutic market and set the price. But even when many brand-name producers enter the marketplace, lower prices do not necessarily follow.

The therapeutic market for ulcer medications in the United States is a case in point. Tagamet (generic name: cimetidine) dominated the market for six years after its 1977 introduction by SmithKline Corporation (now SmithKline Beecham). There was no competition for this breakthrough product. Then, in 1983, Glaxo Pharmaceuticals, the world's largest brand-name producer, entered the field with Zantac, followed in 1986 by Pepcid, produced by Merck Frosst, and two years later Axid, made by Eli Lilly & Co.[47]

One would expect that competition would cause prices for these ulcer medications to fall, but that's not what happened, according to Donald Drake and Marion Uhlman, authors of *Making Medicine, Making Money*. Instead, Zantac came on the market costing more than Tagamet; its producers claimed that the higher price was justified because it caused fewer side effects, a claim that is only true when the drug is used with three other specific drug products.[48] Following Zantac's introduction, the prices of both drugs moved upward in parallel fashion. When Pepcid and Axid were introduced, they too were priced higher than Tagamet.

The only logical conclusion is that brand-name drug companies do not compete on price. Today, Zantac is the best-selling drug in the history of the pharmaceutical industry. But Tagamet continues to enjoy U.S. sales of over $1 billion a year.[49]

Is There a Better Way?

There are three key strategies to address the problems of inappropriate prescribing, the undue influence of drug industry promotion, and inflated costs.

The first is to recognize that the proliferation of multiple products to treat the same illnesses actually represents an opportunity for large purchasers, like government drug programs, to use their leverage to get better prices. Joining forces to maximize bargaining power, the premiers of Atlantic Canada recently announced their intention to jointly purchase fifty drugs common to their drug programs.[50]

In the United States, about one-third of health maintenance organizations (HMOs) have policies favouring "therapeutic substitution."[51] They actively manage their formularies (the lists of drugs they agree to stock and pay for) and prefer to include only one or two drugs in each therapeutic class as the drug of choice for a particular problem. For instance, in deciding which ulcer drug will win first place, the HMO might send out a request for competitive bids. The product that best combines clinical usefulness and safety at a good price will make the A list. The others will be used only in specific circumstances for specific patients. One HMO in the United States managed to reduce its spending on arthritis drugs by 50 percent using this strategy.[52]

However, you do need to have some agreement among doctors and pharmacists to make therapeutic substitution work. Unfortunately, Canadian doctors rarely get together to set guidelines, and even when they do, they are rarely enforced.

Canada could take a tip from New Zealand, where, over the past year, a committee has been developing guidelines for treating common conditions. For example, the report on high blood pressure recommends starting most patients on a generic drug one hundred times less expensive than newer medications for hypertension.[53]

The second strategy to improve the quality of prescribing is to help doctors become more knowledgeable about drugs and drug alternatives. One U.S. study found that face-to-face educational encounters between a local, influential doctor or phamacist and a prescribing physician could counteract the influence of biased promotion by the drug industry. This program of academic detailing didn't just improve the quality of prescribing, it also reduced overall costs. In fact, the savings realized were eight times greater than the costs of the educational program.[54]

The third strategy is to involve consumers, encouraging them to become more aware of potential problems in medication use.

Brown-bag programs conducted in Ontario and in British Columbia, encouraging people to bring old prescriptions to their pharmacists for disposal, are both popular and effective. Toronto's South Riverdale Community Health Centre has been educating seniors to ask questions about their drugs and become aware of alternatives. "By encouraging consumers to speak up," says Elsie Petch, the centre's health promoter, "we are asking them to be active participants in their own health care."

The Drug Industry and Academe: An Uneasy Union

Teaching hospitals have been a particular target of the drug industry's promotional activities. "During medical school, the example of clinical instructors is the most important influence on medical students, interns, and residents," says Dr. Psutka. Instead of learning about medications from physician specialists in drug therapy (clinical pharmacologists), interns and residents learn about heart drugs from cardiologists, arthritis drugs from rheumatologists, and so on.

Drug companies know if they can influence these instructors to favour particular drug products, their prescribing preferences will likely be passed on to the students. That's why the industry concentrates on influencing drug practices in teaching hospitals. They work hard to get their brands on the hospital's formulary. The industry knows that loyalties developed early have a good chance of influencing physician prescribing habits for the future.

"We found this to be a problem in our hospital," says Dr. Gordon Guyatt, a professor of clinical epidemiology and biostatics who heads the residency program for internal medicine at McMaster University. "The industry was sponsoring hundreds of drug lunches,* and senior residents were always in contact with sales representatives. Some students were being sponsored by the industry to attend conferences in exotic locations that we felt had little educational value. In general, we wanted to

---

* Drug lunches typically involve a free meal with the screening of a film or videotape developed by the industry.

reduce the amount of inappropriate interactions, while preserving relationships with the industry that were of mutual benefit."

Although the Canadian Medical Association (CMA) had already established guidelines for physician relations with the drug industry in 1991,[55] Dr. Guyatt and his colleagues believed they needed something more specific to deal with the unique issues that arise in postgraduate medical training. So, after extensive debate with students and faculty, they developed their own set of guidelines aimed at reducing contact between students and sales personnel in a number of ways.[56] Drug lunches and all conferences not seen as having educational priority were out, for example. And no longer would the residency program be a party to residents receiving largesse—food, pens, stationery—from the industry.

Suddenly, much more seemed to be in jeopardy than a few roast beef sandwiches and pizza.[57] Some of the students in the residency program polled the drug companies for their reaction and discovered that about half of those who responded found the guidelines unacceptable. A senior official from the Pharmaceutical Manufacturers' Association of Canada (PMAC) told Dr. Guyatt that the guidelines might compromise drug industry support, not only for education but for research as well: "When I said that sounded like a threat, he denied that it was, but instead reminded me that the relationship between academic medicine and the drug industry is 'like a marriage in which both partners have to compromise.'"

The PMAC official who spoke with Dr. Guyatt also held a senior position at a major multinational drug company. When McMaster's Dr. David Sackett, an internationally recognized clinician and research scientist, applied to this company for funds to sponsor research, he was turned down. The following is an excerpt from the letter he received:

> [Our company] has always had mutually beneficial relationships with many physicians and health care professionals in your institution. Recently, access to many of these key people has become limited, including the medical residents. Without this contact, it is very difficult for a partnership to develop. Consequently, it is not easy for [our company] to justify philanthropic donations to research, when there is limited or no access to researchers,

and no hand in the type of research project selected for
support. Unfortunately, at this time, we will have to
decline your request.

This letter certainly appeared to link the guidelines with the
refusal of funds, even though subsequent efforts to corroborate
an explicit connection didn't succeed. After several letters from
Dr. Sackett asking for clarification, including a final one threatening to bring the matter to the attention of the Royal College
of Physicians' Committee on Health and Public Policy (which
Dr. Sackett was chairing at the time), the company official ultimately denied any link between the decision not to fund the
research and the new guidelines.

Meanwhile, other departments at the medical school, many
of which were much more dependent on industry sponsorship
for research and education than the residency program, were
feeling the wrath of the drug industry. Some drug companies
evidently believed that the guidelines applied throughout the
institution and not just to the residency program, and they were
threatening to go elsewhere with their funding support. Many
faculty members were very worried that these sources of external funding would dry up if they didn't compromise, and they
began agitating for a uniform and much more lenient approach
to the industry for all the programs in the medical school. Ultimately, however, their bid failed.

"I think this shows that attempts by the industry to intimidate
academic decisions are likely to backfire," says Dr. Guyatt,
commenting on the experience. "And even though we might be
tempted to bow to this pressure, the industry will only damage
its own image if they attempt to carry out reprisals."

The Industry and Organized Medicine

The cozy relationship between doctors and drug companies has
found critics in every age, dating from Geoffrey Chaucer's
famous lines from *The Canterbury Tales*:

All his apothecaries in a tribe
Were ready with the drugs he would prescribe,

And each made money from the others guille
They had been friendly for a goodish while

Though ethical issues have often been raised in this regard, organized medicine essentially avoided taking leadership in this area until "the Squibb computer incident" captured headlines across the country. "That was the straw that broke the camel's back," according to Dr. Eike Kluge, a former director of ethics and legal affairs for the Canadian Medical Association.[58]

In the spring of 1988, Squibb Canada Inc. began conducting a post-marketing survey of Capoten, a drug for high blood pressure. Physicians who agreed to participate were asked to monitor ten or more patients on the drug and keep track of how they were doing, using computers supplied by the company. The problem was, when the study ended there was no attempt (initially) to retrieve the computers.

The licensing and regulatory body for Ontario's doctors, the College of Physicians and Surgeons, suggested that accepting the computers might put physicians in a conflict of interest. Dr. Michael Dixon, registrar for the college, expected that the Pharmaceutical Manufacturers' Association would pursue the matter with Squibb. He was astonished when PMAC president Judy Erola took aim at the college instead. "It is unfortunate that the professional integrity of thousands of medical practitioners who participate in this necessary research has been questioned," she said. "It is also unfortunate that this important medical research has recently been portrayed as a form of product promotion."[59]

As the controversy raged on, the CMA appointed Vancouver family physician Dr. Robert Wollard to chair an ad hoc committee to study the issues highlighted by the Squibb program. "There were concerns it overstepped the bounds of propriety by blurring the difference between research and promotion," he said, adding that "it definitely put the development of functional guidelines on the medical agenda."[60]

When the CMA guidelines came out in 1991 they too proved controversial, especially the one suggesting that travel and accommodation arrangements, social events, and venues for industry-sponsored continuing medical education should be in keeping with the arrangements that would normally be made without industry sponsorship. Referring to this item in a speech in February 1992, Dr. Jean Gray, an associate dean of Dalhousie's Faculty of Medicine, said, "This is going to upset the applecart a bit more than anything else in the guidelines. We've all become rather accustomed to being fêted by the drug companies—trips to exotic places, free meals, a little booze."[61]

For example, at the 1993 annual meeting of the CMA, delegates voted against a proposed amendment that would have reduced even further their freedom to dispense free samples. Dr. Noel Doig, who chairs the CMA's committee on ethics, says the feeling that doctors cannot be influenced by free samples or other industry perks is still "fairly prevalent among certain people in the profession."[62] However, he added, "there have been any number of studies done in the United States and in other jurisdictions which have shown that in fact the prescribing habits are influenced by pharmaceutical industry advertising." Dr. Wollard agreed. "The industry has spent and continues to spend millions of dollars a year on the clear assumption it influences physician behaviour. To deny that is to deny something so obvious that it puts us in an embarrassing position."

The Power of the Patent

In February 1993, the federal Tories eliminated compulsory licensing by passing a controversial new law, Bill C-91, which extended twenty-year patent protection to pharmaceuticals. Since most products take an average of ten years to go through the development and approval process, this gives each new brand-name product roughly a decade of freedom from generic competitors—ten years of monopoly.

Drug companies claimed that they needed this protection in order to recoup the money invested in bringing new products to market. The federal government claimed that the move brought Canada in line with the rest of the world, and that international trade agreements such as GATT and NAFTA required these changes in Canada's patent law. Critics of the bill said it would spell financial disaster for provincial health plans, penalize consumers, and threaten the future of the largely Canadian-owned generic drug industry.

"They're driving the first stake into the heart of the Medicare system that they've promised to nurture and protect," said Liberal Senator Royce Frith on the final day of debate on the drug bill. "Compulsory licensing is being destroyed, not for the benefit of the people of Canada or even the sake of people in other lands, it's being destroyed in order to benefit large, very powerful corporations headquartered in the United States, Switzerland, and other far-off lands."[63]

"This whole thing is bizarre," said Barry Sherman, president of Apotex Inc., Canada's largest generic manufacturer. "Normally, governments fight for their own industries, but in the pharmaceutical industry the government is taking up the cause of the American-owned industry."[64]

In a letter to former prime minister Brian Mulroney, U.S. consumer advocate Ralph Nader asked, "When economic policies shaped by pressure from multinational companies clash with procedural fairness and the maintenance of valuable Canadian social services in the process of U.S.–Canada–Mexico 'harmonization,' which is likely to bend?"[65]

Health ministers tried to point out the absurdity of Ottawa trying to criticize provincial governments for rising health care costs when federal policies ensured higher spending on provincial drug programs. Every province except Quebec objected to the changes.

Elizabeth Cull, British Columbia's former health minister and now minister of finance, in her brief to the legislative committee reviewing the bill, noted that extending patent protection for *two drugs alone* (Mevacor, a cholesterol-lowering agent, and Vasotec, a heart drug) would cost the citizens of British Columbia more than $145 million. Louise Simard, Saskatchewan's health minister, said Bill C-91 would cost her province between $3 million and $10 million a year. Former Ontario health minister Frances Lankin called for a national approach to controlling drug prices and predicted an additional expenditure of $1 billion over the next decade in her province.

Meanwhile, some politicians were dismayed at the government's efforts to short-circuit debate and rush the bill through. "I believe this is the first time in Canadian history that closure has been used at every stage of the passage of a bill through the House of Commons and the Senate," said Liberal senator Michael Kirby, "I do not understand it, because there is only a political downside to this.... What is the political payoff here?"[66]

What indeed!

Compulsory licensing, which permits firms other than the inventing company to copy brand-name drug products, had been legal in Canada since 1923. Few companies took advantage of this provision, however, because the patent legislation didn't allow copies of any drug manufactured outside of Canada. This all changed in 1969, when Canada—faced then with some of the highest drug prices in the world—began to allow compulsory licences on imported drug products. This gave a major boost to the Canadian generic drug industry, an industry that thereafter grew very rapidly, reaching sales of about $440 million in 1992.

By 1987, generic companies had applied for about seventy licences, and about thirty copies of the most popular brands of pharmaceuticals were available on the market. The impact of generic availability on prices was considerable. Following the "more the merrier" rule, a study by Dr. Joel Lexchin demonstrated price differences as great as 80 percent when four generic companies competed with one brand-name producer.[67]

The overall economic benefit of generics to Canadian consumers has been calculated by provincial governments, Consumer and Corporate Affairs, Industry, Science and Technology Canada, Statistics Canada, and the U.S. General Accounting Office. While their estimates differ, it is quite clear that the presence of generic competition in the Canadian drug marketplace has produced annual savings that range from $200 to $420 million per year.

The success of generic competition has proven to be particularly embarrassing to our neighbours to the south. A study by the U.S. General Accounting Office of 121 of the most frequently prescribed drugs found wholesale prices were on average 32 percent higher in the United States than in Canada.[68] Clearly, generic competition is a "much more effective way to lower prices than regulatory measures," says Lexchin.

But this level of healthy competition was not welcomed in all quarters. Naturally, the multinational drug industry wants full patent protection. They want the products they invent to enjoy a monopoly for as long as possible. And their lobbyists began working all-out to get rid of this encroachment on "intellectual property rights."

Mastering the two-step

Victory for the multinationals came in two steps—the first in 1987. Even though the government's own Eastman Commission reported that the multinationals' growth and profits had not been hurt by the existing rules for compulsory licensing, Ottawa partially restored patent protection to the drug industry anyway. Despite protests from the usual quarters, the changes gave brand-name producers protection from compulsory licensing for between seven and ten years.

The new provisions also created the Patent Medicine Prices Review Board (PMPRB), mandated to monitor price increases and hold hearings on drug prices considered out of line. But the board was given very weak authority over the entry price of new products, which is a key issue.[69] Between 1982 and 1989, new medications to treat arthritis, high blood pressure, and ulcers were priced 35 to 60 percent higher, on a daily treatment cost basis, than the drugs they were to replace.[70] In a study by GreenShield, one of Ontario's largest group insurance companies, the cost per prescription of new brand-name drugs was 138 percent higher than the cost of existing ones.[71]

Multinational industry spokesperson John Pye said the PMPRB has managed to keep a lid on prices, pointing out that "Canadians pay less than people in a lot of other countries."[72] But the PMPRB's own study of 177 of the biggest-selling brand-name products in Canada and other industrialized nations found that for 43 percent, Canada had either the highest or the second-highest prices in the world.[73]

For its part, the multinational industry promised more investment in new research and development in Canada—a promise that included creating "over three thousand new scientific and research-related jobs" in the industry,[74] although past chairman of the PMAC John L. Zabriskie clarified that one-third of these new jobs would come from increased spending in universities, hospitals, and medical schools rather than within the industry itself.

Critics say this promise was never kept. To create 2,000 research and development jobs between 1988 and 1995 would have required adding 250 new jobs a year, but an internal PMAC survey suggested that only about 150 jobs were added annually between 1987 and 1990.[75] Of a further 939 new jobs created, about 700 were in marketing and sales. Meanwhile, over the same period, the generic industry documented 700 job losses.

Stage two in the battle—the February 1993 passage of Bill C-91—was really the *coup de grâce*. This law completely eliminated compulsory licensing during the twenty-year patent life of drug products. The bill even contains a retroactivity clause applying to any product licence granted after December 20, 1991. According to the Canadian Drug Manufacturers' Association (CDMA), many of their licence applications were filed long before this date and had involved them in research and development costs exceeding $100 million.[76] Now no licence would be granted on these products until they were fully off-patent. Many observers commented that this date was set in an attempt to offer extended protection to Merck Frosst's Vasotec, worth an estimated $700 million to the company.[77] Some even referred to C-91 as the "Merck bill."

To push C-91, the multinational drug companies bought services from nearly every lobby firm in Ottawa. Sean Moore, editor of the Ottawa-based *Lobby Digest,* noted, "It's a rare but classic example of a multifaceted, all-fronts lobby."[78] "There's hardly a consulting company in the country who hasn't been approached to work for the multinational drug industry," says Toronto consultant Ted Ball, who points out that the university sector was also promised rich rewards for its support. Even some voluntary organizations were warned, unofficially, that donations to them from the industry could be contingent on their support for Bill C-91.

Nova Scotia's Dalhousie University, for example, was embroiled in a controversy after a Liberal provincial MLA linked a $1.3 million research grant to the Faculty of Health Professions with a letter from the dean supporting the bill. In fact, explained the dean of the faculty, Dr. Lynn McIntyre, there was no connection. The money had been received before the university even thought of writing the letter. But she acknowledged that "there are cases where drug companies have made contracts conditional on support—for sure."[79]

Certainly the scientific research community in Canada went all out to support the bill. The Canadian Society for Clinical Investigation asked its members to become actively involved in lobbying by phone, fax, and mail. The Canadian Federation of Biological Societies, whose members depend a great deal on drug company grants, also spoke out in favour of the bill.[80] And who can blame them? Through financial cutbacks to the provinces, Ottawa had reduced support not just to provincial health care but also to post-secondary education. And government-support for research has long been declining.

The original position of the Canadian Medical Association was to support the bill provisionally while arguing for a number of amendments, the most important of which was to tighten up the definition of "research and development."[81] It has been pointed out many times that most of the research conducted by multinationals in Canada is not basic research to discover new products but rather clinical trials required to comply with Canada's Health Protection Branch rules.

McGill's professor emeritus John T. Edward wrote an editorial in the *Globe and Mail* staunchly defending the need for more patent protection. He claimed that the industry needed it in order to develop the kind of new breakthrough drugs that in the past forty years had saved Canadians $10 to $20 billion in health care costs.[82] In rebuttal, Dr. Gordon Guyatt pointed out that neither drugs nor vaccines can take credit for the increased longevity experienced since the turn of the century, noting that death rates had fallen substantially long before these products were even available.[83] He also noted that the PMPRB's own assessment found that only 8 of the 162 new drug products introduced to Canada between January 1988 and December 1990 were substantial improvements over what was already on the market. Dr. Guyatt documented the fact that even breakthrough drugs are frequently prone to inappropriate use, "generating cost, but no benefit, and possibly harm." Dr. Guyatt concluded that Professor Edward's estimate of savings was "pulled from the air," since most drugs do not cure disease and many require expensive, long-term administration.

With the passage of Bill C-91, it was pay-back time for the industry's supporters. Merck Frosst, for example, will have continued opportunities to show the industry's gratitude to its biggest supporter, former prime minister Brian Mulroney. After retiring from politics, Mr. Mulroney joined Ogilvie Renault, the Montreal law firm that advised Merck during the Bill C-91 debates. And once again the PMAC promised more jobs and more investment in research and development, including a $200 million commitment over five years to medical research and training.[84]

Twenty million dollars is slated for a "partnership" with the Medical Research Council (MRC), the major source of research funding for biomedical research in Canada.[85] However, the venture will cost the MRC resources in the short term, and the drug companies will retain patent rights for any new products developed.

All the same, expert observers doubt that Canada could ever become a major centre of basic pharmaceutical research. Most parent companies are headquartered in Europe or the United States, and that's where the major research efforts are centred. If this is so, if jobs created will occur more in sales and promotion than in scientific positions, if new drug prices are allowed to elude regulatory control, and if the additional costs to consumers and provincial governments are going to force more cutbacks in provincial drug benefit programs—what's in it for Canada? What was really behind Bill C-91?

Whither Sovereignty?

The answer is both disquieting and embarrassing. Bill C-91 is yet another unmistakable signal that Canada has lost significant sovereignty as a nation. It points to our dwindling ability to enact policies in the public interest when they conflict with powerful commercial interests. Government seems to have lost its capacity to be a good Guardian, as Jane Jacobs describes the role.

There are new masters afoot—unelected lords of commerce sweeping through our global economy looking to maximize profit. As *Montreal Gazette* reporter Nicolas Regush pointed out in *Safety Last,* his critique of Canada's consumer health protection system, "Drug companies, like other multinationals, can pick and chose where they spend their cash. If the economic or political climate in one country becomes unfavourable, they simply move to a sunnier one. This is the bottom line."[86]

During the debates over the 1987 changes to patent legislation, rumours raged about the connection between the new law and the then hotly debated Free Trade Agreement. The government strongly denied any link to the FTA—until, that is, a leaked copy of a signed draft revealed the following passage: "Canada has agreed to pass the pending amendments contained in Bill C-22 in respect of compulsory licencing of pharmaceuticals."[87] Although this clause never appeared in the final version of the FTA, the cat was out of the bag. And U.S. treasury secretary James Baker later talked about Canada's commitment to "review more extensive patent protection for drugs within ten years 'for no U.S. concessions.' "[88] In the end, Bill C-91 fulfilled that commitment. But this time the link to international trade agreements was acknowledged openly. It was, in fact, a principle argument used by government to justify the bill.

Twenty-year patent protection for drugs has implications well beyond Canada and our principal trading partners. Developing nations and even reformers in the United States looked on Canada's former laws concerning compulsory licensing as a beacon of sane domestic policy. Now that we've succumbed to the global agenda, the light in the beacon has been extinguished.

And there may be worse news on the horizon. Bill C-91 will boost costs for provincial drug plans while providing outrageous profits to brand-name drug companies. But, like any glutton worth his jowls, the multinationals are not satisfied; they want even more. Michael Hodin, vice-president of U.S.-based Pfizer Pharmaceuticals, ominously noted, "Things aren't perfect in Canada. There are still problems to be settled." Within two weeks of C-91's royal assent, the industry was talking about the need to eliminate provincial drug programs, calling them "restrictive trade practices."[89]

Democratic governments all over the world know only too well that the multinational drug industry is not accountable to taxpayers, only to shareholders. And it appears that having a big bankroll means the industry can buy (or at least rent) scientists, politicians, and even whole countries. In return, governments are allowed to enjoy the fiction that they are in charge, as long as their policies do not interfere with industry's ability to control the marketplace.

Of course, we have a new government in Ottawa now to put to the test. Will the Liberals, like the Tories before them, continue to "just say yes" to the multinationals, whatever the political costs at home? Do they have any choice?

Chapter 6

Health Care
Goes to Market

IT'S SIX O'CLOCK—the "hour from hell" in many Canadian households. Mary C. rushes home from work to get started on dinner, but before it's ready her husband, Joseph, arrives with their two children. As she stands at the stove, her eight-year-old, Stanley, pulls on her apron strings, complaining of a sore throat. Mary takes his temperature and finds it's 38 degrees Celsius (about 100 degrees Fahrenheit). Now Mary is really fixed. Her doctor's office closed at five, and besides, it usually takes almost a week to get an appointment with him.

When Mary was a child, she was always taken care of at home when she had a cold. But with her own children, she's become more cautious. She always takes them to the doctor, and usually they return with a prescription for antibiotics. On this day, her husband remembers there's a walk-in medical clinic in a nearby mall. He volunteers to take Stanley there while Mary finishes making dinner. An hour later, they're back with a prescription for penicillin.

Mary's older sister, Elizabeth, fell on the ice recently and injured her shoulder. Elizabeth's doctor said she needed physiotherapy but noted that the local hospital had just laid off its physiotherapists and was closing its out-patient department. There is a publicly funded community physiotherapy clinic nearby, but it has a six-week waiting list. She has two other options. She could go to a private clinic and pay $25 for each session, or she could go to a doctor who has his secretary provide the services, even though she has no formal training in physiotherapy. Elizabeth can't afford the private fees and doesn't think she can wait six weeks for free care, so she decides to get her treatments from the doctor's secretary.

Elizabeth and Mary's mother, Grace L., is sixty-two years old. She has heart disease, and her doctor recently prescribed enalapril and lovastatin. These medications are very important for Grace. In fact, enalapril has been found to reduce heart disease deaths by up to 30 percent.[1] But the prescriptions cost $100 a month, which she can't afford from her meagre income. Her children have to pool their scant extra resources to pay the bills.

Stanley is the only one in this family who entered the system quickly and easily, but the care he received was inappropriate. Most of what we call colds or flus are caused by viruses—germs you can't kill with antibiotics. It wouldn't matter if Stanley saw a doctor or not; it wouldn't matter if he took the penicillin or not. People with colds get better on their own, regardless of treatment.

This story begs a question: why was it so easy for Stanley to get care that was useless when Elizabeth and Grace couldn't get the kind of care they really needed?

Health Care: A Market Like No Other

Natalie is a waitress with after-tax earnings that amount to $8 an hour. Suppose that Natalie decides to spend $8 on a movie. Naturally, she hopes the movie will provide enough enjoyment to balance the trouble it took her to earn the money—one hour's worth of work. If the movie turns out to be a dog, Natalie will feel she has wasted her money. If she kept on seeing movies that disappointed her, eventually she might get completely fed up and pick another pastime altogether. Alternatively, she might try to be more discerning about the films she chooses to see. If the movie houses in her town offered a poor selection, she might check out videos. However, if Natalie persisted in going to movies she didn't like, complaining all the while that she had no money for activities she *did* enjoy, we would say she was violating a commonsense economic rule: the value received from each dollar we spend should be commensurate with the cost to us of earning it.

In Canada's health care system, we violate this rule every single minute, aided and abetted by a complicated maze of legislation, regulation, and perverse incentives. Current institutional arrangements in our system mean that doctors can set up walk-in clinics and earn a good living offering useless treatments to people with colds, but we can't seem to guarantee that people like Grace L. and her daughter get essential medications or receive timely services from a qualified provider. This suggests a market failure—the inability to match supply with need.

Some people claim that this failure is due to public financing of health insurance and recommend privatization, and in particular, user charges for doctors' and hospital services. But would user fees really solve anything? This chapter sets out the case against user fees, examines the real reasons why markets in health care fail, and then begins to look at how to make the health care system more responsive to people's needs.

Why User Fees Fail

Alberta premier Ralph Klein thinks that people who can afford it should pay a small fee for their health services. He claims that this would help to pay for the costs of health care and keep people from abusing the system.[2] Quebec premier Daniel Johnson is also on record as supporting user fees.[3] Are they right? Would user fees do what their supporters claim?

Professor Robert Evans of the University of British Columbia and some other economist colleagues recently reviewed the evidence and concluded that user fees are primarily a mechanism for redistributing wealth: the rich and the healthy gain; the poor and the sick lose.[4] What's more, their analysis shows that user fees do not achieve the policy objectives their advocates claim. User fees do not control health costs. Nor do they improve the appropriateness of care. They do, however, have a devastating impact on the health of poor people. Because all this evidence has not managed to "do them in" as a policy option, Evans calls user fees "Zombies"—they should be dead, but they keep coming back from the grave to haunt us. It's time we put them out of their misery.

User fees would not control health care costs

To understand why user fees are unhelpful in controlling health care costs, it helps to know that the costs of health care are largely determined by existing capacity and not by the individual decisions that patients make about how and when to use the system. How much care is delivered and how much it costs are primarily functions of how many institutional beds are funded and how many doctors work in the system.[5]

In the past twenty-five years the ratio of doctors to population in Canada doubled, but workloads per doctor didn't fall. We built too many hospitals and proceeded to overuse them. We've added new technologies to the system all the while, often without rigorous evaluation of their effectiveness. These factors in combination have created conditions for continuous expansion. And the system has clicked along at more or less the same rate of growth, regardless of whether or not user fees have been in place.

We know this because in the 1960s and 1970s Saskatchewan politicians unwittingly devised a magnificent natural experiment into the effects of user fees. In 1962, the Cooperative Commonwealth Federation (the predecessor of the New Democratic Party) implemented Canada's first universal public medical insurance plan in Saskatchewan. The new system had no user fees.* In 1964, however, the CCF/NDP government was defeated by the Liberals under Ross Thatcher, and in 1968 the Thatcher government began charging user fees for physician and hospital services. The charges were relatively small—$6 to $10 in today's terms[6]—and they remained in effect until 1971, when the NDP regained power in Saskatchewan under Allan Blakeney and abolished them.

Economists Glen Beck and John Horne studied what effect these user charges actually had on the utilization of health services in Saskatchewan.[7] Here's what they found:

---

* There are two broad types of user fees: coinsurance and deductibles. Coinsurance is a fee paid at the time of service, either a flat charge, as it was in Saskatchewan, or a proportion of the total cost of the service, as it was in the Rand Health Insurance Experiment. A deductible is the amount that must be paid by the patient directly before he is eligible for insurance coverage. Typically, the deductible portion is calculated on an annual or semi-annual basis.

- The cost of physician services fell by 6 percent overall.
- This decrease in physician costs was due almost entirely to an 18 percent drop in utilization by the poor and the elderly.
- By contrast, higher income groups slightly increased their use of physician services.
- There was no difference in the utilization of hospital services—the most expensive category of care.
- In total, Saskatchewan's introduction of user fees had virtually no effect on the overall cost of health care.

The most sophisticated investigation of user charges for health care was one part of a $136 million (1984 U.S. dollars) study funded by the United States Health Care Financing Administration—the Rand Health Insurance Experiment (HIE). The investigators examined the effect of user charges on the utilization of health services and people's health.[8] The experiment's participants were randomly allocated to fee-for-service plans with different rates of user charges or to plans with first-dollar coverage. As in Saskatchewan, there was an annual limit on how much an individual would have to pay.

Not surprisingly, the HIE found that the use of health services declined with increased user charges—people do respond to financial disincentives. However, the declines were greater among poor people than among middle- or upper-class participants.[9] The total cost of health services was 25 percent lower for the group with the highest user fees compared to those who had first-dollar coverage.

At first glance, this finding appears to contradict what happened in Saskatchewan, where total health care costs remained the same, with or without user fees. However, as Robert Evans points out, "the Rand study did not, and by design could not, show that [user fees] led to an overall system-wide reduction in utilization and costs."[10]

Here's why. In the Rand experiment any single fee-for-service doctor had only a handful of patients who were enrolled in the experiment. Even if all of these patients decreased their rate of utilization because of the user fees, it wouldn't have affected that physician's income. The doctor would simply have had room in his schedule to see other patients not enrolled in the study. The costs of care for these non-enrolled patients were not, of course, tracked by the study and could not influence its results.

In Saskatchewan, however, the user fees affected nearly everyone: all doctors and all patients in the province.* If there had been an across-the-board decrease in utilization, doctors would have lost income. But, of course, only the poor decreased their use of services. Upper-income residents actually increased their use of doctors' services, mostly for the kind of services that are most often initiated at the discretion of a physician, such as complete physical assessments and annual health exams. It is quite likely that most of this increase in physician-induced visits was unintentional. Doctors simply had more time in their schedules (because of decreased visits from their poorer patients) to see those who could afford to pay.

The same thing happened to doctors in southwest Pennsylvania in the late 1970s.[11] The United Mine Workers introduced user fees to their health benefit program in 1977. As a result, the miners and their families reduced their use of doctors' services, and the local doctors faced lower incomes. However, the doctors increased the number of visits for patients covered by other plans, particularly the relatively generous one for members of the United Steelworkers of America.

Evans and his colleagues argue that user fees, "by diversifying and privatizing funding sources, are more likely to lead to higher costs through higher prices (and provider incomes) rather than to lower costs through lower use."[12] To illustrate their argument, they point to the United States, which relies heavily on user fees, as the only system in the world where costs are totally out of control, and to France, which "in recent years has been the least successful of the European countries at controlling overall health care costs," despite, or because of, the implementation of substantial user fees.

User fees don't improve the appropriateness of care

The Rand HIE used expert panels of physicians to determine the appropriateness of care provided. They found the same level of

---

* Social assistance recipients were exempt; the working poor, however, were not.

inappropriate antibiotic use with or without user fees.[13] And, while the user fee group used 24 percent fewer hospital days than those with first-dollar coverage,[14] the proportion of inappropriate hospital admissions and hospital stays was the same in both groups.[15] The authors concluded that "because cost sharing did not selectively reduce inappropriate hospitalization, it is important to develop other mechanisms to do so."[16]

Some proponents of user fees think too many patients abuse Canada's system by seeking care for trivial problems, and that this costs big bucks. This claim is simply bogus. In the first place, patients don't really have much opportunity to abuse the system. Institutional care, prescription drugs, laboratory tests, and physician services amount to nearly 80 percent of the costs of health care and nearly 90 percent of publicly funded health care. But access to the first three of these items requires a doctor's order. Even most of the costs of physicians' services are determined by doctors. You can't see a specialist in most communities without a physician referral, and many visits to family doctors are callbacks. Robert Evans and his colleagues say that less than 10 percent of the health budget is open to patient abuse, and even in this category, they argue that a patient's decision to seek medical advice and treatment is often perfectly sensible. Overall, the authors estimate that the true cost of patient-initiated abuse is almost certainly less than 1 percent of total health spending.

User fees punish the poor and the sick

The Canada Health Act requires that insured services be available according to need.[17] In general, the poorer you are, the worse your health is and the greater your need for health services. It follows logically that in a health system with user fees, services and income are transferred from the poor and the sick to the well-to-do and healthy.

The Rand HIE found that both high-risk and low-income participants who had to pay user fees had an increased risk of dying compared to those who had free care.[18] The reason? It was mainly because participants with first-dollar coverage were more likely to have their hypertension (high blood pressure) diagnosed and treated.[19] All told, a fifty-year-old man at high risk for health problems had a 20 percent increased risk of death over a five-year period if he had to pay user fees.[20]

Other studies have found charges for health care associated with poorer health outcomes.[21] In fact, the United States is the world's best example of who benefits and who doesn't in a health care system rife with user fees. The United States stands alone among wealthy countries in the extent to which it relies on private financing for health care. Only 42 percent of U.S. health care is paid for from the public purse, compared to 72 percent in Canada, 84 percent in Britain, and 95 percent in Norway.[22] In the United States, 20 percent of health costs are paid directly out of people's pockets.[23] One of the effects of this policy is that wealthy Americans get more services than the poor.

This is not the case in Canada. For example, according to a study by Dr. Geoffrey Anderson of Toronto's Institute for Clinical Evaluative Sciences, Canadians in poor neighbourhoods are the most likely to get heart bypass surgery, while Americans in poor neighbourhoods are the least likely to get this type of surgery.[24] Heart disease death rates are much higher for the poor than the rich, so it's safe to conclude that many poor Americans are not getting access to necessary heart surgery.[25]

On the other hand, it's possible that wealthy Americans are actually getting more bypass operations than they need. Dr. Anderson cautions against drawing this conclusion from his study but notes that "in the United States the financial incentives for hospitals to perform surgery are quite attractive, and maybe they do too much."[26]

Who gains from user fees?

Robert Evans and his colleagues make no bones about the distributional effects of user fees. Care flows away from those who need it towards those who might not; income flows away from the poor towards the rich. So the healthy and the wealthy stand to gain from them. Also, for some providers of care, user fees mean more income and less government control over health expenditures. Taken together, these factors help explain why user fees—the Zombies of the health care system—keep breaking out of their crypt.

Some consumers ask: "What damage is done if I pay a little more to get a little better service?" The answer is that user fees can cause a lot of damage. The shift from a system without charges for doctors and hospitals to one with some charges is a major policy departure, not a minor one. Once allowed, user fees, with so many payers and so many recipients, are incredibly difficult to control. Over time, the fee amounts will tend to rise, inevitably creating new demands for private insurance.

To Market, To Market ...

The discussion of user fees highlights the fact that health care is not a normally functioning market, and therefore traditional economic analysis must be tempered when applied to health services.

There are several preconditions necessary for a properly functioning economic market. One is the presence of informed consumers. If consumers are not fully informed, then competitors can't "signal" the advantage of choosing their product over someone else's.

Another essential precondition is that businesses should find it easy to enter the marketplace. If it costs too much for businesses to set up, then you can bet only a few firms will control the marketplace, and the resulting oligopoly will tend to drive prices upward. Other barriers—like licensing and certification—can also interfere with market entry.

Informed choice

In many situations, we can't determine appropriate care until the patient is properly consulted. This is easier said than done. Many aspects of health care are highly technical, which makes it difficult for patients to become fully informed. The extent of this asymmetry of information between providers and patients puts consumers at a distinct disadvantage when it comes to making informed choices.

But beyond this problem is the fact that our health care system often fails to give patients the chance to become informed. Many opportunities are being missed for incorporating patient preferences into the decision-making process.

Harvard radiology professor Dr. Barbara McNeil shook many in the health community with her 1978 article in the *New England Journal of Medicine* suggesting that many lung cancer patients might forego possibly life-extending surgery* and opt for radiation therapy instead if they really understood the trade-offs.[27] Radiation therapy kills very few people, but it doesn't cure the cancer. By contrast, lung cancer surgery offers a better chance for a cure, but it has a death rate of up to 10 percent. That's why radiation therapy patients are more likely to live two years while surgical patients are more likely to live five years.

McNeil argued that if a patient valued the chance for a "cure" very highly, and if he were relatively young, he would probably opt for surgery. Alternatively, if the patient were "risk averse" and relatively old, he would probably opt for radiation.

The main point of McNeil's article was that practitioners cannot determine what treatment a patient should have without first fully incorporating an individual's specific values and preferences. Since this landmark study appeared, the field of eliciting patient preferences has exploded.[28]

In Chapter 4, we discussed Dr. John Wennberg's work with an interactive video to help patients with non-cancerous, enlarged prostate glands decide on the best course of treatment: whether to have surgery or to opt for "watchful waiting."** The video disk is used with a computer, and the patient can tailor the advice to match his own circumstances. For example, a patient using this technology can find out his own specific risks and possible benefits from surgery. He can call up interviews with doctors who had the same condition themselves and hear about the choices they made and whether they were pleased with the results. In about an hour, the patient can provide himself with a second opinion.

The video was first used for patients attending the Kaiser-Permanente Medical Plan in Denver and the Group Health

---

* In fact, only about one-third of lung cancer patients are considered to be candidates for surgery.

** Since the interactive video was first developed, new treatment alternatives have become available for benign prostatic hypertrophy, including thermal microwave treatment and drug therapy. These newer alternatives have been added to the list of choices presented to patients in the video, highlighting the need to continually update this technology to maintain its relevance to clinical practice.

Cooperative of Puget Sound in Seattle. When patients started viewing the video, the rate of surgery dropped in the short term by 44 percent and 60 percent respectively.[29] This technology has won wide acceptance from patients and practitioners alike. Now, new interactive videos have been developed to help patients choose among alternative treatments for low-back pain, early-stage breast cancer, and mildly elevated blood pressure. Future plans for this technology include interactive videos for patients considering hysterectomy, coronary artery bypass surgery, and many other common procedures.

Communicate or die

Of course, good communication is central to eliciting patient preferences. In fact, the quality of clinical communication is also a key determinant of many health outcomes, including (but not limited to) reduced blood pressure, better asthma control, and reduced anxiety.[30]

How good are doctors at communicating? Considerable evidence suggests that this is a problem area for many. Studies have shown that doctors often misunderstand what their patients have really said and are inclined to misinterpret patient preferences.[31]

Consider, for example, research conducted by Professor Richard Frankel of the University of Rochester Medical School. He videotaped a number of physician-patient encounters and found that, on average, it took patients about ninety seconds to raise their chief concerns. The average doctor, however, interrupted after only eighteen seconds. Interrupting too soon can interfere with diagnosis, according to Frankel, since in many cases the first symptom patients mentioned was not the most serious.[32]

Canada is a leader in researching health care communication, and great strides have been made here in improving the communication skills of health professionals.[33] In fact, in 1991, experts in health care communication from around the world met in Toronto to draft the first consensus statement on doctor-patient communication. Three of the seven authors were Canadians.[34] However, there are few incentives for patient education within our current system, and many patients never have the chance to become properly informed because they are unconscious or mentally incapacitated. The point is that without informed patients, you can't have a proper market.

Regulation and red tape

Anything that limits ease of entry into the marketplace contributes to market failure, and health care is rife with regulation that limits who gets to practise in the health care market. Most health care services are restricted to physicians only. And most provinces won't pay—or won't pay very much—for care that is not delivered by doctors.*

On the surface, much of this regulation appears appropriate—the ostensible goal is public protection. Some regulation of health care workers is necessary to protect the innocent from unscrupulous practitioners.

In the nineteenth century, many different kinds of medical practice were in open competition in the North American health care market, including allopaths (precursors to modern medical doctors), naturopaths, homeopaths, and many others.[35] There were awful episodes in which unqualified or poorly trained doctors did serious damage to innocent victims, taking their money and sometimes their lives. In response, allopathic doctors convinced provincial and state legislatures to restrict the right to practise medicine to members of their group.[36]

Though its aims may be worthy, there are major flaws in our current regulatory system. Certain health professionals have been shut out of the marketplace merely because they threaten the interests of other professions. We often use more costly professionals, with extensive training, when less expensive personnel could do the job as well or even better. Specialist doctors in some communities spend much of their time providing care that could be delivered by family doctors. Family doctors spend much of their time providing care that could be provided by nurses or social workers. Registered nurses spend much of their

---

* Public coverage for non-physician services varies considerably across the country. Some provinces do provide limited coverage for chiropractors, optometrists, dentists, massage therapists, podiatrists, naturopaths, and osteopaths. Public coverage for midwives and nurse practitioners is also gradually becoming more available in some provinces.

time providing care that could be provided by practical nurses or health care aides. And health professionals of all types provide care that could be provided by patients and their families.

One of the best examples of inappropriate regulation is the extent to which the practices of nurses have been limited. We have known for years that nurses are competent to perform many services normally delivered by family doctors.[37] There are even studies showing that specially trained nurses can substitute for specialists.[38] For example, Drs. Jerry Avorn and Daniel Everitt of Harvard University surveyed five hundred doctors and three hundred nurse-practitioners (nurses with enhanced training) to investigate their interviewing skills and therapeutic decision-making for patients complaining of abdominal pain and insomnia.[39] They found that physicians were less likely than nurses to take a complete medical history and more likely to prescribe drugs. The conclusion? These nurses were providing a higher quality of care.

Why don't we act on this information? Why don't nurses get the chance to provide these kinds of services more often? There are two major factors working against this type of policy shift: 1) the presence of restrictive regulation, and 2) the perverse incentives created by fee-for-service medicine.

Perhaps the most famous study of nurses substituting for physicians was conducted by McMaster University in the wealthy suburban community of Burlington, Ontario.[40] The investigators randomly assigned patients to receive primary care* from either a family doctor or a nurse-practitioner. The study found no differences in health outcomes, quality of care, or patient satisfaction with care, but it did find huge financial differences for the practices involved. In fact, practices employing nurse-practitioners lost 5 percent of their gross income and up to 10 percent of net income. Provincial governments allow doctors to bill the system directly, but not nurses. Nor can doctors receive

---

* Primary care is first contact care including family doctors, primary care nursing, and some rehabilitation and social services. Secondary care includes first level specialty care (e.g. pediatrics, general internal medicine, general surgery, psychiatry, and obstetrics). Tertiary care includes sub-specialty care (e.g. cardiology, thoracic surgery, and ophthalmology).

additional resources from government to pay for care provided by nurses.* Under these structural limitations, doctors have little incentive to hire nurses to provide services that the physicians can perform and bill for themselves.

Dentistry is also rife with inappropriate regulation. In the late 1960s and early 1970s, Saskatchewan developed a children's dental program based on a ratio of ten specially trained dental therapists for every dentist. (The program for training therapists was based in Prince Albert, and it not only helped to educate therapists for the province, it also trained many for work in the Third World.) The dental therapists did preventative work as well as basic restorative work (fillings and crowns). In 1976, three outside dental specialists evaluated the quality of care of 410 children who had received dental care either from dentists or dental therapists. The therapists' work was judged to be far superior to that of the dentists.

- 47 percent of the therapists' work was judged to be superior compared to 17 percent of the dentists' work.
- 4 percent of the therapists' work was judged unacceptable compared to 21 percent of the dentists' work.[41]

However, by the late 1980s some of the province's dentists were concerned that they were losing work because of this program. Their lobby fit well with provincial policy—Saskatchewan's Conservative government was bent on finding public services to cut. On June 11, 1987, Premier Grant Devine announced the program's demise at the annual meeting of the Saskatchewan Dental Association. Within a year, the dental therapists were unemployed and the training facility dismantled.

The Fee's the Thing

The majority of doctors in Canada are paid on a fee-for-service basis, a system that provides payment for each billable

---

* A minor exception to this rule is the allowance for doctors to bill government when nurses working for them give allergy shots.

service doctors provide. But research evidence suggests that fee-for-service adds to the costs of care without improving overall health outcomes.[42] The incentives appear to encourage doctors to do too many unhelpful things.

It's also pretty clear, however, that fee-for-service actually penalizes some doctors, especially family physicians who are trying to deliver high-quality care. Let's see how this works by checking in with Toronto physicians Drs. A. and B.

Dr. A. sees about 140 patients each week. To provide better service to her patients and reduce their reliance on walk-in clinics, she always keeps some room open in her schedule so she can see sick patients the same day if necessary. She also works two evenings every week and on Saturday mornings.

Dr. A.'s patients usually don't see her when they have minor illnesses. They've been trained to handle these problems on their own—although if they have any questions, they've been encouraged to telephone for advice about whether or not they need to schedule an appointment. Dr. A. enjoys obstetrical care and she delivers about four babies a month. But the deliveries often play havoc with her office schedule and personal life. Besides that, a complete course of prenatal care plus the delivery pays her only about $500 per patient, even though it can take up more than ten hours of her time. Dr. A. also has fifty patients who are HIV-positive and twenty with full-blown AIDS; at any given time, she's looking after two patients dying at home with AIDS. Dr. A. shares after-hours call with a group of seven other doctors. However, she has given her home phone number to her dying patients so they can reach her directly for urgent help. Dr. A.'s gross billings to the Ontario Health Insurance Plan (OHIP) are $140,000, and her pre-tax net income, after expenses, is $85,000.

Dr. B. sees over 400 patients each week. Monday to Friday, he works from 9:00 a.m. to 6:00 p.m. After hours, he is completely unavailable, and patients who call then hear a recorded message referring them to a walk-in clinic or the local hospital's emergency department. Dr. B. isn't in the habit of purposely leaving room in his schedule so he can see patients who really need to be seen the same day. The best his receptionist can do is offer them the first available opening—often days away. Those who feel they can't wait may go to a walk-in clinic or emergency department for care. About ten of Dr. B.'s patients each day get allergy shots. About twenty patients a day come in with minor illnesses—colds, flus, stomach upsets. For these patients, Dr. B. prescribes drugs and orders lab tests, which are often not needed. He also books a follow-up appointment to see these patients four or five days later; follow-up visits account for twenty of Dr. B.'s appointments in a given day. Almost all these patients will have recovered from their minor illnesses by then and they will spend a total of about thirty seconds with the doctor to find out their test results—almost invariably normal. A further twenty patients each day are either people with chronic conditions, such as high blood pressure or diabetes, or people who are perfectly well coming in for services like well-baby visits or checkups. The balance of Dr. B.'s patients are immediately referred to a specialist, without first doing a prior examination or lab work-ups; these are patients with potentially very serious medical conditions. Dr. B.'s gross billings to OHIP are $370,000, and his pre-tax net income, after expenses, is $270,000.

As you can see, doctors in our system are well rewarded for seeing relatively healthy patients with minor illnesses. However, physicians caring for patients with serious chronic illnesses like AIDS and schizophrenia don't enjoy nearly the same level of earning potential. Treating very sick patients in the community pays doctors very poorly.

In addition, fees for specific services differ widely. In general, invasive procedures—surgery, fibrescopic endoscopy, catheterization, and so on—pay the most. As a result, doctors are encouraged to spend their time cutting and prodding rather than listening and thinking. What's more, fee-for-service doesn't recognize different skill levels or experience among practitioners. Recently the Ontario directors of family practice training programs and the Canadian College of Family Physicians criticized the fee-for-service system.[43] The College's discussion paper claims that fee-for-service penalizes family doctors.

Fee-for-service hikes costs

In one part of the Rand Health Insurance Experiment, over 1,600 patients were randomly allocated to receive their health care from either the Group Health Cooperative of Puget Sound—a

Seattle-based, non-profit health maintenance organization (HMO) with salaried doctors, governed by a community board—or from fee-for-service physicians in the Seattle area.

The experiment found no significant differences in the health of the two groups of patients but a very large difference in how much their care cost. Average costs for the HMO patients were 25 percent less than those seeing fee-for-service doctors, due almost entirely to the fact that the HMO patients spent 40 percent fewer days in hospital.[44]

In the United States, HMOs are funded on capitation—subscribers and/or their employers pay a fixed amount each month to cover all care requirements, whether or not services are actually provided. Capitation funding, especially when combined with salaried group practice, appears both to attract more conservative doctors and to reward more conservative practise.

Of course, these financing and reimbursement methods may also encourage underservicing—an incentive that may be heightened in for-profit organizations. However, in the Rand experiment, there was no evidence overall that patients enrolled in the non-profit Group Health Cooperative were receiving less care than they needed. There are additional caveats to interpreting the results of the Rand Health Insurance Experiment but they don't change its overall message.[45] Fee-for-service reimbursement costs more without producing more health payoffs.

Doctors on salary

Canada has been slow in developing alternatives to fee-for-service medicine. The exception is Quebec, and to a lesser extent Ontario, where doctors working in community health centres, or CHCs, are paid on salary.

There are about 250 CHCs across the country. Most encourage multi-disciplinary teamwork, and some incorporate an expanded role for nurses. Consumer participation and community governance are other commonly-found features.

Quebec began to develop its network of primary care clinics in 1972 as part of the reform of its health and social services system. Known as CLSCs (*centres locaux des services communautaires*), the network now boasts about 170 centres throughout the province combining primary health care, social services, home care, and other programs, depending on local priorities.

In 1988, about 5 percent of the population was receiving primary care from CLSCs.[46]

Ontario has about fifty community health centres, largely dedicated to serving poor or marginalized communities. Saskatchewan and Manitoba have about half a dozen each, and the other provinces have even fewer, if any.

The health service organization, or HSO, is another alternative to fee-for-service for doctors working in Ontario. The province funds about ninety HSOs offering primary care, and in some cases specialty care as well. HSOs, like the HMOs in the United States, are funded on capitation, meaning that they receive a fixed payment each month for every patient on their roster, regardless of whether or not patients actually use any services. However, unlike the HMOs, Ontario's HSOs only provide out-patient services; they are not financially responsible for providing hospital care.

In addition, Ontario is also trying to develop a Canadian version of the American HMO called the Comprehensive Health Organization, or CHO. The CHO will receive capitation payments to provide out-patient and also in-patient services across the full spectrum of primary and secondary care. Most of the community's funding for hospital and community care will be rolled into these capitation payments. The first CHOs are slated to open in 1994 in the northern communities of Fort Frances and Wawa.

There is relatively little evidence on how well community health clinics in Canada perform. However, controlled studies in Saskatoon, Prince Albert, and Sault Ste. Marie have shown that they are less expensive than fee-for-service practices without any apparent compromise in quality.[47] Studies from Quebec have demonstrated that CLSCs provide higher-quality care for patients presenting with headaches,[48] more appropriate cancer screening,[49] better cancer prevention services,[50] and more complete childhood immunization.[51] Quebec research also indicates that CLSC doctors have different attitudes and practice styles, probably because the system attracts doctors who already demonstrate these attitudes and behaviours rather than because the model itself fosters them.[52]

Hospital Funding: Tell Me the Rules and I'll Play the System

If fee-for-service doctors have incentives to increase the numbers of services they provide to patients who don't really need care, hospitals paid on a global budget have an incentive to admit patients who don't need to be there and keep them as long as possible.

There are some key differences across the country in how hospitals are funded, but most provinces rely on global budgets. Under this system, hospitals receive an overall amount of money to fund all their activities for the year. It's more or less up to hospitals to decide how to spend these resources—although, as we've discussed, most of the costs are driven by referral patterns and clinical decisions made by doctors.

Historically, all hospitals in a given province receive annual across-the-board percentage increases to their budgets, although some provinces adjust specific allocations to reflect population growth, special high-cost services, or to redress historical inequities.

Global budgets provide rather perverse economic incentives. A 1988 study showed that patients with uncomplicated heart attacks could leave hospital after three days[53] but the length of stay in most Canadian hospitals for heart attack patients is about ten days. The explanation is that the first three days of a hospital stay for heart attack patients are the most expensive. That's usually when patients receive the most tests and other procedures. It's also the time when they are likely to require the most intensive kinds of nursing care—more or less continuous monitoring. The last seven days are mainly for rest and recovery. Expenses incurred by the hospital during this period are mostly for "hotel costs" (e.g., food and laundry services) rather than for actual care.

If the hospital routinely discharged heart attack patients after the first three days, what would happen? Other acutely ill patients would come in to take their place. Over the year, the hospital would be providing more days of relatively expensive service, and its costs would almost certainly go up. A former deputy minister of health once joked that a smart hospital would specialize in patients with skin diseases because they need few expensive services.

Alberta is the only province in Canada to have abandoned global budgeting. Hospitals there receive funding according to the type of patients, or case mix, treated over the course of the year. Each patient is slotted into one of several hundred categories upon admission, depending upon the diagnosis and related conditions. The hospital receives a fixed sum based on the patient's designation and must provide all necessary care for that fee. Under this type of system, heart surgery patients are "worth more" than those getting hysterectomies, who in turn are "worth more" than those being treated for pneumonia, and so on. This case-mix approach to hospital funding now predominates in the United States, where it is called DRG (diagnosis-related group) reimbursement.

Case-mix funding avoids the perverse incentives inherent in global payment but replaces them with new ones. For example, case-mix funding encourages Alberta hospitals to discharge their patients "sicker and quicker." Because the hospital is paid for each new case, they have an incentive to speed up throughput, off-loading cases and costs to home care, other community services, and families. There is some evidence that case-mix reimbursement in the United States has caused health problems when arrangements for post-discharge care have not been made.[54]

In the late 1980s, a few Ontario hospitals began their own limited experiment with case-mix funding, based on methods developed in New York State. This system rates patients for the severity of their illness and assigns a "resource intensity weighting" factor, or RIW, to adjust funding. However, the system has some specific limitations. For example, the lowest-ranked RIWs are for newborns and postpartum women. True, these patients require relatively little physical care. Still, first-time mothers usually do need significant help learning how to care for their newborns and how to manage breast-feeding. Unfortunately, New York's RIW system did not consider these services part of hospital nursing care.

Ontario hospital managers soon figured out the new rules of the game under RIWs. Lengths of stay for mothers and babies fell off sharply, in some communities by 35 percent or more within a matter of months. Soon, emergency room nurses reported seeing a lot of young parents who didn't know how to look after their new babies. Eventually, a few pilot programs were developed to help these mothers, but many hospital nurses still worry that public health departments and home care programs have not been able to pick up the slack.

There's a lesson here. When it comes to changing economic incentives, it's hard to do just one thing. A push one place creates a pull somewhere else. Monitoring these pushes and pulls and responding appropriately are key challenges for health care managers.

The management muddle

Managing human services is like navigating a swamp without a map. There are few clear objectives. Even those we have are often obscured by loud and competing demands from clients and providers.[55]

The impact of recent health system reforms has been devastating for some health care workers. Roughly 75 to 80 percent of hospital spending goes to labour, much of which is unionized. Health care is a human service—it takes people to care for people. In most parts of the country, unionized health care providers have a limited right to strike. Collective bargaining over wages, working conditions, pensions, and other benefits is handled by a number of different unions. In some cases, the same type of health care worker may be represented by a number of different unions, depending on where he or she works. Even within the same establishment, two identically classified workers might belong to different bargaining units. Also, depending on the province, bargaining may occur locally (within each establishment), regionally, or even provincially.*

Hospitals present one of the most complex environments in the working world. Rigid and multilayered hierarchies have tended to be the norm. Sharing power with workers to help solve problems cooperatively has not. Although there are exceptions, the consequence is a rigid system with little ability to tap the knowledge and experience of front-line workers.

Hospital managers: hang together or hang separately?

"The Prisoner's Dilemma" is a classic story from economics. It

---

* In some provinces certain issues (e.g. wages) are negotiated centrally and others (e.g. working conditions) are negotiated locally.

concerns two robbery suspects being interrogated separately. The police offer each prisoner a better deal if he confesses and agrees to testify against the other. There are three possible outcomes:

- If one prisoner confesses and the other doesn't, then the one who pleads guilty gets a two-year sentence—the other gets ten years.
- If they both plead guilty, the police won't need their testimony and they'll both get six years.
- If neither confesses, each gets four years because the police have a harder time proving their case.

The best choice for the robbers *collectively* is for both to remain silent. That means eight years in total—the best overall scenario. But the best choice for each robber *individually* is to confess and hope that his friend keeps quiet. Of course, if the suspect thinks his friend is likely to confess, he'd better confess too or he could face ten years.

Larger communities with multiple hospitals are trapped in a kind of prisoner's dilemma. Suppose the province offers a new magnetic resonance imaging (MRI) scanner to the community. It's in the community's overall interest for the hospitals to cooperate and plan the most appropriate location for the new MRI. However, each individual hospital has an incentive to fight hard to get the scanner for itself. Seen in this light, the hospitals stand to lose a lot if they cooperate.

This problem is particularly acute in the United States, where each hospital has to have each new gadget or risk losing its competitive advantage. That's why almost every American hospital with more than two hundred beds has an MRI scanner, even though this increases the per-unit cost for diagnostic imaging. It is also why so many hospitals have heart surgery units, even though the staff may perform too few operations to keep their skills sharp.

The prisoner's dilemma helps to explain why voluntary cooperation is so difficult to achieve among health facilities. What's good for the community as a whole almost always risks harming individual facilities. It's no wonder that most hospitals have tended to remain lone wolves—they figure they'll do better in the long run by remaining aloof.

Where's the Plan?

Until recently, there was very little planning for health services. Some provinces did create local planning agencies—District Health Councils, for example—but no one pretended that these had much authority over how resources were allocated or who got to work in the system. Nor have provincial governments had much success with planning; centralized plans are usually too late and too distant from local realities to cut the mustard. Instead, provincial ministries of health zero in on those few items—capital budgets for buildings and equipment, for example—that they can control.

Given that over 80 percent of total health spending is decided by doctors, it is clear that our current pattern of resource allocation is really the sum of individual decisions made by individual doctors about individual patients. Doctors choose who to treat and who to refer. They decide who needs hospital admissions, drugs, tests, and, in many provinces, who needs nursing home care. If health care were a perfect market, we'd expect a perfect pattern of resource allocation, but of course this isn't the case, and our pattern of resource allocation is similarly far from ideal.

Doctors multiply like rabbits

Of course, some aspects of our system are planned. For example, Canadian governments have been planning physician resources for decades.

In the late 1950s and early 1960s, there was concern that Canada wasn't training enough doctors. Justice Hall's Royal Commission on Health Care in 1964 recommended expansion, based on a projection that Canada's population would reach 30 million by 1986. Governments responded by building new medical schools and expanding enrollment in the existing ones. However, Hall's predictions turned out to be wrong. The postwar baby boom ended abruptly in 1966, and by 1986, Canada's population stood at only 25.4 million.

As a consequence, Canada has witnessed a staggering increase in the physician-to-population ratio. Between 1975 and 1989, growth in the supply of doctors ballooned by 51 percent—three times faster than the 16 percent growth in our population over the same time period.[56] These figures don't tell the whole story, however. Reference to the total number of physicians doesn't reveal how many hours they work, or what kinds of patients they see. Overall supply numbers also mask real shortages in certain specialty areas and totally ignore the poor geographic distribution of doctors. All the same, there is no question that unfettered growth in our physician supply presents a serious problem for our health care system.

Despite this, until quite recently planning commissions have repeatedly recommended that Canada train even more doctors. The problem is the method they've traditionally relied on for determining need.

Consider, for example, Ontario's Macdonald Task Force, which reported in 1983.[57] This study, like most others, used a "utilization-based" approach to planning. This method assumes that all the health care currently provided is necessary and appropriate. Then the impact of changing demographics is factored in (older people need more health care) and doctors' practice styles are considered (female doctors, who now make up a larger than ever number of those being trained, tend to work shorter hours). It's hardly surprising that this planning strategy invariably leads to the conclusion that more doctors are required. After all, if the doctors we have now are working flat out to perform necessary services, then it seems logical that we'll need more of them to meet future needs as the population grows and ages.

Of course, the assumptions behind the utilization approach are more than a little faulty. We have already reviewed evidence that substantial amounts of unnecessary care are being provided. What's more, many services currently delivered by doctors could be provided by other, less expensive personnel.

A much better way to plan human resources in health care would be to use a "needs-based" approach. This is really a variant of zero-based budgeting. It doesn't assume that current levels of utilization or current structures for delivering care are optimal. Instead, it begins with an analysis of the population and the kind of care it needs.

The U.S. Graduate Medical Education National Advisory Committee (GMENAC) pioneered this approach. GMENAC began with estimates about the rates for different illnesses likely to be encountered in 1990. It then investigated the most effective ways to diagnose and treat these ailments. Finally, GMENAC calculated how many full-time equivalent doctors were needed to perform these services. Not surprisingly, this method led GMENAC to conclude that the United States had an impending surplus of doctors.

There's an important lesson here for Canada. We could, in fact, organize health care services very differently and get much better efficiency with fewer doctors. For example, according to a growing body of research evidence, better primary care services can substantially reduce the need for specialist doctors and institutional beds and a better use of nursing talent can reduce the need for family doctors.

Dr. Nancy Hall is the director for health promotion at the North Shore Health Unit in British Columbia. She studied the impact of a "wellness" program developed and delivered by public health nurses for elderly persons, who had already signalled their need for help by applying to the province's long-term-care program.[58] In this randomized, controlled trial, participants in the experimental group initially spent up to two hours with a nurse developing a specific list of goals and a plan for action. The nurse then followed up with her clients on an as-needed basis to assess any changes that might require revisions in the plan. After thirty-six months of follow-up, seniors visited by these nurses had one-third the likelihood of entering an institution compared to those who had applied for long-term care but did not have access to this special program.

Several experimental studies in the United States have shown that teaching patients how to manage their own minor illnesses can reduce clinic visits for minor problems by up to 50 percent.[59] Teaching greatly reduces costs and consumption of care for patients with chronic illnesses like asthma and other respiratory conditions.[60] But once again, Canada's health care system provides no incentives to physicians or others to educate patients. Given fee-for-service reimbursement, it would be like asking them to steal from themselves.

Several other studies demonstrate that other, rather minor changes in primary care can produce big pay-offs for the frail elderly and chronically ill.[61] For example, a Veterans' Administration clinic in Vermont found that simply keeping closer track of patients by phone could reduce overall costs by 30 percent.

Their study documented 20 percent fewer clinic visits, 15 percent fewer medications, 30 percent fewer hospital days, and 40 percent fewer days spent in the intensive-care unit among the group receiving telephone contact.[62] The study also documented a 65 percent decrease in deaths among those with the poorest health![63]

These kinds of results fly in the face of criticism that prevention can't produce short-term pay-offs. On the contrary, research increasingly indicates that more comprehensive health care for people with the most serious health problems can achieve major economic and health benefits.

Unfortunately, our system is not currently structured to support innovation. Doctors spend too much time with patients who don't need to see them, like little Stanley, and too little with people who are really sick. Even in a city like Toronto with thousands of family doctors and more than one hundred walk-in clinics, public health nurses find few physicians willing to make home visits to the frail elderly or to take on patients with AIDS, schizophrenia, or other difficult medical problems. The great British general practitioner and primary care theorist Julian Tudor Hart referred to this phenomenon as the "inverse care law": "The availability of good medical care tends to vary inversely with the need for it in the population served."[64]

Cracking down on physician supply

It wasn't until the 1990s that governments in Canada began to get serious about the doctor supply issue and its impact on provincial expenditures. Finally, slashed federal cash transfers and burgeoning debt forced provincial action on a number of fronts.

For example, until very recently doctors had access to a government budget category that had no upper limit. Provincial governments did, and still do, negotiate the overall fee increase with medical associations—in other words, together they agree on the price. But until very recently the volume of services provided was not subject to negotiation. Since overall spending on physician services depends on both price and volume, the overall budget couldn't be predetermined.

Over the years, the volume of services escalated faster than population growth, and even faster than the growth in physician supply. And despite the dramatic growth in the physician supply, fee-for-service reimbursement has meant that there are no unemployed doctors in Canada.*

Gradually, provincial governments have begun to impose more control by negotiating or even imposing ceilings on the total amount available to pay doctors. These are referred to as global caps on physician billings.** In 1992, the provincial and territorial health ministers met in Banff, Alberta, and unveiled a national physicians' strategy known as the Banff Declaration.[65] The ministers agreed to reduce medical school enrolment and postgraduate positions by 10 percent and to establish predictable budgets for doctors' services.***

Setting limits on the size of the resource pie for physician reimbursement created a new receptiveness among doctors to the idea of restricting growth in their numbers and rationalizing their geographic distribution. In fact, by 1993, provincial medical associations were practically leading the charge for change. That winter, the Ontario Medical Association Council gave their negotiators the go-ahead to discuss paying newly registered doctors less than those already established in practice.[66] The negotiators were also told to consider penalties or other restrictions on young doctors who wanted to set up practices in well-doctored areas of the province.

In April 1993, Ontario's government responded to the OMA by proposing measures that would have barred young doctors from practising in most parts of the province. That's when the

---

* By contrast, almost 20 percent of Europe's doctors are out of work, and this proportion is expected to climb in the next few years. ("European doctors struggle on the dole," *Medical Post*, 12 January 1993.)

** An overall ceiling on the budget for all physician services should not be confused with the so-called individual caps or limits on individual doctors' billings that have also been implemented in some provinces, notably Quebec and Ontario.

*** There were other points of agreement including moving away from the fee-for-service method of payment and developing policies to encourage physicians to serve rural areas.

fat really hit the fire! The Professional Association of Interns and Residents of Ontario (PAIRO) went public with their out-rage and frustration and found a sympathetic ear. The OMA quickly retreated, doing their best to make it look as if the whole idea had originated with government. In August 1993, a new doctors' deal was signed that put no restrictions on new doctors as long as they were "made in Ontario" practitioners. Doctors without at least one year of Ontario training, however, were barred from billing the province.

Medical associations and ministries of health from other provinces were apoplectic. Even though most observers viewed Ontario's move as unconstitutional,* other provinces felt they couldn't wait for a court decision. Concerned that they were about to be engulfed with out-of-province doctors, they quickly began constructing their own moats, dictating who could and who couldn't be paid for practising medicine in their jurisdictions.[67]

Professional Education

Early in this century, North American medical education under-went a revolution after the release of a blockbuster report by Abraham Flexner.[68] Flexner was a noted educator and was commissioned by the Carnegie Foundation to review how doc-tors were being trained. His report singled out the many med-ical "diploma mills" of the day for the harshest criticism. Within a few years, two-thirds of North America's medical schools had closed down.**

Surviving schools had to conform to the Johns Hopkins model of medical education—a style patterned on German medical schools of the late nineteenth century. The core of the curriculum was hard science and included anatomy, physiology,

---

* Section 6 of the Canadian Charter of Rights and Freedoms protects mobil-ity rights and appears to expressly prohibit the type of restrictions imposed by the OMA agreement.

** Many of the schools that closed trained women, blacks, or non-traditional practitioners like naturopaths.

and the developing field of biochemistry. Students seldom saw patients in their first two years. Up to one thousand hours or more were spent painstakingly dissecting cadavers. There was no discussion of social issues or communication skills.

Today, the training and educating of health professionals are once again facing increasing criticism. In particular, there's a growing concern that physician education is totally out of step with the real needs of our health care system. Decades' worth of planning documents call for services delivered by multidisciplinary teams.[69] This ideal of team-based practice in a mutually respectful state of interdependence doesn't mesh well with the fact that doctors are trained in virtual isolation from other health professionals.

Reports on primary care talk about "collaborative" practice models and a flattened hierarchy in which doctors and nurses each function to their full potential. But most family practice training programs continue to represent nurses as handmaidens—a completely outdated and much resented role.

Most provincial health care inquiries have called for humanizing the practice of medicine and moving towards a more holistic approach that pays more attention to the psychosocial concerns of patients. And yet, much about medical training tends to desensitize students to patients' real needs.

In fact, a number of studies in Canada and the United States demonstrate an alarming level of abuse and harassment in medical school.[70] In a study at the University of Toronto, 85 percent of female medical students and 64 percent of male students said they had experienced problems with harassment and abuse.[71] A survey from the Department of Psychiatry at the University of Illinois showed that 72 percent of medical students claimed some form of abuse during their four years of training.[72] Over half were yelled at and one-quarter were sworn at by their teachers. In addition, over one-third of women reported unwanted sexual advances from their teachers.

For years medical professors have shown slides of naked women in provocative sexual postures to illustrate their lectures. Could the purpose have been to make female students uncomfortable? In the fall of 1991, a professor at the University of Toronto was merely following this time-tested tradition when he was challenged by a group of outraged students. The students in this group call themselves the Trotula Collective after an eleventh-century female Sicilian doctor. They are determined to counter the sexism they believe is ingrained in the medical school. In response to their pressure, the committee accrediting the university's medical school insisted on action, and the uni versity struck a gender issues committee in 1992. In a survey of its first- and fourth-year students, the university found 46 percent of women and 19 percent of men said they had been subjected to sexual harassment—everything from unwanted advances to sexual intercourse.[73]

Dr. Catherine McKegney, a professor of family practice at the University of Minnesota, equates the process of medical education to living within a dysfunctional family.[74] According to Dr. A.M. Hayton of St. Albans, England, "The inevitable consequence of putting doctors through several years of hardship is that they are forced to adopt long-term coping mechanisms usually reserved for [sufferers of] post-traumatic stress syndrome."[75]

In some ways, the techniques of modern medical education resemble the kind of initiation rites used by cults to captivate their followers. Hazing rituals are still quite common, particularly during clinical training, which usually begins in the final year of medical school and continues throughout postgraduate education. Although generally informal, these hazing practices are key "brainwashing" techniques used to socialize young students into the medical profession. It's almost as if medical students were training for the Marines. Military brainwashing starts by separating the person from everything that's familiar. The victims have to remove their clothes. They can't see their family or friends. They are persistently deprived of sleep. Come to think of it, this is pretty close to the life of a senior medical student or intern. Chronically tired, typical student doctors have little time for normal social interaction with family and friends. They practically live at the hospital, where everyone wears a uniform.

A better way?

In 1967, McMaster University in Hamilton, Ontario, opened its new medical school. Under the leadership of Dr. John Evans, its first dean, the school's mission was to produce doctors in a new way. They began by changing the criteria for selecting students—half were accepted for reasons other than their science marks. The school also adopted new methods for teaching based on adult learning theory, which employs small, self-directed groups to help each student master the material.

Although these changes represent a significant departure from business as usual, McMaster remains fairly traditional in a number of other ways. There's almost no opportunity for multi-disciplinary education, and students mainly see nurses functioning in quite traditional roles. However, research does indicate that McMaster's medical grads are different in some important ways and are, for example, more likely to keep up to date with recent medical advances than their counterparts from the University of Toronto.[76]

This kind of success enhanced the reputation of McMaster. By the 1980s, faculty members were busy teaching their tricks to Harvard's medical school. But they weren't having much of an influence on the rest of Canada. At first, only the schools at the University of Calgary, Sherbrooke, and Memorial University adopted the small-group learning approach. However, now other medical schools are slowly moving in McMaster's direction. Even the stodgy University of Toronto is using some of "Mac's" tactics to revamp its medical curriculum.

Planning for other health professionals

In the late 1980s, Ontario's Premier David Peterson and Health Minister Elinor Caplan were taking serious heat for letting heart patients die on waiting lists. At the time the delays were blamed on a nursing shortage, although subsequent investigation showed more serious management problems were really responsible.

During the boom years of the 1980s, a good nurse could make a lot more selling real estate or setting up a fitness centre than working in a hospital. In 1989, over one thousand openings for nurses in Metropolitan Toronto were unfilled. Hospitals all over the country were reporting similar difficulties recruiting and retaining nursing staff.

Provincial governments struck task forces to study the issue. Ironically, by the time most had finished their reports, the problem had evaporated. A serious economic downturn led to the closure of thousands of hospital beds and the layoff of nurses across the country. In fact, by 1993, employment prospects for nurses were very grim. Thousands of nurses were collecting unemployment insurance in Ontario alone. Entire classes of graduating nurses were looking outside the country for employment.

Nursing wages did increase dramatically in the early 1990s, but these improvements appear to have only accelerated the layoff rates. Instead of relying on more costly RNs, employers began looking at alternatives—substituting registered practical nurses and even health care aides.

In 1994, the situation for new nursing graduates is grave indeed. Less than 10 percent can expect to find full-time work in Canada. Government has adopted its usual position of ignoring the problems of nurses: we've seen little evidence of the shift promised to community care, and few new nursing jobs have been created. And, for all the press stories eliciting sympathy for the *potential* problems of young doctors, there's been little media attention about the *actual* disappearance of job opportunities for young nurses. Some nursing educators are speaking out, however. For example, Dr. Dorothy Pringle, from the University of Toronto's School of Nursing, recently called for reduced enrollment in nursing schools as the only sensible policy.

Other health care workers are caught in an economic squeeze play. For example, depending on the hospital, registered practical nurses are either benefitting from tough economic times with an expanded role and heaps more respect or finding themselves out on the street, victims of turf protection waged by RNs. "All kinds of lame excuses are given for restricting what RPNs can do,"* says Verna Steffler, executive director of the Registered Practical Nurses Association of Ontario, "but the bottom line is that nurse managers are invariably RNs and they naturally tend to protect their own."

In the 1980s, a perceived shortage of occupational therapists and physiotherapists led to expansion in their training programs. However, once hospitals had to produce balanced budgets or else, they found it easiest to begin eliminating positions that weren't yet filled; PT and OT job openings started to disappear.

---

* RPNs are also known as licensed practical nurses (LPNs), registered nursing assistants (RNAs), or certified nursing assistants (CNAs) in other provinces.

Right now, it's very difficult for these "scarce" therapists to find work in Canada.

Planning for Institutions: A Built Bed is a Filled Bed

Is our planning for institutional facilities any better? In short, the answer is no. Until recently, the method for planning new hospitals or long-term-care facilities was utilization-based—the same flawed process used for planning physician resources.

In the late 1950s, Dr. Milton Roemer taught at Cornell University in Ithica, New York. He coined the rule that bears his name—"a built bed is a filled bed"—to describe a universal phenomenon in health care.[77] Canada—where hospital utilization is even higher than in the United States and where lengths of stay continue to be longer than necessary for many conditions—provides a strong illustration of this rule. Institutional occupancy levels here continue to run at 85 to 90 percent.

As we built up our system, Canada made some key decisions that locked in patterns of high institutional use. For example, we insured hospital care before out-patient medical care—a fact that created an over-reliance on in-patient services from the very beginning. Most provinces provided at least some coverage for nursing homes before funding home care programs.* As a result, our institutional over-capacity helped create a mind-set among providers, patients, and family members alike that the best care was in-patient care.

These excess beds should be treated as money in the bank to fund a new system. That is, we could withdraw funding from institutions and reallocate it to develop more community and home care. But we may be missing the boat. Many beds have already closed, but few of the resources saved have been reinvested in community care.

---

* Long-term care institutions are called by many different names, including nursing homes, homes for the aged, intermediate care, and extended care facilities.

The Answer: Planning by Need

The present mix of health care personnel, services, and facilities is clearly out of line with what communities really need. Our system provides public payment for useless or dangerous services, and yet needed services are often unavailable. In other words, you can get what we have on offer, but if you need something else, forget it.

For example, in 1993, a long-term, multicentred, randomized controlled trial to test new techniques for managing insulin-dependent diabetes found that very strict control of blood sugar—involving a comprehensive package of diet, exercise, counselling, frequent blood-test monitoring, and, when indicated, more frequent insulin injections—could reduce serious complications like kidney failure, stroke, heart attack, and blindness by 50 percent.[78]

Sari Simkins, a dietician participating in the research, worries about how the health care system will respond to this new information. "We're not sure yet that all family physicians in Ontario are even aware of these results," she said. "Besides, the study suggests a need for expert dietary counselling and patient support—doctors currently don't have the training or the time to provide this. Nor are there enough dieticians in our system to do it." But of course, the issue goes well beyond human resource concerns. Patients opting to try this regimen will also need much more equipment than conventional management of diabetes requires, including monitors, more insulin, more needles, and a much larger supply of test strips to check blood sugar. The system hasn't even begun to plan how to respond adequately to the results of this study.

But imagine what would happen if we built a system that dramatically expanded the chances for patients to become informed and make real choices based on their preferences? Then we could really do some definitive health care planning.

In fact, if we let the informed choices of patients and families drive the planning process, then we could simply construct a system based on the sum of their individual choices.

If fewer patients opted for prostate surgery and other elective procedures, then we could naturally get by with fewer hospital beds and surgeons. If more patients had the option of dying at home with home care support and palliative services, then fewer institutional beds would be necessary. If more patients were taught how to manage their own minor illnesses and could get advice from a nurse over the phone, then we'd need fewer family doctors, walk-in clinics, and emergency rooms. And if patients with serious chronic illnesses were taught how to monitor their conditions and had access to primary care nurses or other health professionals, then we'd need even fewer hospital beds and medical specialists. The system's priorities would change overnight. In fact, if patients were really in the driver's seat, we'd be much more confident that our health spending was worth its cost to society.

This new system would almost undoubtedly have fewer doctors, although we would need to change their specialty mix and geographic distribution. The system's backbone, however, would be comprehensive primary care* based on a few simple principles:

- a focus on whole-population primary care;
- collaborative practice between family doctors and primary care nurses, and in some cases, social workers;
- integration with secondary and some tertiary health care services and community health and social services;
- mainly non-fee-for-service payment; and
- meaningful involvement in governance by patients and communities.

The relationship among primary, acute, and long-term care would be continuous. The entire spectrum of services would be seamless, with no gaps in care as patients move back and forth between their homes, community care settings, and institutions.

An informed community plans its health care

But how would communities create new structures to deliver the kind of care desired by informed consumers? Well, first they'd need the authority to actually restructure the delivery system, and then they'd need to control the resources.

The way health services are organized now didn't come about because of a plan. What we find today has largely been

---

* More detail on this will follow in Chapters 9 and 10.

determined by history and the power of vested interests. The system's evolution over the past hundred years is comparable to a one-room shack transformed by successive additions into a twenty-room mansion—now we have to walk up a few flights of stairs and then down a few just to get from the kitchen to the dining room.

To develop a more rational delivery system, we need to pool all existing health care resources going into a community. Only then can we fund services according to the need for care—as determined by patients' informed choices—and the best scientific evidence concerning what works best.

Professors Stephen Birch and John Eyles and their colleagues at McMaster University have been developing a formula for funding health care according to needs.[79] The McMaster group is using the standardized mortality ratio (SMR) for people aged zero to sixty-four (the SMR is the death rate in a particular community compared to the provincial average) to adjust per-capita funding for the community. Scotland uses this method to allocate hospital funds in its system.[80] Manitoba researcher Professor Noralou Roos and her colleagues have recently suggested further refinements to recognize social and economic risks in per-capita payments.[81]

Given these resources, primary care facilities could then allocate funding to support both existing and new providers of care. In general, the dollars would follow the individual patient, based on his or her informed choices.

Explaining the basic economic principles affecting health care financing and delivery leads to conclusions that seem counterintuitive: public health insurance is more efficient than private insurance; the knowledge gap between caregivers and patients almost eliminates price as an effective signal in the market. It's easy to see how anyone—including politicians—could go wrong.

To make it simpler, just remember—if anyone tells you health care is just like any other commodity, ask them if they'd like to buy the Peace Bridge. Anyone who'd believe that free market economics is a sound basis for health policy would probably fall for the offer.

Chapter 7

Lies about Canada, Myths about America

ON TUESDAY, FEBRUARY 20, 1990, Vancouver General Hospital's cardiac unit was even more hectic than usual. A crew from the U.S. Public Broadcasting System was busy filming Dr. Victor Huckell as he performed the ultimate diagnostic work-up for heart problems: cardiac catheterization. Almost all of the patients seen that day were men with coronary heart disease, the most common cause of death in Canada, the United States, and most other developed countries.

The film crew was shooting scenes for *Borderline Medicine,* a documentary comparing similar patients in the Canadian and U.S. health care systems. Mr. Albert Mueller was one of the patients filmed in that day's sequence.

Roger Weisberg, the show's producer, is well known for his liberal views concerning America's social problems, and *Borderline Medicine* was right up his alley. "The documentary tries to debunk some of the myths that are emerging about the Canadian system in the United States. On balance, the Canadian system comes off looking extremely attractive and puts our system to shame," Mr. Weisberg told Paul Taylor, medical reporter for the *Globe and Mail.*[1]

The show featured a number of stories illustrating how much harder it is to get access to care in the United States. It showed that many pregnant women arrive at the hospital in labour without having had any prenatal care at all, and how an upper-middle-class American woman with breast cancer found herself dying in penury, impoverished by health care bills after her insurance company cut off her benefits.

Still, most of the key Americans debating health care reform in the United States aren't candidates for either pregnancy or breast cancer. The majority of these decision-makers—like the president and most members of Congress—are white, middle-aged men. What they worry about is heart disease and whether they'll be able to get surgery right away if their doctor says they need it. If these people were going to identify with *anybody* in the documentary, it would almost certainly be with Mr. Albert Mueller, the heart patient.

The documentary informed viewers that, a few months prior to his catheterization, Mr. Mueller had developed angina—chest pain caused by blockages in his coronary arteries. That day's test confirmed that he was in big trouble: both major coronary arteries were completely obstructed. His heart was already showing signs of damage as a result.[2] Dr. Huckell told his patient that his condition was very serious and that he needed surgery urgently.

Towards the end of the program, Walter Cronkite—the show's narrator and arguably the most trusted man in America—announced ominously: "Five months later, Albert Mueller is still waiting for surgery, despite the fact that 25 percent of patients with left main coronary artery disease die within a year."[3] Americans who might have been interested in knowing more about the Canadian system were now forced to think: "Well, that's that. Canada may have a system for everyone at a fraction of what it costs us, but I guess they have to compromise quality to pull it off. We'll just have to look elsewhere for solutions."

The only problem with this story is that it wasn't true. Mr. Mueller didn't have to wait five months for his surgery. He could have had the operation almost right away. He just didn't want it.

A year after the program was filmed, Dr. Huckell told us that he knew Mr. Mueller's heart problem was urgent. He wanted to get him to a surgeon immediately.[4] But Mr. Mueller wasn't interested. The patient simply refused to have surgery or even see a surgeon to discuss it. As the months passed, Dr. Huckell advised his patient several times that he needed the surgery, but Mr. Mueller remained adamant.

About four months after his catheterization, the Vancouver General Hospital also contacted the patient twice and offered him the surgery. Mr. Mueller refused both times. As far as he was concerned, the drugs he was taking for his angina were working. He was feeling better. So much better, in fact, that he spent the spring and summer of 1990 driving around the western United States and Canada, visiting relatives. But Mr. Mueller's heart problems did grow worse and his condition deteriorated. He had surgery in February 1992.

How did an excellent crew of American journalists end up slandering Canada's health care system? In their defence, they did talk to officials at the British Columbia Ministry of Health and the province's Royal Commission on Health Care and Costs. So how did they end up getting the facts of Mr. Mueller's story wrong?

The answers to these questions go a long way towards explaining why the United States, more than any other country in the industrialized world, relies on private funding for health care. In this chapter we'll look at the relative performance of our two health care systems. We'll try to explain the policy gridlock south of the border and demonstrate why reforming the American system is so important to preserving our own.

Canada versus the United States: Who Has the Better Health Care System?

When the Toronto Blue Jays competed with the Atlanta Braves for the 1992 World Series, American attention was riveted northward. Journalists covering the games singled out many things to praise about Toronto, "the cleanest city in North America." And when hundreds of thousands of Torontonians took to the streets until dawn to celebrate the Blue Jays' victory, American sportscasters marvelled that the crowd's exuberance never once erupted into violence.

Though Canadians are very conscious of the differences between our two countries, these are greatly outweighed by the similarities. In fact, Canadians and Americans are more alike than any other two peoples in the world. Visitors from the United States usually feel right at home here—able to speak the same language, eat the same food, drive the same cars, even catch their favourite television shows. And if, for example, during the 1992 World Series, Ted Turner, owner of the Atlanta Braves, or his wife, Jane Fonda, had needed health care while they were in Toronto, neither would have found much difference in the quality of service. Toronto's downtown hospitals rate with the world's best—they have the latest in equipment and highly trained and talented doctors and nurses.

In spite of these similarities, in the past thirty years our two countries have taken a very different approach towards social programs, and in particular how we each finance health care. In Canada, health care has become one of the important ways in which we distinguish ourselves from our southern neighbours. Indeed, fears that the Canada–U.S. Free Trade Agreement might somehow jeopardize Canada's health care system threatened to erupt into a major election issue during the 1988 federal campaign, with Opposition leader John Turner and NDP leader Ed Broadbent fanning the flames of debate. It took Justice Emmett Hall—considered the Father of Medicare—to provide reassurance that nothing in the FTA immediately imperilled the system.[5]

By contrast, in the 1993 federal election campaign, Justice Hall warned that the Reform Party's platform endangered Medicare.[6] Both Preston Manning and then prime minister Kim Campbell were at pains to reassure the voters that their parties were "pro-Medicare." They knew what the polls said: Canadians love their health care system.

In the competition for the world's best health system, Canada and the United States are only two of many contenders.

It's been said that a health care system can be fast, cheap, or good—and that a given system can display any two of these characteristics, *but only two*. For example, the British system is very cheap by international standards and has pretty good quality. But it's also very slow. The American system is very fast and has excellent quality—that is if you define quality as having the highest of high-tech and ignore the access problem of having 35 million people without health insurance. But the U.S. system is also the world's most expensive.

How does Canada's system stack up? How well do we compare with the United States? Let's look at the issue in terms of cost, access, and quality.

Comparative Costs

No matter what measure you choose, America's system for delivering health care is the world's most expensive. There are many

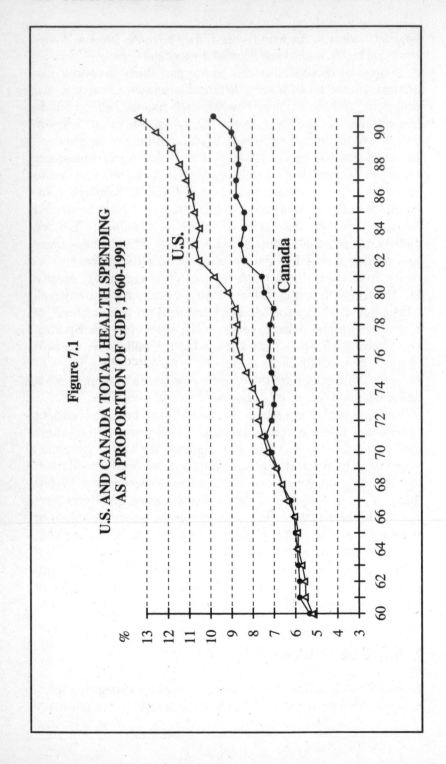

Figure 7.1

U.S. AND CANADA TOTAL HEALTH SPENDING
AS A PROPORTION OF GDP, 1960-1991

ways to approach international cost comparisons,[7] but the best is to look at what share of a nation's income (as measured by the Gross Domestic Product, or GDP) is spent on health care. This method lets you compare costs at a given point in time but also shows how well each country controls costs over the long term.[8] Because it looks at total health spending, regardless of the method of financing, the comparison is valid.

It is important, however, to remember that this statistic is a ratio involving two separate measures, both of which change over time. An ever-increasing share of GDP going to health care might mean rising health care costs, poor GDP growth, or both.

As you can see from Figure 7.1, Canada and the United States were both spending about the same share of their respective national incomes during the 1960s. In both countries, health care costs were rising steeply throughout the decade. But the cost trends began to diverge significantly after 1971. By then Canada had fully implemented national health insurance, but the United States continued with its mainly private system.

The divergence sharpened over the next twenty years. Health care costs as a share of national income stabilized in Canada but not in the United States, where the pattern set in the 1960s continued unabated into the 1990s. Health spending slowed significantly in Canada during the 1980s. The sharp increases in health expenditures as a share of GDP at the beginning of the 1980s and again into the 1990s were almost entirely due to falling GDP during the recessions that bracketed the decade. By 1991, Canada was spending 9.9 percent of its GDP on health care while the United States spent 13.3 percent.[9] (A study commissioned by the American health insurance industry tried to claim the opposite—that costs rose faster in Canada than in the United States[10]—but it has been soundly refuted by Canadian analysts.[11])

Three factors account for most of the difference between American and Canadian health care costs:

- Canada has much lower costs for administration; in 1985, the United States spent 0.59 percent of GNP* versus 0.11 in Canada on administrative overhead.

---

* GNP is the same as GDP except it includes profits of national corporations that are repatriated.

- Canada spent less on hospital services—3.48 of GNP versus 4.18 in the United States.
- Canada spent less on physician services—1.35 percent of GNP versus 2.07 in the United States.[12]

Administration: paper trail travails

Each province in Canada operates a single, large health insurance plan, and this federal-provincial single-payer system is the main reason our administrative costs are so well controlled.[13]

By contrast, there are more than 1,500 "payers" in the United States, which means 1,500 sets of actuaries, 1,500 computer systems, and 1,500 sets of high-paid executives. The cost and complexity are further compounded by the fact that each company offers a multiplicity of plans. Plans differ in terms of premiums, coverage, and in the cost-sharing arrangements with patients. America's system is drowning in paperwork, as President Clinton declared in his speech to Congress introducing his new health care reform package.

Hospital hoopla

When it comes to hospital services, Canada spends less, even though wages for Canadian hospital workers are, if anything, higher than in the United States.[14] And we find that Canadians actually use more hospital days per capita than Americans.

- In 1989, Americans used 814 hospital days per 1,000[15] while the comparable figure was 1,164 days per 1,000 in Ontario.[16]
- In 1987, the rate of major surgery* for residents of Ontario was 35 percent higher than in California and 15 percent higher than in New York State.[17]

What accounts for the cost difference is the fact that U.S. hospitals provide more services to their patients than Canadian hospitals. However, this higher level of service intensity doesn't

---

* Defined as a procedure that was not performed on a not-for-admission basis in 1987.

appear to produce better results. For example, a recent study of heart attack patients in the United States and Canada showed that Americans were twice as likely to have heart x-rays (coronary angiography) or surgery, but found no differences between the two countries in the patients' survival rates [18]

Physician costs: yearning for earnings

Canada spends less on physician services, even though Canada and the United States have almost the same number of doctors per capita.[19] Costs for physician services here are lower partly because fees (and salaries) are lower and partly because a much smaller proportion of Canadian doctors are specialists.

While it's generally true that U.S. doctors earn more than their Canadian counterparts, the overall figures hide some important details.

For example, the U.S. General Accounting Office (a nonpartisan agency that reports to the U.S. Congress) found that the average gross income of self-employed U.S. physicians was $256,000, nearly double the $129,000 earned by Canadian physicians in 1987.[20] But because Canadian doctors spent much less on overhead ($46,000 versus $124,000), their net incomes wound up being only about 35 percent lower.

There are two main reasons why overhead expenses for American doctors are so much higher: malpractice insurance costs more, and the process for billing and collecting fees is much more complex.

Consider Dr. Rupert P., a family doctor in Chicago. He has a busy family practice looking after about 1,200 patients, who are covered by several dozen different insurance companies. Each company has its own reporting requirements, for both the physician and the patient. Just to keep all the office paperwork straight, Dr. P. has to employ two full-time people to process his billings and track his receivables.

By contrast, Dr. M. practises as an family doctor in London, Ontario. He also sees about 1,200 patients in his practice, but billing and collecting fees for Dr. M. is much more straightforward. Once a month, Dr. M. submits a computer disk outlining all the services he has provided; 98 percent of his payments usually come within four weeks. He has never needed to hire special people to handle billings; the clerk who works in his office easily handles the task, which takes about four hours of her time a month.

Much of the remaining difference in average net incomes for physicians relates to the mix of specialist and generalist doctors in each country. Over half of Canada's doctors are family physicians, but only 13 percent of American doctors are in this category. One study found that the net incomes of U.S. family doctors were only slightly greater than those of Ontario family doctors.[21] Ontario pediatricians and internists actually had slightly higher net incomes than their American counterparts. American surgeons enjoyed the biggest difference in earning capacity, netting much higher remuneration than Canadian surgeons.

In fact, the sky's the limit for the earning potential of popular U.S. surgeons, which is one reason why some of Canada's star surgeons are wooed south of the border. Almost all the reports about Canadian doctors moving south concern sub-specialist surgeons. But most choose not to leave: Dr. Tirone David of Toronto and Dr. Wilbert Keon of Ottawa, both world-renowned cardiac surgeons, recently turned down offers of $1.2 million and $2 million respectively to move south.[22]

Eligibility and Access to Care

All Canadians are eligible for health insurance as a right of citizenship. Landed immigrants, established refugees, and foreigners claiming refugee status are also covered. By contrast, in the United States, at least 35 million Americans have no insurance whatsoever.[23] In fact, during a three-year period, over 60 million Americans—one-quarter of the entire population—lacked health insurance for at least one month.[24]

Even with health insurance, some Americans may still have trouble getting the care they need. At least 20 million and perhaps as many as 50 million Americans are inadequately insured. They may lack coverage for certain illnesses like AIDS, heart disease, or cancer. Also, some insurance policies have a lifetime limit on benefits that might be lower than the cost of treating serious illness.[25]

For example, Bob L. is a fifty-two-year-old professor at a southern state university. He has high blood pressure. His wife

Carolyn, forty-three years old, is the manager of the university bookstore. How could Bob and Carolyn have health insurance problems? Last October, the family doctor who had been treating them for ten years decided to stop dealing with Bob and Carolyn's insurance company. Because the university, like other employers, offered a variety of plans, Bob and Carolyn were able to switch to a plan their doctor would accept. But the new insurer would not cover Bob for any diseases related to his high blood pressure for one year. In private insurance lingo this limitation is for "a pre-existing condition" and it is routinely used to deny coverage to people with a higher risk of falling ill. In Bob's case, stroke and heart attack are the most likely complications of his hypertension. If Bob has either this year, the family's savings will be wiped out and Bob will never again qualify for private insurance.

Even without a "pre-existing" condition, many people still face high costs for insurance. For example, Randy and Denise Sadler of Kernersville, North Carolina, spend almost $3,000 a year on health insurance and have to cough up an extra $200 each month in copayments for care. For Tom and Deb Winslow of Lincolnville, Maine, health insurance and out-of-pocket costs eat up 20 percent of their income. Even so, they're only covered for $84 a day in hospital care, while their local hospital charges $500 a day![26]

When Vancouver real estate investor Stephen Sander announced in 1990 that he had established an international charity to aid the sick and the homeless, he never expected to hear from people in the world's wealthiest country, but almost every letter came from Americans facing life-threatening medical problems with little or no insurance coverage.[27]

In his state of the union address in January 1992, President George Bush claimed (incorrectly) that people couldn't choose their own doctors in countries with national health insurance. He was quite wrong, of course. Canadians, for example, are free to see any doctor they like; what we cannot do is choose our insurance company. It's rather ironic that in the United States, people have some choice of insurer but less and less freedom to see the doctor of their choice.

President Clinton's reforms may address some of these problems by guaranteeing universal health coverage and by regulating against limits to coverage for people with pre-existing conditions. But his health reform package still links "choice" with ability to pay. And the choice being offered is still a choice among insurers and plans rather than among doctors and hospitals.

Access and use of non-high-technology services

Canadians have much better access to primary health care than Americans and, in fact, use more. For example, in 1987, Canadians used 50 percent more physicians' services than Americans.[28]

There are two reasons for this. The first has to do with the availability of providers. As already mentioned, more than half of Canadian physicians are family practitioners; only one-eighth of American doctors are. A second factor is that preventive care, including vaccinations and Pap smears, is available without charge in Canada. Most U.S. insurance plans don't cover these types of services.

Lack of coverage for immunizations in the United States has had a dramatic impact on the health of Americans. During the late 1980s, as U.S. vaccination rates fell, the country experienced a resurgence of vaccine-preventable diseases, including measles and whooping cough.[29] By 1991, the United States, along with Haiti and Bolivia, had one of the lowest rates of immunization for children under two years of age in the western hemisphere.[30]

Treatable infectious diseases like syphilis and tuberculosis have also been on the rise in the United States,[31] and the problem is made worse by lack of access to health care for those who need it most—the poor and the destitute. A study done at a Harlem hospital in New York City showed that 90 percent of new tuberculosis patients got "lost" in the system before completing their treatment. Dr. Allyn Nakashima of the prestigious U.S. Centers for Disease Control deplores the result: "This is like going back to the pre-penicillin years."[32]

Access and use of high-technology specialized services

Let's begin by admitting that Canada offers less high-technology service than the United States. In Canada, hospitals are not free to develop services such as open-heart surgery and transplantation, or to purchase expensive equipment such as magnetic resonance imaging (MRI) scanners, without specific prior approvals from provincial governments. Provinces have strict control over these kinds of major capital investments, which also have high long-term operating costs associated with them. This has meant that high technology has diffused more slowly in Canada than in the United States, and access to it is more limited.

However, provincial governments don't have nearly as much influence over spending on medical care and pharmaceuticals. No provincial approval is necessary for a doctor to open an office or prescribe most drugs. Perhaps the provinces' tight grip on high-tech is simply a matter of controlling where they can. The danger here lies in being "penny wise, pound foolish." For example, the Ontario government pays doctors over $200 million a year to treat people with colds but the province has fewer MRI scanners per capita than even Britain's much maligned National Health Service. Questions of need don't seem to have carried much weight—the government's refusal to purchase additional MRIs appears to have been based mainly on financial grounds.

Dr. Robert Kane, the chairman of the School of Public Health at the University of Minnesota, claims that Americans suffer from "galloping health care technophilia"—an almost fetishistic worship of medical high-tech. Various surveys show that American doctors are also much more likely than their colleagues in other countries to believe that a particular diagnostic or therapeutic technology is appropriate.[33] Perhaps for that reason, media stories suggesting that Canadians have trouble getting high-technology care—like the story of heart patient Albert Mueller—strike a responsive chord among American audiences. More than anything else, Americans see this limitation as the Achilles' heel of Canadian health care.

In a war, truth is the first casualty. The debate over health care reform in the United States has been like a war, with various combatants battling over the trillion-dollar prize that is the U.S. health care system. Opponents of publicly funded insurance have used every opportunity to discredit Canada's system by presenting a host of misleading information about the lack of high-technology in Canada.

For example, the American Medical Association and the insurance industry have taken great trouble to point out that the United States has eight times as many open-heart surgery units as we do. They imply that Canada doesn't have enough capacity to perform heart surgery, never even hinting that maybe Americans have more than they need.

It is seldom mentioned, for example, that heart surgery in the United States is very profitable—a major reason why so many centres are in operation. When new heart units open, it's rarely because the other heart units in the community are overloaded. Peoria, Illinois, for example, has four heart units for a total referral population of about 500,000; Hamilton, Ontario, has only one unit serving a total population of about 1.25 million.

In Canada, almost all heart surgery is done in university hospitals. This concentration of service within a smaller number of centres keeps the skill level of our surgical teams high, which provides an added measure of safety for Canadian heart patients. Studies in the United States have shown that surgical death rates are much higher in hospitals with low volumes.[34]

And even though the United States does more heart surgery than we do, the right people may not be getting the operations. Studies have shown that Americans who are poor or poorly insured are much less likely to get bypass surgery or other heart procedures, even though they have higher rates of heart disease.[35] By contrast, rates of bypass surgery in Canada are actually higher among people coming from low-income communities, where one would expect to find the greatest need.[36]

More than any other single example, the opponents of public health insurance in the United States have used heart surgery to play on the public's fears. In particular, they have taken advantage of widespread misperceptions about the urgency for bypass operations.

Many people are under the impression that once heart surgery is recommended, it must be performed right away or the patient is at great risk of dying. In fact, this is only true for a minority of patients—typically only 15 to 20 percent of the patients seen in any one centre.[37] Only high-risk patients—those with blockage of their left main coronary artery or blockage of the three major arteries, with very unstable angina—have more than one chance in three hundred of dying for each month they remain on a waiting list.[38] Having the operation itself is ten times riskier.[39] But even though the majority of heart surgery patients are not at risk of losing their lives while waiting, they may suffer physically, psychologically, and economically, and these concerns are certainly not trivial.[40]

Sometimes, Canadian doctors and hospitals engage in what McMaster University professor Jonathan Lomas calls "orchestrated outrage."[41] That is, they embellish or concoct circumstances to create the impression that someone has suffered because of shortages of staff or equipment. In Ontario, in 1988 and 1989, media stories about patients dying while waiting for heart surgery began to appear as doctors and hospitals upped the pressure on government.[42]

Dr. Charles Wright, the vice-president for medicine at the Vancouver General Hospital, says heart surgeons often like to give the impression that waiting lists are more severe than they really are, because they want more facilities for what they do.[43] Dr. David Naylor, the director of the Institute of Clinical Evaluative Sciences at Sunnybrook Hospital in Toronto, agrees that some surgeons play to the media. He says some doctors prefer to keep long waiting lists instead of referring patients to other surgeons with shorter lists, "on the grounds that the queues illustrate the inadequacy of government resources for cardiac surgery."[44]

At any rate, at the end of the 1980s, heart surgery in Ontario became a political hot potato. In response, the Ministry of Health launched an investigation, appointing a panel of cardiologists, cardiac surgeons, and epidemiologists to study the issue and recommend solutions. What they found were several serious management problems.

For example, it was found that at the height of the perceived crisis in 1989, the Toronto General Hospital's department of surgery took 1.5 days of operating-room time away from cardiac surgery and gave it to general surgery. Had this not occurred, almost 10 percent more open-heart procedures could have been done in Metropolitan Toronto.[45] Was this a management mistake or an example of "orchestrated outrage"?

It also turned out that although some hospitals had long waiting lists, others didn't. The investigation showed that some surgeons with long lists didn't use a formal system for assigning priority to patients. Other surgeons, sometimes even in the same hospital, had lots of openings. The expert panel recommended a number of specific changes in the management of heart patients and called for a modest increase in resources. Their recommendations were implemented.

By 1990, a new triage system and a registry were in place to priorize patients and re-route them to other surgeons or hospitals if necessary.[46] The Ontario government also added 10 percent to the resource base for cardiac surgery. Together, these measures went a long way towards solving the problem of waiting lists.

On August 11, 1992, Canadian media mogul Ted Rogers had bypass surgery at the Mayo Clinic. His doctor in the Bahamas made the diagnosis and recommended he have his operation in the United States. But there was no need by then for anyone from Ontario to go south for heart surgery. According to Dr. Tirone David, chief of cardiac surgery at the Toronto Hospital, waiting times were down to two weeks at the most.[47]

Access to high-technology: the plight of the uninsured

The U.S. system is plagued by a persistent paradox—the more you need care, the harder it is to get.

Dr. Beverley Morgan is a doctor at the University of California Medical Center at Irvine in Orange County, south of Los Angeles. Orange County is one of the wealthiest communities in the United States. Dr. Morgan had heard that a large increase in the number of free-standing MRI scanners—most co-owned by doctors and located in private clinics—was dramatically improving access to this service in Orange County. By October 1992, the country had forty-one MRI scanners to serve 2.4 million residents.

Dr. Morgan called each of the seventeen free-standing MRI facilities three times over a three-month period. During the first call, she pretended to be a well-insured person with a minor orthopedic problem. She was offered an immediate scan.

The second time, Dr. Morgan said she was a Medi-Cal patient (Medi-Cal is the state's public insurance plan for the poor) and said her doctor thought she might have a brain tumour. This time eleven centres refused to see her, and the other six would only see her in two to three weeks after her physician completed a complicated form.

On the third call, she pretended to be a patient with no insurance and a possible brain tumour. This time, none of the seventeen centres would see her without a minimum down-payment of $500 and proof she could pay the balance of the $1,000 fee.[48]

As of October 1992, the United States had over two thousand MRI scanners; Canada had only twenty-two.[49] Dr. Morgan's little experiment shows, however, that even if MRI scanners were as numerous as McDonald's outlets, those with no or inadequate insurance—one person in four in the United States—would still face big obstacles to getting a scan when they needed one. And because there are so many scanners in the United States operating below peak capacity, the price per unit of service goes up, leading to even higher prices and more compromises to access.

Quality of Care—Quality of Proof

Doctors with practice experience in both countries maintain that the general patterns of treatment and quality of care are quite similar in both settings. In 1991, Dr. Michael Johnston moved from Denver, Colorado, to head up the division of thoracic surgery at Toronto's Mount Sinai Hospital. He says Mount Sinai is a "premier location" for doing the work he wants to do—lung cancer surgery. "When it comes to academic surgery, Canada and the United States are very much one."

- The development of medical education followed a similar pattern in both nations. Advice from American Abraham Flexner, who conducted a major review of all North American medical schools during the first decade of this century, was implemented in both Canada and the United States, with the result that today, medical education in both countries is very similar.
- Hospitals in both countries were accredited by the same organization until the 1950s.
- Credentials for doctors and nurses are accepted across the border. *

But there's still a lot of confusion about whether Canada compromises quality to achieve its lower costs. George Bush contributed

---

* About half the state licensing agencies accept Canadian medical credentials directly. The other half ask Canadian doctors to write an examination.

to the controversy by claiming that "post-operative mortality is 44 percent higher in Canada than the United States for high-risk procedures."[50] But the former president got it wrong. The evidence he was citing actually showed that most surgical outcomes were better in Manitoba than in New England.[51]

In fact, the researchers looked at short-term and long-term mortality from ten surgical procedures that were grouped into low-risk, moderate-risk, and high-risk operations. In almost all cases the Manitoba patients fared better. The major exception was in short-term mortality for the two high-risk conditions: hip fracture repair, and heart valve replacement concurrent with coronary artery bypass surgery.

With respect to Canada's higher short-term mortality rates, one of the study's authors, University of Manitoba professor Leslie Roos, says that the finding is mainly unexplained, especially since the figures for longer-term mortality—deaths occurring one year after hip fracture repair—were virtually identical in both countries. We note that these data are also consistent with Manitoba doctors tending to be less aggressive than their American colleagues in treating patients who are likely to die soon.

Other studies suggest that the quality of outcomes in the two countries are very similar. For example, as mentioned earlier, Canadian and American heart attack patients had similar short-term and longer-term survival, even though American patients were twice as likely to have heart x-rays or surgery and Canadian patients were slightly more likely to have activity-limiting angina at the end of the study.[52]

Health status and quality of care

As a general rule, living conditions have much more impact than health care on outcomes like life expectancy and infant mortality. Nevertheless, if Canada's health care system were really as bad as some American critics have suggested, it should show up in these conventional measures. But it doesn't. Canadians live longer than Americans. Our newborns are less likely to die and less likely to be born underweight (see Table 7.1).

How do financial barriers to care in the United States affect health status? Mary D. is a widow who lives in New York City. She is sixty years old and has had high blood pressure (hypertension) since she was forty. There are numerous complications associated with hypertension, including heart disease and stroke. Hypertensive patients require medication and regular primary care to monitor their condition. But Mrs. D. can't afford to see her doctor, and sometimes she can't afford her medicine. Although she's been a garment worker all her life, her employer doesn't offer health insurance benefits and her income is barely enough to cover food and rent. Although she can't afford to pay for care on her own, she isn't poor enough to qualify for Medicaid.*

A couple of months ago, Mrs. D.'s cat got sick, and $100 to pay the vet meant she didn't have any cash left over for her pills. Although she didn't know it, Mrs. D.'s blood pressure rose dangerously. One evening she got up to get her cat a snack and suffered a fatal stroke.

Recent U.S. studies have documented decreased access and poorer outcomes linked to income and/or insurance status for newborns,[53] glaucoma,[54] childhood immunization,[55] mammography, and pap smears.[56] One study found that people without insurance were more likely to die after hospital admission.[57] Another has shown that poorly insured elderly people were less likely to receive needed follow-up care.[58]

Public health insurance gives Canada a competitive edge

In Canada, there's no need for management and labour to negotiate for basic health benefits, since these are already provided publicly. Instead, Canadian negotiations over health care relate to those parts of the system where public insurance is not available. Sometimes called "extended health benefits," these include items such as dental care, preferred (single room or double room) hospital accommodation, and prescription drugs.

But in the United States, it's another matter entirely. Negotiating basic health insurance benefits is a major preoccupation. The stakes and the costs are both enormous. For example,

---

* Medicaid is publicly funded health insurance for the poor in the United States.

Table 7.1

RECENT HEALTH STATUS INDICATORS IN CANADA AND THE UNITED STATES

	Canada	United States
Infant mortality	**0.68%** 1990	**0.91%** 1990
Low birthweight (< 2500 grams)	**5.1%** 1989	**7.05%** 1989
Very low birthweight (< 1500 grams)	**0.84%** 1989	**1.28%** 1989
Life expectancy at birth		
Male	**73.4 years** 1988	**71.5 years** 1988
Female	**80.3 years** 1988	**78.3 years** 1988
Life expectancy at 65 years		
Male	**15.0 years** 1988	**14.9 years** 1988
Female	**19.6 years** 1988	**18.6 years** 1988

Sources: G.J. Scheiber, J.P. Poullier, L.M. Greenwald "U.S. health expenditure performance: An international comparison and data update"; Statistics Canada, 1991; National Center for Health Statistics, *Health United States, 1991.*

Chrysler estimates it spends $700 (1988 U.S. dollars) on health benefits for every car it produces in the United States. The comparable figure for cars produced in Canada is only $233.

Health benefit negotiations in the United States have also become increasingly acrimonious. In 1990, health care was the number-one issue in 83 percent of negotiations and the key factor in 55 percent of strikes and lockouts.[59]

The United States health insurance system puts an enormous burden on business. This is particularly true for the manufacturing industry, which has a relatively high proportion of unionized employees and a relatively old workforce. To quote Ontario Premier Bob Rae, "The cost advantage for us in manufacturing in terms of the health care issue is enormous and it's growing. The longer the Americans take to resolve this, the happier I'll be."[60]

In summary, a direct comparison of the Canadian and U.S. health care systems concludes:

1. The Canadian system costs substantially less than the U.S. system and the difference is getting bigger.
2. Low-income Canadians have much better access to health care services than low-income Americans.
3. For urgent conditions, Canadians and Americans have similar access to high tech services.
4. For elective services, upper-income Americans have better access than Canadians.
5. There is little difference in the quality of patient outcomes between the two countries.

The United States and the World

We've looked at how the Canadian and U.S. systems compare, but how does the United States stack up against the rest of the world? A look at the health care systems developed by the twenty-four member countries of the Organisation for Economic Cooperation and Development (OECD) shows that the United States is a striking anomaly to the rest of the industrialized world.

Twenty-two of the twenty-four OECD countries, including Canada, rely mainly on public financing for health care. The exceptions are the United States and Turkey. In Canada in 1990, 73 percent of health care expenditures were paid from the public purse, almost exactly the OECD average of 74 percent. By contrast, in the United States only 42 percent of expenditures were paid publicly.[61] The proportion of public spending among the remainder ranges from Portugal at 62 percent to Norway at 95 percent.

While there are some important differences among publicly funded systems, they all have much more in common with one another than with the U.S. system. Germany has attracted considerable American interest because health insurance there is managed through 1700 private "sickness funds" organized according to occupation. Some Americans find this system analogous to their own private insurance system. But there are big differences. For one thing, Germany's "private" funds are really quasi-public, non-profit organizations that mainly channel money from workers and employers to physicians and hospitals. When it comes to determining prices in the system, Germany's federal government sets a very tight framework for the negotiations between providers and the "sickness funds." Germany does have a very small private system, but it's used by less than 3 percent of the population. And, once you decide to leave the public "sickness fund" for the private system, it's very difficult to come back—there is little bouncing back and forth between the two.[62]

Political reasons for policy gridlock

Why is the United States the only wealthy industrialized country that still relies mainly on private financing?

Analysts put forward a number of possible explanations. For example, America's rather narrow and right-of-centre political landscape has never produced a significant national labour or social democratic party. Dr. Vicente Navarro of Johns Hopkins University suggests that this may be a key factor hampering the development of public health insurance in the United States.[63]

Others point to America's governmental structure itself. The elaborate system of checks and balances between Congress and the president makes major policy reforms—like public health insurance—much more difficult to accomplish than in parliamentary systems with a majority government.[64]

In Canada, when a political party wins a majority of seats in the House of Commons, major policy changes can occur within a relatively short period. Party discipline is strictly enforced for Canadian Parliamentarians. Members of the House of Commons on the government side must vote in favour of the government's legislation unless a "free vote" has been specifically proclaimed.

This contrasts sharply with the American experience, in which party discipline is almost nonexistent. To win support for controversial legislation, the president is often forced to use up scarce political capital in convincing reluctant members from his own party to vote in favour. As a rule, major policy changes can occur only when the president's party holds significant majorities in both the House of Representatives and the Senate. That's how Lyndon Johnson managed to pass his "Great Society" programs and how they came to be repealed under Ronald Reagan's presidency.

Another problem with the U.S. system of government is that it is very difficult to hold any one party accountable for the health policy gridlock. The president blames Congress. Congress blames the president. Democrats and Republicans blame each other. Although Canada's parliamentary system has its own problems, at least our voters know who to blame for the failure to implement a specific policy—the governing party.

Also, because provinces have constitutional authority over health care, it was possible for Saskatchewan to implement hospital insurance in 1947 and medical insurance in 1962 without any interference from the federal government. But in America, the U.S. federal government has such tight control over the regulation of employee benefits—including health benefits—that individual states need Congressional waivers to make significant changes in health insurance.[65]

Interest groups and institutional gridlock

Lobbying by interest groups is common in both countries. In Canada, however, the focus is almost always on the prime minister, cabinet members, and senior bureaucrats. There's little point paying much attention to backbenchers, especially if they are opposition members.

But in the United States, every vote in Congress is up for grabs. The lack of effective party discipline and the complex system of checks and balances give far more scope to the well-funded lobbyists. Between 1981 and 1991, health industry political action committees (PACs) contributed over $60 million (U.S.) to congressional candidates.[66] Over $18 million went to members of only four congressional committees that oversee health-related issues. The American Medical Association alone contributed nearly $12 million during this period, while the insurance industry kicked in $19 million. And this is only the tip of the iceberg. Both the American Medical Association and the insurance industry have spent millions trying to discredit Canada's health care system since 1991.

American Values: The Evolution of Differences

What are the philosophical roots that underlie American attitudes towards social programs? How did Canada and the United States come to diverge in their values and beliefs?

U.S. and Canadian health care systems used to be almost indistinguishable from one another. Private financing was the norm in both nations. Both countries introduced federal programs to help build hospitals after the Second World War.[67] The United States even took a crack at a national health insurance program introduced by President Harry Truman in the late 1940s, but it failed in Congress, thanks to a massive crusade against it financed by the American Medical Association (AMA). The AMA invested a staggering $1.5 million in this lobby effort— easily making it, at the time, the most expensive campaign ever mounted by an interest group.[68]

The tactics used in this initial battle played on a deep-seated fear of anything that smacked of socialism. A pamphlet produced for the campaign asked, "Would socialized medicine lead to socialization of other phases of American life?"[69] Forty years later, the AMA and the Health Insurance Association of America were using the same ploy—decrying "socialized medicine" and raising fears that a Canadian-style solution would inevitably compromise an individual's freedom to choose.

But while public health insurance foundered on the shoals of ideology in the United States, it found a welcoming harbour in

Canada's developing social policy. Although the CCF/NDP played the major role, Liberals and Conservatives also contributed their support. For example, in 1984, when federal Health Minister Monique Bégin, a Liberal, was fighting to pass the Canada Health Act, Brian Mulroney, who was then Opposition Leader, made sure his fellow Conservative MPs voted in favour of the bill. Indeed, the measure was passed unanimously by all three parties in Parliament. Publicly financed health insurance has not been a particularly partisan issue here for twenty-five years.

While it seems strange to many American observers, prominent Conservatives have not only supported but fought for public health insurance. For example, in 1961 Conservative Prime Minister John Diefenbaker appointed former Saskatchewan Supreme Court Justice Emmett Hall to head the Royal Commission on Health Services. At the time, opponents of the scheme—the Canadian Medical Association and insurance companies—were pleased, believing that Hall would come out against the idea. They were wrong. Hall's report strongly recommended public insurance—and not just for doctors' care but also for dentistry, drugs, and a range of other services.

Hall's basic reason was essentially a "small-c conservative" argument: public insurance, in his view, would involve less administrative cost and would therefore be more efficient.[70] He knew that having a single payer in each province would mean less paperwork and fewer clerical staff. So while U.S. Republicans were calling public health insurance a communist plot,[71] Canadian Conservatives were making the sensible and prudent public policy decision to implement it.

In this contradiction lies much of the explanation for the difference in health insurance financing. Canada provides publicly financed insurance for all while the United States provides public funding for only the poorest and the elderly—those the private sector won't take care of.

American author Seymour Martin Lipset has been a constant observer of Canadian politics ever since he journeyed to Saskatchewan to study the new government of Tommy Douglas in 1944. In a recent book, *Continental Divide: The Values and Institutions of the United States and Canada,*[72] he reconsiders the similarities and differences between the two countries and traces essential characteristics back to the time of the American Revolution.

Significant differences in values and institutions were evident even in the late eighteenth century. The Americans were suspicious of government authority. In developing their constitution, they were very careful to avoid concentrating political power and instead apportioned it among the executive (the president), the legislature (the House of Representatives and the Senate), and the judiciary (the Supreme Court).

By contrast, the northern British colonies continued to respect the absolute power of the monarch and his or her advisers. The monarchy was retained and Canada adopted a parliamentary system of government modelled on Britain's. Canada's first constitution, the British North America Act (1867), was an act of the British Parliament. It wasn't until 1982 that Canada acquired the legal right to change its own constitution, without reference to Britain's Privy Council.

You pay for what you value

The institutions and interests developed by a nation will inevitably reflect the values held by its people as a whole. Canada and the United States emerged with and have defined themselves according to different political values, and those values are in turn reflected in their approach to health care and other social programs. Some observers maintain that American values are not that different from those of countries that do have public funding for health insurance.[73] Others maintain that American values are very different from the rest of the world and quite incompatible with a publicly funded health care system.[74]

Professor Daniel Fox of the State University of New York puts forward three values that have guided the financing of the U.S. health care system:[75]

1. Individual rights and individual welfare matter more than the common good.
2. Private or public-private solutions to social problems are almost always superior to public remedies.
3. Wealth and poverty are mainly the result of economic factors rather than status conferred by social background, gender, ethnic, or geographic characteristics.

This world-view makes it much more difficult for America to develop the kind of single-payer, single-tiered system we enjoy in Canada.

Evidence from international surveys suggests that Americans do differ somewhat in their attitudes about health care from people living in countries with public health insurance. In 1991, the Lou Harris polling organization surveyed Americans and residents of Canada, France, Great Britain, and West Germany about their attitudes towards health care and health insurance.[76] Lou Harris president Humphrey Taylor and Princeton University economist Uwe Reinhardt reported that "the relevant social ethic is not very different in the United States from that in the other countries surveyed." For example, the poll showed that Americans were similar to Canadians in agreeing that health care costs should not bankrupt the sick.

However, Americans were much less likely than Canadians to agree that the healthy and the rich should pay for care for the sick and the poor. And 35 percent of Americans polled, but only 11 percent of Canadians, believed that if you have more money, you should be able to purchase better care. As Professor Reinhardt has noted elsewhere, "Americans believe in first class and steerage for hospitals as well as cruise ships."

Cognitive dissonance: get your facts out of my values

"Thinking's a dizzy business, a matter of catching as many of those foggy glimpses as you can and fitting them together the best you can. That's why people hang on so tight to their beliefs and opinions."[77] As this quote from Dashiell Hammett affirms, people don't find it easy to change their minds. The appearance of an odd fact here and there isn't enough to bring about a major change in beliefs. Psychologists call this conflict between facts and values "cognitive dissonance." They point out that it's much easier to ignore or change the facts themselves than it is to change deep-seated opinions. But over time, if the facts keep coming and are really compelling, cognitive dissonance reaches a crisis point. That's precisely the point when the values of an individual—or even a society—can and do change.

Americans have been experiencing a steadily increasing level of cognitive dissonance when it comes to their health care system. For example:

- How can Canada and other countries provide health care for everyone, while America—the world's wealthiest nation—leaves millions unprotected?
- Why do systems that mainly rely on public financing end up costing less?

America's system leaves so many citizens without coverage because the private insurance industry does its best to maximize its profits, which leads to pre-insurance screenings, exclusions, and prohibitive pricing for small group and individual policies. The U.S. system costs so much more because private insurers impose a heavier administrative burden than public insurance and yet don't have enough leverage to negotiate better prices from health care providers. But neither of these facts fits the core belief that America has the world's best system. The result: cognitive dissonance.

Meanwhile, the American Medical Association and the insurance industry have been more than ready to provide alternative explanations better adapted to American beliefs. In short, they "change" the facts to match conventional wisdom. Thus we hear that Canada's system costs less because it doesn't provide the care that people need. Former President George Bush claimed that citizens in countries with national health insurance couldn't chose their own doctors. Newt Gingrich, the Republican Whip in the House of Representatives, claimed that it was illegal for Canadian seniors to get most operations. Even 1992 Democratic presidential hopeful Paul Tsongas got into the act when he claimed that he couldn't have received his life-saving bone marrow transplant in Canada. All of these assertions are wrong. But they served a key purpose: to keep Americans confused about public insurance.

A 1992 editorial in the *New Yorker* magazine made an ironic observation: once conservative American politicians admitted that Canada's health care system was actually better than America's, they would also have to admit that governments could do other things for their citizens besides fighting wars: "The compulsion that drives President Bush to distort the facts about Canadian health care suggests that official American policy is in the process of becoming what conservatives, in discussing the Soviet Union, used to call a 'total ideology'—a system blindly convinced of this absolute truth, and yet so fragile in its relationship to reality that it is incapable of considering even the most obvious reform."[78]

The Tunnel at the End of the Light

George Bush is no longer president of the United States. But the American health care industry still has lots of friends in the House of Representatives and the Senate. In September 1993, after eight months of work by a task force led by Hillary Rodham Clinton, President Bill Clinton presented Congress with a 1300-page proposal for reforming the U.S. health care system. The plan he offered differed little from the one he originally proposed—so-called "managed competition."

Privately, the President and First Lady admitted that they preferred a single-payer, Canadian-style plan. They acknowledged that single-source funding was essential to ensure cost control and access. They also recognized that any monopsonist (single purchaser) of health care needed to be accountable to the public. However, the Clintons and their advisers believed that Americans would never accept a plan where government directly funded the system. They also feared the Republican accusation that the Democrats were making a big tax grab to finance the reform.

That's mainly why their plan continued to attach health insurance to employment, with employers contributing 80 percent of the financing, and employees contributing 20 percent. The plan did allow businesses with fewer than 50 workers to receive government subsidies and permitted self-employed people to deduct premiums from their taxes. The President's plan concretely defined what was included as "basic coverage," but also permitted consumers the option of paying more for a richer basket of services. The plan included user fees of $10 to $20 for a doctor's visit.

Because the President's scheme shunned government finance, an entirely new mechanism was proposed for obtaining insurance coverage. All citizens in a given geographic area were to join a "health care alliance," the idea being that these alliances could leverage better prices and services from competing health plans. The alliances were supposed to be democratically controlled by their members, which made them look suspiciously (to Republicans) like government structures. And, in fact, some Democrats even hoped that states (like Vermont) with great interest in the single-payer option would choose to become "alliances" themselves and allow a Canadian-style model to develop.

The plan exempted some groups from alliance membership. Big

corporations with more than 5,000 employees could have opted out and dealt directly with insurers or run their own plans. Concerns raised by seniors and their advocates led the Administration to exempt Medicare, the U.S. public program for the elderly, even though many hoped it would eventually be folded into the package.

Clinton's plan also proposed regulatory measures to control premium increases and to outlaw risk-rating practices that currently set lower prices for healthier people. The President acknowledged that financing the plan might require major cuts in Medicare. Other financing was to come from a dramatic increase in tobacco taxes.

Critics were quick to point out that this "made in America" solution had never been tried anywhere else. Had it been implemented, the number of insurance companies would almost certainly have fallen. The largest firms would have had the advantage—a feature which led most of the big companies to break away from the Health Insurance Association of America, which was intent on fighting the plan.

Most policy analysts agreed that the plan would have improved access. But cost control was another matter. Canada and other countries with national health insurance can set overall budgets for health care, but the President's plan didn't allow this. What's more, the poorest 20 to 40 percent of Americans were likely to find themselves sequestered in the "basic coverage" plan. This worried some advocates for better access. Evidence of other "targeted" social programs in America suggests that funding for them inevitably erodes over time. Political and public support dry up because most people don't derive any benefit from the program. Groups like the American Public Health Association were also troubled about the sizable user fees proposed, fearing that these would compromise access further.[79]

As the battle over Clinton's plan raged on into the Spring of 1994, it was clear that the President and First Lady had made major miscalculations. They counted on avoiding a clash with the insurance industry by allowing private insurance companies to sell their products to the alliances. But this compromise didn't work. The Health Insurance Association of America launched an all-out assault against the package as if the industry's very existence was at stake. Another serious drawback was the plan's extraordinary complexity—it was such a Rube Goldberg-type of package that even minor changes could have rendered it completely unworkable. And changes are always demanded in America's political process. Compromise is how U.S. policy develops.

By the summer of 1994, it was clear that Clinton's plan was on its last legs. True, the President's party, the Democrats, controlled the House of Representatives and the Senate. And, true, the American people wanted change. But lack of party discipline mixed with millions of dollars in political donations proved toxic to the Clinton reforms. Conservative Democrats joined with Republicans to scuttle the President's plan and propose much weaker reforms in their place. Eventually, the President and his allies were forced to concede defeat in September 1994. The Republican sweep in the November 1994 mid-term elections appear to have killed off any prospects for health reform for the forseeable future.

Do It Right or Do Us Wrong

Canadians can't afford to be disinterested spectators in the debate over America's health care reform. The outcome has grave implications for the future of our own health care system, which is already vulnerable to the workings of the U.S. system. The explosion of largely unevaluated U.S. technology, driven by incentives for private profit, has created pressure for similar expansion here. Very high incomes for some American doctors—particularly surgeons—have put pressure on certain specialities in Canada. Both of these factors are a strain on Canada's health budget. Most importantly, will America's rejection of a Canadian-style health care system now lead us to doubt the fundamental soundness of our own approach to health care financing? Will it prey on our growing fear that we can't afford it after all? And will we continue to suffer from the misinformation generated by the U.S. propaganda war?

Canada, France, Germany, Sweden, Australia, and the other wealthy countries have demonstrated that they can provide all their citizens with the fruits of modern health care. The United States has more of this "fruit" than anywhere else, but fewer and fewer of its people have the chance to partake of it. And its cost is crippling to government, business and individuals.

There's one main lesson the rest of the world has failed to teach America: public finance is a necessary precondition for cost control.

The deep-seated belief in the boundless potential of the individual and America's commitment to personal liberty don't mesh well with proof that collective problem-solving via public health insurance actually works. America's Lone Ranger mentality will not be able to solve the problems of health care access and cost.

It's such a shame. Affordable health insurance with public financing would have so many positive spin-offs in the United States. For one thing, it would demonstrate concretely that collective action can effectively deal with issues other than national defence. Also, reducing the cost to manufacturers of providing health benefits to their employees would be a real boon to the competitiveness of American industry.

Winston Churchill once said that Americans could be relied upon to do the right thing, after trying everything else. Americans have just about tried everything to make their health care system more accessible and affordable. They've tried a private system. They've tried a mixed system—a public one for bad risks (the poor and the elderly) and a private system for everyone else. They've tried regulation and deregulation. They've tried better management and various competitive approaches. Nothing has worked so far. And the number of uninsured is rising by one million people a year.

Now the most recent reform plan has met its end and American politics have taken a nasty, brutish turn to the right. But the problems with America's health care system won't go away; they're going to get worse. The persistent trend in the U.S. economy towards "McJobs"—low-paying service sector employment without health benefits—guarantees that the number without insurance will continue to grow. Health costs are bound to follow suit because, even though cost increases did moderate somewhat during the debates over reform, the inflation drivers remain embedded in the current system. Poor access and cost escalation—the dual demons of American health care—are set to bedevil the system for many years to come.

One day, we have to hope, Americans will move beyond the fact-values barrier and make a real commitment to solving their health care miseries collectively. As long as our neighbours remain stuck in the quagmire, we risk being pulled in ourselves.

Chapter 8

So This is Reform, Eh?

"MARVELLOUS THOUGH HEALTH care services are in Canada in comparison with many other countries, there is little doubt that future improvements in the level of health of Canadians lie mainly in improving the environment, moderating self-imposed risks and adding to our knowledge of human biology."[1]

"We cannot afford the inefficiencies, the escalating cost increases, the inequities of access to and quality of health care services in Canada. The current financing programs for the 'non-system' not only allow these, but in some cases, actually promote them."[2]

Although both of these statements could easily have been made last week, these quotes actually hail back two decades. The first was made by the Honorable Marc Lalonde when he was federal minister of health and welfare in 1974; the second, by his deputy minister, Dr. Maurice Le Clair, in 1972.

For more than twenty years, Canada has been a world leader in health policy, enriching the field with new conceptual models to help improve our understanding of health and health care. The World Health Organization's "Ottawa Charter for Health Promotion" and the "Toronto Consensus Statement on Doctor-Patient Communications" are two concrete examples of this leadership. A decade's worth of royal commissions and other provincial health care reviews has produced remarkably consistent findings.[3] As a result, there is now broad agreement among politicians, bureaucrats, academics, and even most health care providers that: 1) health care services play a relatively minor role in determining health; and 2) how we organize and finance health care services have created major inefficiencies and inequities in our delivery system.

All the same, despite near-unanimous agreement about Medicare's problems and substantial agreement about the solutions, the pace of implementing reform has been frustratingly slow.

Consider this excerpt from the Ontario Health Review Panel's 1987 report:

> There is a remarkable consistency and repetition in the findings and recommendations for improvements in all the information we reviewed. Current submissions and earlier reports highlight the need to place greater emphasis on primary care, to integrate and coordinate services, to achieve a community focus for health and to increase the emphasis on health promotion and disease prevention. The panel notes with concern that well-founded recommendations made by credible groups over a period of fifteen years have rarely been translated into action.[4]

In other words, we know why and what to do, but we've found it terribly difficult to get on with the job. This chapter will look at why it has been so difficult to introduce fundamental reform and will review current federal and provincial policy initiatives across the country.

Muddling Through: The Status Quo

There are good reasons why the status quo in any policy area has sticking power. For one thing, it's familiar—nurtured by society's values and beliefs and propped up by society's rules and institutional arrangements. As a result, changes to policy usually do not alter the underlying structures of a system. Instead, new policies focus on making successive minor adjustments that, if anything, both reflect and reinforce these beliefs, rules, and arrangements.

Over thirty years ago, American policy analyst Charles Lindblom summed up bureaucratic policy development as "the science of muddling through."[5] His analysis contrasts two quite different approaches to policy development and identifies them as "root" and "branch":

- The root style of policy development begins by clarifying values and identifying goals. This is followed by a comprehensive analysis of all the various policy options that could be implemented to achieve the goals.
- The branch style of policy development uses the values and goals of the day to guide a much more restrictive analysis of policy options. In order to reduce conflict between government and key stakeholders and to be consistent with the experience of decision-makers, the search is limited to policies that are likely to be supported by key interest groups.

The root approach to policy development is rather like a needs-based planning approach or the accountant's zero-based budgeting. There is no assumption that existing institutional arrangements are necessarily the best way to achieve policy objectives. The root approach almost always leads to recommendations for fundamental change.

Lindblom points out that government officials almost always apply the branch approach to policy development, for quite pragmatic reasons. Busy administrators have neither the time nor the resources for the more comprehensive root approach so often favoured by government-appointed commissions. When we ask why task force reports wind up gathering dust on a shelf, part of the answer relates to these fundamentally different starting points for analysis.

Why root solutions don't take root

The following list of issues (summarized from Chapter 5) related to the cost of medications, the quality of prescribing, and the undue influence of the pharmaceutical industry helps illustrate how difficult it is for governments to undertake major reform.

1. Drug costs are escalating faster than any other category of health care expenditure and will likely rise even more rapidly in the future, because federal

     policies to expand patent protection for brand-name
     producers will delay the entry of generic competition.
2. There is evidence of massive overprescribing, mainly
     due to inadequate training of doctors in pharmacol-
     ogy, aggressive promotion by the drug companies,
     and a lack of quality assurance. Every year, poor pre-
     scribing kills thousands of Canadians and causes over
     50,000 hospital admissions.
3. Educational programs for doctors, pharmacists, and
     consumers can improve the quality of prescribing and
     reduce costs.

Despite this familiar analysis, substantive drug policy reform
has stymied provincial governments. Most have responded to
the increased costs of public drug programs by decreasing eligibility, reducing the number and type of drugs covered, thereby
shifting costs to consumers and private insurers.

In 1987, Dr. George Carruthers, one of Canada's best known
clinical pharmacologists, wrote a scathing report on prescription
drug use for the Ontario Ministry of Health. In it, he criticized the
Ontario Drug Benefit Plan, the province's publicly funded drug
program, for wasting money and endangering the public's health,
and he recommended a series of policies to improve quality and
reduce costs. When nothing happened, he resigned as chair of the
province's Drug Quality and Therapeutics Committee.

His report posed a thorny communications problem for the
Ministry of Health. Officials knew that the public didn't understand the nature or extent of the problem. Despite some pointed
questions by then opposition leader, Bob Rae, there was no public outcry for better prescribing or more physician education.
Those who stood to benefit from these kinds of reforms were
not organized in any way. Besides, although better prescribing
would produce enormous savings overall, the average benefit
per person would be tiny, something less than $30 a year. On the
other hand, meaningful prescribing reform would certainly pose
a threat to the more concentrated and powerful interests of doctors, drug companies, and pharmacists.

Back in 1987, Ontario's economy was growing faster than
Japan's or West Germany's. Money was plentiful. And during the
1980s the bill for Ontario's Drug Benefit Program grew at a rate

of more than 18 percent per year.[6] In 1989, the Liberal government of David Peterson appointed Dr. Fred Lowy, a former dean of medicine at the University of Toronto, to study the issues in medication yet again. After Lowy submitted his report in 1990, the new NDP government sat on it for nearly two years before appointing its own Drug Reform Secretariat to involve stakeholders in yet another review of the policy options. Australian health policy analysts Palmer and Short cynically observe that part of the reason governments establish ad hoc enquiries "is the symbolic [purpose] of giving the appearance of taking action on an issue."[7]

By 1992, of course, government revenues in Ontario had collapsed. Controlling the deficit had become a major provincial priority and many areas of government spending were targeted for cuts—including health care. As a result, the Ontario Drug Benefit Plan dropped a number of drugs from the list of products that it would cover. For two years in a row the cabinet seriously debated whether to impose user fees on senior citizens. (The "nays" won.) In early 1994, action plans for better-quality prescribing were still on the drawing board, as various pilot projects to test alternative strategies were running their course.

It's an odd and familiar pattern. Whenever concerns about overprescribing were raised strongly (sometimes by a commission or task force), the Ministry responded by appointing yet another group of experts to "study the problem." Each successive commission used Lindblom's root approach for policy analysis, exhaustively examining every aspect of the issue and carefully screening all possible policy options. The result inevitably produced a damning critique of prescribing practices and a comprehensive set of recommendations for change.

Despite all this advice, government officials took no action until external economic pressures forced them into cost control. Time was of the essence—dollars needed to be saved now. Is it any wonder that the Ministry chose to delist some drugs rather than to take necessary steps to improve the quality of prescribing?

The Rules of the Game

By now you are already familiar with many of the institutional arrangements governing our health care system. For example, we have federal legislation to set the ground rules for health insurance, but all the arrangements for health care delivery are under provincial jurisdiction. Provincial governments pay most physicians on fee-for-service, and most hospitals are financed with global budgets.* For the most part, these arrangements remain unchanged by the "health reforms" so far introduced by individual provinces.

A key factor in the stability of the status quo is the relative power of the various groups who work in or are served by the system. Political scientists commonly analyze policy change by studying how all these different stakeholders work to promote or block new directions. For example, American policy analyst Robert Alford classifies interest groups in health care along several dimensions.[8] First, he identifies the "structural" interests, those people who have a direct stake in the health care system. Using Alford's approach, everyone working in health care has a structural interest in how the system is organized and financed. However, some people are better served by these arrangements than others, and to make this distinction Alford further subdivides structural interests into three categories: dominant, repressed, and challenging. Dominant structural interests have no need to organize for change—the system as currently set up serves their members well. By contrast, repressed structural interests are not well served by current institutional arrangements but have enormous difficulty organizing for change "unless extraordinary political energies are mobilized." Challenging structural interests are created when major developments in the structure of society occur— for example, when new technologies, shifts in the division of labour, or new incentives emerge to produce pressure for "a new way of doing things around here."

Not surprisingly, Alford characterizes medicine's professional monopoly as the dominant structural interest in health care. Other dominant interests include universities, hospitals, long-term-care institutions (both non-profit and for-profit), drug companies, private laboratories, equipment manufacturers, private health insurance companies, and other self-employed

---

* The main exception being Alberta, which uses case-mix funding. See Chapter 6 for details.

health professionals paid on fee-for-service, such as dentists, pharmacists, and optometrists.[9]

Repressed structural interests include most other health care workers and patients. As for challenging structural interests, Alford points to the "corporate rationalizers"—planners, administrators, government officials, and researchers who are increasingly contesting medicine's professional monopoly.[10]

Medicine as a dominant structural interest

Few would disagree that physicians, given their longstanding legal monopoly over health care services, are the dominant force in our system.[11] Individual doctors and their organizations make the key decisions in virtually every area of health policy, including the approval of new drugs and which medical procedures or therapies should be eligible for insurance coverage. Society has also delegated to doctors some types of authority normally reserved for the police and the courts. For example, a physician may order the arrest and detention of a person with a suspected mental disorder. Public health doctors can impose quarantine on individuals and households, and even stop cargo ships from unloading.

Physicians are not only the best-paid workers in health care, they also have the right to define what "health care" actually is, and—equally important—who besides themselves can deliver it. For example, for most of this century, Canadian doctors opposed midwifery. In 1931, Dr. William Hendry, an obstetrician who chaired the Canadian Medical Association's maternal mortality committee, called midwives "a menace to the health of any woman whom they might attend."[12] By the end of the 1980s, organized medicine had shifted to a position of cautious tolerance. Ontario, for example, proclaimed self-governing legislation for midwives in the fall of 1993. All the same, when asked whether midwifery should be legalized in Quebec, Dr. Augustin Roy, former president of the regulatory agency for Quebec doctors, said, "You might as well make prostitution legal. More people are asking for prostitutes than midwives."[13]

Medicine's approach to self-regulation provides another example of the typical behaviour of a dominant structural interest. Like medieval guilds, doctors run their own courts and mete out their own justice. By and large, licensing organizations for doctors discipline their members behind closed doors.* Kate Dunn, a former medical reporter for the *Montreal Gazette*, has criticized the licensing body for not giving complaints an adequate airing and for hiding the disciplinary process from the public. She recently described a professional misconduct case in which the complainant was given no opportunity to present her side of the story during the proceedings.[14]

Other institutional arrangements also support the primacy of the medical profession. The main method for paying physicians in Canada is fee-for-service—an arrangement that reinforces their self-employed professional status and their authority to set their own conditions of work.** By contrast, other health professionals, like most nurses and most physiotherapists, are salaried employees. These payment rules have enormous implications for resource allocations. In other policy arenas—education, for example—budgets are usually quite explicit and set in advance. The process for allocating resources is therefore open to public input and public scrutiny. As things stand now, how health care dollars get spent is mainly determined by the decisions that individual doctors make regarding individual patients. The sum of all these individual decisions sets the pattern. Budgets for health care are therefore set implicitly, not explicitly, and this makes the allocation of health care resources highly resistant to change—especially to change imposed from outside the medical fraternity.

Perhaps an illustration would help explain how health care's various institutional arrangements frustrate change. As you already know, Canadian doctors, together with their colleagues throughout the western world, have two main strategies for dealing with coronary heart disease: drug treatment or surgery. These are examples of what the late physician-philosopher Dr.

---

* In Ontario and the western provinces, these bodies are known as Colleges of Physicians and Surgeons, while in other provinces they are known by different terms—Medical Boards, Corporations, etc.

** Fee-for-service reimbursement and self-employed professional status are also common among some other health professionals, including dentists, optometrists, chiropractors, and pharmacists.

Lewis Thomas called "halfway technologies." Neither option stops or reverses the progress of heart disease.[15] Neither offers a cure, even though patients may benefit through increased life expectancy or better symptom relief for a time.

Now, however, there is good evidence of an effective alternative to drugs and surgery. A comprehensive rehabilitation program that includes a strict low-fat, vegetarian diet, yoga, stress management, smoking cessation, exercise, and emotional support can actually *reverse* coronary artery blockages. The program was pioneered by San Francisco cardiologist Dr. Dean Ornish, and evidence of its benefit comes from a randomized controlled study known as the "Lifestyle Heart Trial."[16] While some might be sceptical about the ability of heart patients to make these dramatic changes, Dr. Ornish says, "Paradoxically, it may be easier to make big changes than to make small ones."[17]

Despite this evidence, we haven't seen any significant change in how Canada's health care system treats heart disease. There has been no public debate about whether we should keep spending hundreds of millions of dollars every year on drugs and surgery to treat heart disease or whether we should shift some of these resources to support a massive rehabilitation and health promotion program for heart patients.[18]

So many structural forces favour the status quo. For example, the prescription of a new drug requires no new infrastructure. Surgery is already supported by an existing network of facilities and staffing. By contrast, setting up a new comprehensive rehabilitation program would require new funding for training, new facilities, and new staffing. And, of course, even though some doctors try to set the record straight, the public still thinks that there's a pill for every ill and that surgery cures heart disease. The values underlying these ideas are not easy to shake.

Is it any wonder the old way of doing things continues?

Repressed and challenging structural interests

The repressed structural interests in health care include nurses, other salaried professionals, non-professional health care workers, health care unions, community service agencies, and patients. None of these groups is very well served by the present system and they are extremely difficult to organize as an effective counterweight to the dominant interests.

In Alford's model, a challenging structural interest began to emerge during the 1970s in the United States when controlling the cost of health care was attracting public attention. Over the next twenty years, a new force, which Alford calls "corporate rationalizers," gained sufficient momentum to challenge the medical profession's traditional monopoly over the production and distribution of health care.

In Canada, these "rationalizers" include senior officials in ministries of health, the administrators of some hospitals and other health agencies, and some academics and consultants. One of the most powerful rationalizers to emerge during the late 1980s and early 1990s is the Conference of Deputy Ministers of Health. First created in 1973 as a successor to the previous Dominion Council on Health, the Conference of Deputy Ministers is chaired by the federal deputy minister of health and includes a separate committee of provincial and territorial ministers and deputies alone. There used to be over fifty committees and sub-committees reporting to the Conference, but recently the deputies downsized them to meet the needs of the 1990s. Today, five key committees advise the conference on:

- health human resources;
- health services delivery;
- population health;
- public education; and
- the National Health Information Council.

After months of hard work by the Health Human Resources Committee chaired by Bonnie Hoyt-Hallett of New Brunswick, the provincial and territorial deputy ministers prepared the National Physicians' Management Plan (also known as the "Banff Declaration") for their ministers in an unprecedented move to control key policies relating to doctors.

What's Belief Got to Do With It?

We've seen the influence of institutional arrangements and structural interests in blocking change, but there is another important factor at work. The fundamental ideologies and beliefs of the population also define the amount of manoeu-vring room available for change and reform. By ideologies we mean those core values that describe how people think the world "ought to be." Values, in this sense, are not "right" or "wrong"; there is no objective way to assess their "correctness," just as there is no objective basis for preferring vanilla over chocolate. On the other hand, we use the term "beliefs" to describe a person's understanding of how the world actually "is." Unlike ideologies, a belief can be tested to see if it corresponds to objective evidence.

An example might help clarify this point. Some people hold the ideology that users ought to pay a fee for medical care; others are firmly opposed to this idea. We can't conclude categorically that either position is "right" or "wrong." What we can do, however, is test people's beliefs about what user fees can accomplish by looking at their effect in the real world. When we did so in Chapter 6, it became clear (hopefully) that user fees would not help and could seriously harm vulnerable groups.

A key problem for governments today is the fact that public beliefs are somewhat out of synch with those expressed by the various Canadian commissions that have recommended fundamental health care system reform. Academics, employees of ministries of health, and leaders of health care organizations have all come to share the views of Marc Lalonde and Maurice LeClair, cited at the beginning of this chapter. But too many Canadians still think that:[19]

- experts don't know very much about what causes ill-ness or what keeps people healthy;
- as long as people have access to health care, there's no need to understand what causes health and illness;
- medicine is a precise science—almost devoid of discretion;
- it's easy to define the necessity for medical care.

Although we now know that these beliefs are largely incorrect, they helped to shape the system we have today. And even though new information is moderating them somewhat, they remain dominant among most members of the public and severely limit the reform process.

The Role of Central Agencies

Over the past twenty years, federal and provincial health ministers and their departments have come to accept new ways of looking at health and health care. Unfortunately, this enlightenment has not necessarily extended to the central agencies of our federal and provincial governments. This term refers to the most powerful government offices and departments: the premier's office, the policy and priorities committee of cabinet, cabinet office, finance ministry, and, in many provinces, the treasury board or management board. The people who work in these areas—civil servants and politicians—are the key decision-makers in government.

Unfortunately, these officials are not necessarily up on the latest developments in health policy. Some may even be ideologically opposed. In fact, finance department officials in particular have quite a long history of opposing progressive health policies. For example, when the Medical Care Act passed in 1966, the plan was to proclaim it for implementation on July 1 of the following year—a Centennial Day bonus. But Mitchell Sharp, who was finance minister at the time, didn't buy the arguments in Justice Hall's report. He and many of his department officials were convinced that public health insurance for physician care was a bad idea. And so on September 8, 1966, when Prime Minister Pearson was out of town and Sharp was acting P.M., he seized his chance to try and scuttle it. Rising in the House, he announced to the amazement of all that the proclamation of the act would be delayed for one year. He was hoping to use the interim to find other delaying tactics. But it wasn't to be. In July 1968 the act was proclaimed.[20]

Twenty years later, finance officials gave health a drubbing again when Treasurer Michael Wilson decided to cut federal transfers for health care under the Established Programs Financing Act (EPF). When federal and provincial health and finance ministers got together in June 1992 to discuss the negative impact these cuts were causing, the feds offered to open up the Canada Health Act then and there for renegotiation.

Sometimes it is difficult for these central agency players to recognize how different policies interrelate. Recently, a senior official from a premier's office confided in a children's advocate that his government's priority had to be jobs, not children. Like most Canadians, he didn't automatically link children's health with ensuring that at least one parent has a satisfying, adequately paying job, even though this is one of the best predictors of a child's health. Similarly, most civil servants know that education for women is the best strategy for creating sustainable development and protecting health in developing countries,[21] but they forget this truth applies to Canada as well.

The Role of Information

We've argued that the rules set by our institutions and people's beliefs are both barriers to health care reform. When people are confronted with scientific evidence that runs contrary to their beliefs or interests, they aren't likely to discard their outdated thinking, quit their jobs, or ask for a pay cut. When facts collide with values, it's usually the facts that get bruised.[22]

What role does information play in Canada's developing health policy? McMaster University health services researcher Professor Jonathan Lomas says research information has been virtually shut out of the policy process since the inception of Medicare in the 1960s.[23] Lomas says this may have happened because so much of the evidence from health services research runs counter to public beliefs and the interests of dominant groups, especially doctors.

You can teach old dogs new tricks: policy-oriented learning

Political scientist Paul Sabatier, of the University of California at Davis, has outlined a detailed theory of the policy process.[24] He argues that beliefs will only change under certain circumstances, most of which have been lacking in Canada's health policy development. Sabatier claims that a prerequisite for what he terms "policy-oriented learning" is public debate between at least two coalitions with adequate resources to put forward their views. The term "coalition" is used here to mean a group of individuals and organizations who tend to act together within a policy subsystem over an extended period of time.

Sabatier suggests that it is a common ideology that holds coalitions together. Groups with common financial interests might be able to work together for a short time, but over the longer term a shared ideology is the real glue. He further suggests that learning is more likely to occur when the coalitions debate beliefs, rather than ideologies. Arguments about ideology produce more heat than light, with both sides shouting past each other to the media or to decision-makers.

Of course, individuals and organizations don't have to be in formal coalitions to act in concert. For example, there is no need for an official coalition of doctors and drug companies to keep non-drug alternatives from becoming popular. As long as medical students learn little about these alternatives, and drug companies, which fund the bulk of postgraduate medical education, spend few resources in this area, it's business as usual.

Sabatier also identifies another group of key actors in policy systems, whom he calls "policy brokers." These people can be politicians, judges, civil servants, consultants, or, occasionally, even a member of a coalition. Brokers are responsible for moderating the level of political conflict and working towards a "reasonable" solution—usually a compromise. For example, Justice Emmett Hall became a very important policy broker when his 1964 Royal Commission won sufficient support to expand public health insurance.

Public health insurance: a classic health policy debate

To gain a better understanding of why it is taking so long to implement health care system reform, let's examine more closely a successful policy initiative—the implementation of public health insurance—and how Sabatier's analysis applies to a real debate.

In the 1930s and 1940s, the Canadian Medical Association actually advocated public health insurance. After the Second World War, organized medicine, with support from the insurance industry and some Liberal and Conservative politicians and civil servants, openly opposed it. On the other side of the debate was a coalition in favour of public health insurance with organized labour, nurses, church and social justice groups, consumer organizations, the CCF/NDP, many Liberal politicians, and some Conservatives (like Justice Emmett Hall) as members. The two coalitions were reasonably balanced in terms of resources.

There were many opportunities for policy forums where the two coalitions could debate the issues: conferences sponsored by academic institutions and government and also literally thousands of radio and television debates.

There were also opportunities to discuss evidence. For example, data presented to Justice Hall's Royal Commission in the 1960s showed that administration would cost less in a public insurance system than in a mainly private system. During the 1970s and 1980s, physicians' groups maintained that doctors only extra-billed patients who could afford to pay, but evidence from Alberta and Ontario showed that at least some doctors were routinely billing patients on welfare.[25] These pieces of evidence, presented in debate after debate, shifted beliefs in the public and even among medicine's senior leadership.[26] Of course, in addition, the Canadian public valued high-quality health care services as a right of citizenship. This translated into strong political support for Medicare.

Health Care System Reform: In Whose Interest?

When it comes to health care *system* reform (in contrast to health *insurance* reform) the situation is very different. There is no strong coalition advocating change. The same repressed interest groups that fought shoulder to shoulder to win public health insurance have had a devil of a time developing a joint agenda for health care system reform. Nurses' organizations and unions representing health care workers have taken strong positions in favour of community care and health promotion, but most of their members still work within institutions and are threatened by the downsizing of hospitals.

Of course, the stakes in the debate are very different for different groups. Consumers have only a diffuse interest in health care reform. For example, only a small percentage of Canadians have surgery in any given year. Even over a lifetime, most of us will (thankfully) experience little surgical intervention. The net result is that most Canadians have no compelling or immediate interest in the overall quality of surgery. Indeed, given its highly technical nature, few people are in a position to judge the quality of surgical care. We just hope it's good.

On the other hand, doctors have a dominant and concentrated interest in any change that might affect their incomes and working conditions. The roughly ten thousand doctors who perform surgery have a clear financial, professional, and personal interest in what form quality assurance programs take. What's more, they have the financial wherewithal and organizational capacity to fight for their interests. Yale University political scientist Professor Ted Marmor has pointed out that concentrated interests, although small in number, can usually overwhelm the diffuse interests in health care, even if the latter are very large in number.[27]

In keeping with the weak-to-nonexistent coalition for reform, Canadians find few policy forums to debate the issues. When doctors complain they need more resources for health care, critics who point out that our current system actually encourages waste and inefficiency don't often get equal air time.

Journalists mirror and influence the public's values and beliefs. Accordingly, reporters tend to think hospitals and doctors manage the health system's resources efficiently. While health policy experts always look for signs of poor management and outdated institutional arrangements as the cause of various health care "crises," journalists, like the public, are more likely to accept the complaints of health care providers at face value.

Sometimes the media refuse to listen, period. For example, in the fall of 1993, an Ontario study showed wide variations in whether breast cancer patients received breast-conserving surgery. During a radio interview, Dr. Tom Dickson, president of the Ontario Medical Association, tried valiantly to clarify that these kinds of variations show up for all kinds of different procedures and tests. But the journalist kept the focus on breast cancer alone, as if the problem was confined to this condition only. As a result, the systemic nature of quality problems in our system remained unaddressed.

Reinventing the Wheel: The Lack of a National Focus for Health Policy

Even when a province comes up with a new way to deliver health care that is better and cheaper, the idea rarely spreads beyond the borders of the province where it originated, according to Professor Leslie Roos of the Manitoba Centre for Health

Policy and Evaluation. Provinces rarely display interest in what their neighbours are doing. For example, Manitoba's immunization registry and British Columbia's Pap smear screening program—two innovations well worth emulating—have not spread across the country.

Dr. Miles Kilshaw is a relaxed, British-trained physician who used to be the vice-president of medicine for the Greater Victoria Hospital Society—a position he ultimately left because his defence of the public's interest made him unpopular with his fellow doctors. Since then, Dr. Kilshaw has acted as a consultant to several provincial governments. In 1992 his study of laboratory services in Saskatchewan traced major inefficiencies to the presence of too many laboratories and too many orders for tests. His report recommended consolidating all laboratory services for the province—a move he estimated would generate a net savings of 20 to 30 percent annually.

While Saskatchewan was mulling over Dr. Kilshaw's report, British Columbia's Ministry of Health appointed him to chair a review of its diagnostic services. Meanwhile, Ontario also set up a task force to investigate lab services. Each of these reviews has different terms of reference, in spite of the fact that most of the issues are similar across the entire country. How much more sensible it would have been to institute a national review of diagnostic services with a panel composed of experts from across the country. That way, each province could strike its own implementation task force after the national report was submitted. A single national inquiry could also serve to heighten awareness of the key issues in the debate and build public support to implement change based on its findings.

When instead, each province does its own thing, we lose the chance to expose the systemic nature of the problems unearthed. This, of course, sets the scene for the dominant interests to prevail. It's much easier to manage several small battles in different locations. In the case of British Columbia, the province's medical association (BCMA) refused to cooperate with the government's inquiry into lab services. Presumably, the BCMA will also oppose any recommendations that might threaten the financial interests of its members. The reason? Could it be that restructuring laboratory services might threaten some BCMA members, who own and make a profit from private labs?

No dough and no show

Since the 1970s, the federal government has steadily withdrawn from the health policy arena. Some analysts point to Marc Lalonde's 1974 report, *A New Perspective on the Health of Canadians*, as the starting point for this retreat. By exposing health care's limited role in determining health status, Lalonde's critique gave Ottawa a good excuse to abdicate its funding responsibility for health care.

In 1984, federal Health Minister Monique Bégin was hoping to introduce new cost-shared programs to foster the development of community services. Her cabinet colleagues, however, rebuffed these overtures. When the Mulroney government came to power later the same year, Ottawa took a meat cleaver to the health care transfer payments.* Ever since, federal leadership in health policy has been compromised. The Conservatives even disdained investigating possible breaches of the Canada Health Act because they didn't want to antagonize the provinces any more than they had already. The provinces aren't interested in federal leadership without money, but even the new Chrétien government seems unlikely to roll back the Mulroney cuts. New federal Health Minister Diane Marleau has hinted that she's interested in a more proactive, Guardian role in policing user fees, for example, but whether Ottawa can retain its moral authority over health care policy without some kind of financial guarantees is an open question.

There's even scant federal support for the Conference of Deputy Ministers of Health. The federal health department does little more than convene their meetings, arrange teleconferences, and supply coffee. There is no permanent secretariat of technical and professional staff.

Expert advice for the conference mainly comes from senior provincial civil servants. These officials already have sixty-hour high-tension work weeks back in their home provinces. Little wonder progress has been slow in most areas.

We think a greater federal presence in health policy is essential. A national strategy for health care system reform could be an enormous help to provinces that are all struggling with the same issues. And it would forestall the increasing balkanization of Canada's

---

* See Chapter 2 for the details of these cuts.

health care. This is something we return to in our final chapter when we examine the politics of health reform in greater detail.

Much Ado about Nothing: Health System Reform, Eh?

In Canada in the 1990s we have witnessed the most severe economic downturn since the Great Depression. In the private sector, industries have been forced to restructure or go under. We wouldn't have a steel industry in Canada today if the major companies had just paid everyone a little less and made a little less steel. The recession forced the sector to re-examine its manufacturing and marketing processes very closely. Some companies decided to retool with more productive technology; others to reorganize work processes to reduce labour costs and boost quality.

So far, the economic recovery has been largely jobless—Canada's gross national product is growing but there are still very high rates of unemployment. The impact on provincial and federal treasuries has been severe.

The consequence for health care policy is no less painful. However, instead of a major restructuring, health reform in Canada has largely confined itself to tinkering around the edges of the system by imposing cutbacks and cost-shifting. The understanding seems to be that the best strategy is to cut everyone just a bit and hope that each hospital or program can handle it by making a few small efficiencies. Because the public does not realize the extent of inappropriate care and wasteful spending in the system, it is likely to view equal cutbacks as the fairest alternative.

In a similar vein, the public is primed to accept decreased eligibility for drug or dental programs, or even a formal rationing exercise, like the one held in Oregon.[28] Most provinces are already having discussions with their medical associations about which services should be dropped from public coverage, forcing the public to consider which patients should be thrown out of the lifeboat. Should it be infertile couples hoping against hope that in vitro fertilization (IVF) will work for them? Should it be people who want cosmetic surgery for disfiguring tattoos? The government and the Ontario Medical Association are fixated on removing whole categories of services, in spite of the fact that almost any service is appropriate for some individual at some time. One deputy minister complained that whenever he asked for advice on more efficiency, all he got back were recommendations to cut services on sex organs (e.g. neonatal circumcision, sterilizations, breast augmentation, testicular prosthetic insertions, etc.).

The organization and funding rules also limit what policies can be implemented, or even contemplated. For example, the Canada Health Act only covers hospital and physicians' services; the provinces cannot allow user fees for these services. But the Act does not apply to publicly funded drug and dental programs, or to a wide range of community services. Because there is no federal restriction against withdrawing public funding from these programs, they are very vulnerable.

Other facets of the system's institutional arrangements protect revenues for physicians and hospitals. Until recently, the provincial budgets for physicians' services were open-ended. The doctors negotiated the *fee* increase, but the overall physicians' budget was obtained by multiplying the fee (the price) times the number of services (volume). Gradually, most provinces have negotiated a total budget for doctors, which sets a ceiling on payments to physicians. But the ceiling also acts as a floor. Despite the recommendations from various health care commissions and inquiries that dollars should be reallocated to health promotion and non-physician services, the budget for doctors in many provinces is now written in stone, off-limits to poachers.

These expert commissions have also recommended shifting dollars from institutions to community services, but once again structural barriers have been getting in the way. There is no mechanism for reallocation. Individual hospitals still have their own budgets, and most provincial health ministries have a separate division for institutions that jealously guards its resource base. Even regional health authorities, where they exist, are reproducing these functional chimneys.

Hospitals: bed cuts and closures

As a result of the above analysis, one would expect the provinces to respond to the fiscal crisis of the 1990s with across-the-board cuts. And, in general, that's what they did.

In Manitoba, the Conservative government of Gary Filmon promised health care reform in 1992. By late 1993 the main reform was to cut hospital funding. There was virtually no reallocation at all.[29] The same story could be told about Nova Scotia, Newfoundland, and most other provinces. A review of health spending by provinces shows little change in the funding patterns over the past six years. (See Figure 8.1.)

In Ontario, 20 percent of hospital beds have been cut since 1986.[30] In Metropolitan Toronto, 30 percent of beds have gone out of service over the same time period. Similar trends are occurring across the country. But few of the resources attached to these acute-care beds are finding their way into the community. According to Almerinda Rebelo, executive director of Toronto's Parkdale Community Health Centre, "Too much money is coming out of the system all at once, and too little is being reallocated to the community to offset the impact."

Retreating from twenty years of party policy, the Rae government in Ontario actually cut back the number of community health centres slated to open, from the six per year planned by the Liberal government of David Peterson to only three. Now the provinces are talking about "magic numbers" for their bed supply. Ontario is aiming for 3.5 acute-care hospital beds for every 1,000 people. British Columbia has targeted 2.75 beds per 1,000. Do these numbers contain some magic property? Obviously not. It's pretty clear that the numbers of beds in a given community should relate to the amount of illness seen in that community and the evidence suggesting that institutional care would improve patient outcomes.

But the "need" for beds also depends heavily on how available alternative sources of care are: areas with less extensive primary and community care will be hard pressed to close beds without causing real harm. The availability of informal care provided by family and friends is another key factor often left out of the equation. As much as 90 percent of all long-term care is provided informally and without compensation, usually by women. Many consumer organizations and unions are warning that the current approach to "health reform" will place an intolerable burden of expectation on families struggling to cope with a loved one's illness or disability.[31]

British Columbia has one of the most extensive and effective home care programs on the continent, a factor that makes it less

Figure 8.1

PROVINCIAL GOVERNMENT HEALTH SPENDING 1987–88 TO 1991–92

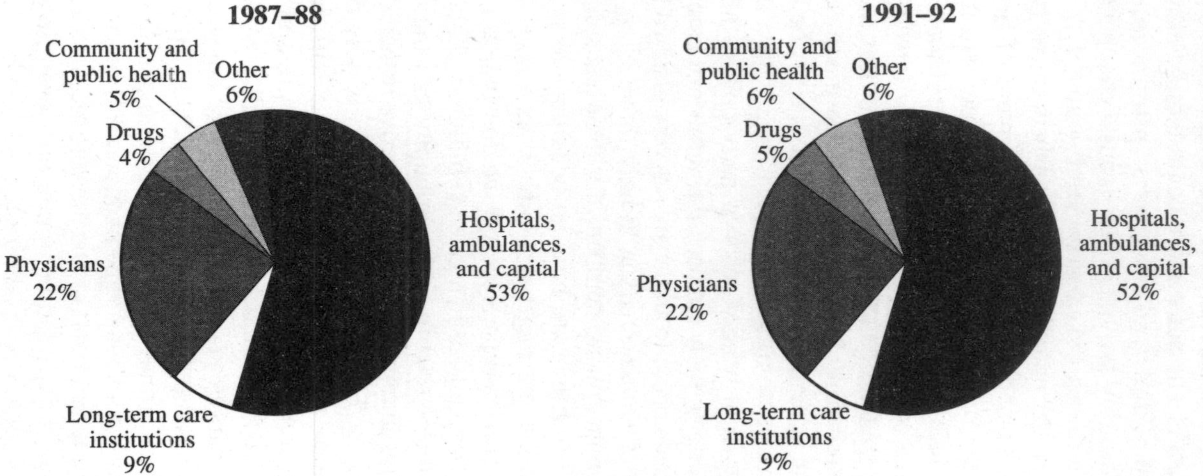

1991–92

Hospitals, ambulances, and capital 52%

Other 6%

Community and public health 6%

Drugs 5%

Physicians 22%

Long-term care institutions 9%

1987–88

Hospitals, ambulances, and capital 53%

Other 6%

Community and public health 5%

Drugs 4%

Physicians 22%

Long-term care institutions 9%

Sources: Self-reports from all provinces except British Columbia.

risky to cut institutional beds there. Indeed, according to the Hospital Medical Records Institute, British Columbia also appears to lead the country in switching to same-day surgery, so patients recover from minor operations at home rather than in the hospital, and receive supports from visiting nurses and homemakers. By contrast, Nova Scotia has been very late in developing these kinds of community care programs. One can expect that sudden bed cuts without reallocation to community services there will create major problems for patients, families, and caregivers.

In fact, however much fat there is in our hospital system, it's a sure bet that it isn't evenly distributed. Historically, more efficient hospitals in our system have been penalized for good management. Indeed, until the mid to late 1980s, hospitals actually had an incentive to run deficits, since they could usually count on provincial governments to bail them out. Hospitals could dramatically boost funding with this strategy. Even though bailouts are no longer allowed, the inequities in base budgets remain. As a result, balancing a reduced budget is easier for some hospitals than it is for others.

In a lot of communities, it makes sense to close a whole hospital rather than impose cuts on each one. In Chapter 2, we noted that many Canadian cities have too many hospitals. The situation is analogous to a company that has several factories all operating below peak capacity. The most efficient solution is usually to close one plant rather than continue to cut production across the board. But few Canadian politicians have had the courage to actually close a hospital.

An exception is Elizabeth Cull, the former minister of health in British Columbia, who managed to pull off this feat when she closed Vancouver's Shaughnessy Hospital in the fall of 1993. Her ministry knew the city of Vancouver had a relative surplus of beds while the high-growth suburban areas needed more. Most of the Shaughnessy Hospital's budget and staff were reallocated to suburban hospitals and community services.

But without effective political leadership, Ministry of Health officials can only squeeze all hospitals and hope the "right" ones give up first. In her address to the 1993 annual meeting of the Ontario Hospital Association, Health Minister Ruth Grier warned that hospital closures in Ontario were very likely, particularly in over-serviced areas. However, she is taking a voluntary approach to the issue, hoping hospitals will offer to close themselves for the good of their communities.

Windsor, Ontario, has been struggling with this issue for more than a year, trying to decide which of four hospitals serving the area should close. The issue is further complicated by the fact that two of the hospitals have religious affiliations; one is owned and operated by a Roman Catholic religious order and one by the Salvation Army. The decision-makers in this process are community volunteers serving on a steering committee. They're trying hard to make the most logical decision and to protect as many jobs as possible, but consensus has been very difficult to achieve. Finally, in February 1994, a plan was brought forward to close two hospitals, but the plan hinges on stakeholders' continued commitment to a complete system-wide reconfiguration.

Donald Schurman, president of the University of Alberta Hospitals in Edmonton, says most administrators nowadays acknowledge the need to close hospitals in Calgary and Edmonton, but individual boards and staff aren't volunteering to be first. Recently Dr. Alan Hudson, president of the Toronto Hospital, suggested that one of the city's hospitals should close, but he certainly didn't offer his own institution as a candidate or finger another for the honour.

While no province except British Columbia has actually closed a big city hospital, small hospitals are another matter. In the summer of 1993, Saskatchewan Health Minister Louise Simard discontinued acute-care funding to fifty-two small rural hospitals. For years, it was known that these facilities—which often had no acute-care patients—were not, and could not function as, true hospitals. They didn't have the volume of patients, the equipment, or the staffing to provide a full range of services. But until the province's finances reached a crisis, these tiny hospitals managed to hang on to political support.

Small hospitals elsewhere in the country will likely close as well. Some, like Ontario's Burke's Falls Hospital, might get transformed into other types of centres, offering, for example, respite care, or giving needed space to community service providers.

Regionalization

Most provincial commissions on health care in the past decade have recommended some form of regionalization or decentralization of provincial control. In a system organized this way, each region would receive all the funds to provide all health care in a particular geographic area. By drawing from an envelope of pooled funding, individual regions could then reallocate resources according to the needs of the population served. In general, this would mean more for health promotion and community services and less for institutions and doctors. Sometimes this pooling of resources is called "vertical integration of funding."

Quebec has had a regional health care system since the early 1970s, and the most recent reforms have strengthened regional autonomy somewhat. However, Quebec has seen little reallocation to community care from the institutional sector, the implication being that regionalization does not necessarily lead to a transfer of resources. The province of New Brunswick wiped out fifty-one separate hospital boards in March 1992 and consolidated hospital governance by creating eight regional boards. Here, too, there has been little movement so far of funds from institutions to community care. Prince Edward Island has also implemented a regional system.

The province of Ontario has been flirting with regionalization for twenty years. The redoubtable Dr. Fraser Mustard, who now directs the Canadian Institute for Advanced Research, headed a task force in 1974 that recommended the devolution of "funding envelopes" to regions. The province used Dr. Mustard's report to create District Health Councils (DHCs), but these are only voluntary planning agencies with no spending authority at all. British Columbia, Nova Scotia, and Alberta all intend to create regional systems, but as of early 1994, the key issues (roles, governance, funding) remain fuzzy.

So far, only Saskatchewan has moved ahead with a system-wide regionalization plan. By October 1993, the province had established thirty health districts that cover the southern part of the province. Districts for Regina, Saskatoon, and Prince Albert were set up first in 1991 and 1992. Today, each district receives the funds for all health care services except drugs and doctors, and has considerable discretion over how to spend these resources. Already some districts have plans to consolidate acute care in one facility, long-term care in another, and to close other facilities in the district and use the freed-up resources to fund community programs.

Paying doctors

There is considerable evidence that fee-for-service payment hikes costs without producing benefits for patients. The fee schedule penalizes doctors (especially family doctors) who want to practise high-quality medicine and makes it difficult for them to be effective members of multi-disciplinary teams. Government commissions have long recommended the community health centre model as the basic building block for the health care system—a model that encompasses team-based delivery and salaried doctors.

Nevertheless, despite these recommendations, most doctors today are paid on fee-for-service and do not work in group practices. The only exception is Quebec, where CLSCs (*centres locaux des services communautaires*) operating throughout the province offer a well-established alternative. Today, about 10 percent of all Quebec family doctors work in CLSCs, and as of 1993, doctors in private practice with less than ten years' experience must agree to work a minimum number of hours each week in a CLSC or emergency department.[32]

Other provinces, however, have balked at introducing new arrangements for doctors. In fact, new contracts with provincial medical associations appear to make reform even more difficult. Ontario got off to a bad start in 1991 when the province negotiated a disastrous deal with the Ontario Medical Association. The contract gave the OMA the right to veto any movement of funds from the overall budget for doctors to non-fee-for-service practice, *even if the doctors paid on fee-for-service wanted to change how they were paid.* The 1991 agreement also established a new Joint Management Committee (JMC), with membership from the OMA and the Ministry of Health. The deal appears to give the OMA veto rights over any policy change that might affect doctors. In 1993, as Ontario began to consider major reforms in primary care, the government's new agreement with the OMA specifically said that the JMC would decide such policy. One can imagine the limitations likely to be imposed.

Spreading like measles, an identical agreement was signed in Nova Scotia (1992) and similar ones were inked in Newfoundland

(1991), Alberta (1992), British Columbia (1993), and Manitoba (1994). The most serious problem with these committees or commissions is the fact that they meet behind closed doors and hide the decision-making process. Even Michael Decter, Ontario's former deputy minister of health and one of the JMC's chief architects, admits that the JMC has "hardly been a hotbed of reform."[33] We agree.

Nurses and workers: picking up the pieces of health care reform

Approximately 75 percent of hospital budgets are for personnel, meaning you can't make deep cuts all at once without laying off employees. Without a careful strategy to reallocate budgets and redeploy personnel to community services, nurses and hospital workers end up on the street. And that's exactly what has been happening. As of April 1993, over ten thousand nurses had been laid off and nearly twenty thousand other hospital workers were collecting unemployment insurance.[34]

In the meantime, the nurses who still have jobs are run off their feet. Vera Chernecki, president of the Manitoba Nurses Union, claims that the budget cuts have made it even more difficult to provide good patient care. The union documented 230 cases in which it claimed patients had been put at risk in the first year of the "reform" process.

Mental health reform

Over the years our system for dealing with mental illness has changed substantially. In 1964, Justice Hall's Royal Commission recommended that the provinces should transfer patients from provincial psychiatric hospitals to the general hospital system. As a result, the number of beds in psychiatric hospitals in Canada fell by two-thirds between 1960 and 1976.[35] Even though the general hospitals did increase their supply of psychiatric beds, the overall number of psychiatric beds fell by 27,000. Unfortunately, the resources freed up were never transferred to community care, leaving many patients on their own and without support.

Dr. Tyrone Turner, chief of psychiatry at the Doctors' Hospital in Toronto, says that Medicare in Canada facilitated a massive shift of resources from "the neediest to the squeakiest." As support for provincial psychiatric hospitals dried up, more and more psychiatrists and family doctors began setting up lucrative psychotherapy practices. The psychiatric hospitals used to treat people with severe mental illness—caused, for example, by schizophrenia or head injuries—but psychotherapists mainly see the "worried well," people who, despite their social or psychological problems, are usually able to work and function in society.

Today, Ontario offers the most generous coverage for traditional Freudian psychoanalysis in North America. Patients receiving this type of psychotherapy have to see the analyst nearly every day for years, at a cost of over $20,000 a year each. Meanwhile a family with a schizophrenic child who's addicted to cocaine is told that there are no services available. A survey of the homeless in most Canadian cities would reveal large numbers of seriously ill psychiatric patients with no access to treatment and no homes to go to.

All told, Ontario pays doctors over $300 million each year for psychotherapy at $90 per hour. There is no evidence that physicians are better at psychotherapy than social workers or psychologists. Either of these professions could do the same job for far less money.

Over the years many experts have recommended pooled funding for mental health, just as other commissions have called for pooled funding for physical health programs. The intention is the same—pool existing resources for community and institutional care and then pay out according to needs. New Brunswick is the only province to do so, however, through a provincial mental health commission and four regional boards that plan and fund programs. The provincial board has representatives from professionals, consumers (patients), and their families.[36]

Still Muddling, Not Yet Through

Earlier in this chapter we talked about a seminal article by Yale professor Charles Lindblom called "The Science of Muddling Through." In it he concludes that fundamental changes in policy are rare because the focus of most policy analysis is on minor, incremental adjustments (branch analysis) rather than on radical alterations (root analysis). In 1979, Lindblom revisited this original article, then twenty years old, with a new piece called "Still Muddling, Not Yet Through."[37] His explanation of incrementalism's resilience calls to mind the positions taken by any number of Canadian health policy decision-makers: "Of course we know we should be moving faster (approaching reform more comprehensively, dealing with big problems instead of little ones, etc.), but we are doing all we can *in the current circumstances*."

We mean no disrespect to the people working in Ministries of Health and health organizations across the country. These people have very hard jobs that have become even harder in recent years. However, we think that their jobs would become less onerous and more interesting if their political masters could only engineer a few key policy breakthroughs. Incrementalism won't work. Without major change to the rules for funding and organizing health care we simply cannot create the kind of system experts have been recommending for years.

However, one thing is certain: the status quo is no longer tenable. Unless our system becomes more responsive to people's real needs, Medicare will be jettisoned like an expensive kitchen machine that can't be made to slice tomatoes. A little more political know-how and a little less muddling could deliver us from policy gridlock into the promised land of health care reform.

Chapter 9

New Rules, New Roles:
Reforming the System

THOMAS C. IS AN EIGHTY-SEVEN-YEAR-OLD man who lives in the North Beach area of San Francisco. Mr. C. came to America just after the First World War to work in his uncle's laundry. He eventually ran his own grocery store in San Francisco's China-town, married, and raised a family. But his children moved to Los Angeles when they grew up, and his wife died ten years ago. Mr. C. managed to get by on his own for a while but in 1990 a stroke partially paralyzed him and left him with a speech deficit.

When the hospital social worker discussed Mr. C.'s discharge with him and his son Michael, she presented two options. Mr. C. could enter a nursing home with all the costs of his care covered by government.* Or he could stay in his own apartment above his old store and join the On Lok Seniors' Health Services. Mr. C. chose On Lok.

The Cantonese words "on lok geui" mean "abode of peace and happiness," and the name reflects the philosophy of this program. On Lok Seniors' Health Services opened its non-profit operation for the "frail elderly" in 1973 with a day health

---

* Mr. C. qualified for both the U.S. Medicare program (because he was over sixty-five years old) and the Medicaid program (because he lives far enough below the poverty line). In the United States, Medicare pays hospital and medical service costs for the elderly. Medicaid provides coverage for the poor of all ages.

centre located in a renovated downtown nightclub. Today, from three such centres, On Lok serves 325 high-risk seniors, with an average age of eighty-three.

On Lok gives Mr. C. some services in his own home, but four days each week he is picked up by a van and taken to the day centre, where he can eat a nutritious lunch, do some Tai Chi, and enjoy the company of friends over a game of cards. His blood pressure and general medical condition are checked regularly there by his On Lok doctor and nurse-practitioner. These centres are the hub of On Lok's programming; all of their participants must agree to come in to one of them at least once a week. Most choose to come more often, on average three times a week.

Clients at On Lok are very frail. To participate, applicants must be over fifty-five and be judged by a state assessor to need nursing-home-level care. Three-quarters of On Lok's participants are incontinent and 63 percent have some type of chronic mental disturbance, including Alzheimer's disease. In addition, many are at special risk because of poverty and isolation. Like Mr. C., 60 percent of On Lok participants live alone, and 40 percent are poor enough to qualify for Supplemental Security Income (SSI). Many of those who belong to On Lok are Chinese (75 percent), although Filipinos, Italians, other Caucasians, and Blacks also use its services.

About a year into the program, Mr. C. developed diabetes, but careful attention to his physical activity and diet (with the assistance of a Chinese-speaking dietician) has generally allowed good diabetic control without the use of additional medications. Recently, however, Mr. C.'s diabetes became uncontrolled while he had the flu and he spent two days in one of On Lok's transitional apartments, where he was given intravenous insulin and fluids and monitored very closely until the crisis passed.

Health promotion is the centrepiece of On Lok's programming. To stay healthy, everyone needs proper nutrition, exercise, and socialization. These are even more important for the frail elderly. Regular attendance at the day centre by participants means the staff have frequent opportunities to monitor their clients and catch problems early, before they become so serious they require hospital care. This monitoring is a key factor in preventing acute flare-ups of chronic conditions.

Another important distinguishing characteristic of On Lok is the multidisciplinary team in each day centre: doctors, nurse-practitioners, nurses, social workers, audiologists, podiatrists, physiotherapists, speech therapists, and drivers work very closely together. A doctor from On Lok is always available to the program participants and their families; the program has two salaried, full-time physicians as well as two half-time doctors for night call. The teams meet frequently, and each member plays a valuable role. For example, On Lok works very closely with clients and families to develop a "health wish"—a kind of "living will." On Lok's founder and executive director, Marie-Louise Ansak, says that many times it is the program's drivers who know about the participants' desires for care should they fall acutely ill. Just as a stranger will often open up more readily to a taxi driver, some of On Lok's clients turn to their drivers to engage in this kind of weighty discussion. This is just one way in which the drivers have come to be key members of the team.

Unlike a nursing home in Canada, On Lok is not confined to using all of its revenues for institutional care. The program can use its resources in whatever way seems most appropriate to meeting a participant's needs. In other words, the program has the ability to conduct zero-based planning for health and social services. Funding is *attached to the person* rather than to any specific institution, community service agency, or program.

On Lok has taken full advantage of this flexibility. The program uses only 16 percent of its budget for institutional services, including acute hospital care. More than half of its resources go to home care and day programming.

For nearly twenty years, On Lok has operated in the black. On Lok's lowest wages are 50 percent higher than minimum wage, and all workers have generous benefits that include full health care coverage (worth $2 to $3 per hour for California workers). The staff turnover is less than 5 percent per year. The California government pays On Lok 95 percent of what it would have paid a nursing home for care of its participants through the U.S. Medicare and Medicaid programs. In the 1990-91 fiscal year, On Lok spent approximately $2,500 (U.S.) a month ($83 per day) for each program participant. This is about what a nursing home in Ontario receives for ward care. However, On Lok either directly provides or pays for long-term community care, medical care,

prescription drugs, nursing home care, *and* acute hospital services. In other words, the program is at full financial risk—once
a person has joined On Lok, the program is completely responsible for the cost of the individual's care for the rest of his or her
life. No one can be cut off from coverage. Participants can drop
out at any time, but only 2 percent ever do so. The other 98 percent eventually die within the program.

On Lok's record of success speaks for itself. On any given
day, only 6 percent of its participants are in an institution: 5
percent in a nursing home and 1 percent in an acute-care hospital. Only the most demented and/or incapacitated are placed in
nursing homes. As for acute care, On Lok has managed to
nearly eliminate hospitalizations due to flare-ups from chronic
conditions. What *can* be prevented by health care *is* being prevented by health care.

When you compare On Lok's 6 percent institutionalization
rate for such frail, elderly people to Canada's record, where at
least 16 percent of *all people over seventy-five* are in institutions, you can see that the scope for improvement in Canada is
very large indeed.[1]

Right now, this kind of service package is impossible in
Canada because of present organizational and financing rules.
In our system, we generally do not fund services unless they are
provided by a doctor or by someone working in an institution,
such as a hospital or nursing home. We have no way of pooling
all the resources for nurses, doctors, drugs, social workers, labs,
hospitals, and nursing homes and spending where the needs are.
The vast majority of the spending in Canada's system for the
frail elderly goes to institutional, pharmaceutical, and medical
services, not community care.

The On Lok program is limited to middle-aged and older persons with chronic disease, the types of patients responsible for a
majority of overall health care costs. As Canada's population
ages, this is a model of health care delivery that we should be
looking at very closely. On Lok does have some critics, however, and no doubt some features (like its charismatic executive
director) cannot be duplicated easily,[2] but there has been a randomized controlled trial in the Bronx that has confirmed the On
Lok model's superiority over conventional long-term care.[3]
Besides, we are convinced that the On Lok program has features

that could vastly improve *any* health care delivery system, including ours:

- The care provided is based on patients' and families' informed choices.
- The services are delivered by multidisciplinary teams, which are less hierarchical than traditional models of health care delivery. As much as possible, the team member delivering any specific service is determined by objective evidence of cost-effectiveness.
- The doctors have clear collective responsibility for their tasks. The physicians are not paid primarily on fee-for-service.
- Services that promote health and prevent disease, including self-help and mutual aid, have a very high priority.
- The various levels in the delivery system (e.g. primary, secondary, tertiary) are integrated in that their financing comes from the same source. The dollars are attached to *persons*, not *services*.

The question is, how can we use these key features to reinvent Canada's health care system? How would we go about creating a more responsive and more efficient system?

Transforming Health Care's Rules

The first step in rebuilding our health care system is to change the rules that govern how it is organized and financed. In political science jargon, these rules are sometimes called "institutional arrangements." As the rules change, so will the roles of the various players in the system. More than anything else, that's what this chapter is about. New rules, new roles, and some new tools—all are needed to make Canada's health care system the best in the world.

Defining roles: Guardians and Traders

Jane Jacobs's discussion of Guardians and Traders is pertinent in deciding on the appropriate roles for government and the private sector in a reformed health care system. You will recall that Jacobs describes two basic ways humans make their living—taking and trading—and that each has its own separate and distinct moral system.*

Governments, by definition, must maintain and protect territory, so our provincial governments are stuck with their Guardian role. They can't change it any more than a leopard can change its spots. But health care is much more of a Trader activity. At their best, health care delivery organizations are innovative, efficient, and open to making changes.

For example:

- A program to get hospital patients up and about more quickly after heart surgery was first implemented in Oxford, England, in 1992. The Toronto Hospital tried this program with 130 patients in a three-week pilot project in May 1993 and demonstrated savings of about $3,000 per patient. On June 2, 1993, the hospital announced the program as a new policy.[4]
- In 1989, the Vancouver General Hospital saved over $100,000 when it substituted one antibiotic regime for another.[5] A careful evaluation showed no disadvantages to the new policy.

Too often, health care organizations are blocked from innovation by the inappropriate intrusion of Guardian values into their regulation. For example, a recent U.S. Veterans' Administration study showed that substituting frequent telephone calls for clinic visits with chronically ill middle-aged men reduced health care costs by 28 percent.[6] Such a program couldn't happen in most parts of Canada. Almost all our family doctors are paid on fee-for-service and can't bill for phone calls. As a result, most avoid telephone communication with patients. In fact, in the American study, nurses made a lot of these calls. However, because we largely finance health care through doctors and hospitals, we find few nurses in primary care settings.

---

* For a complete listing of Guardian and Trader values as outlined in Jane Jacobs's book, *Systems of Survival: A Dialogue on the Moral Foundation of Commerce and Politics*, see Chapter 1.

In our view, health care delivery in Canada needs to be much more entrepreneurial.* But if this is going to happen, the system's institutions and providers will have to give up some cherished Guardian values that interfere with progress. For example, in order to respond quickly to changes, the delivery system cannot adhere to tradition. It is tradition—often bolstered by strict laws and funding rules—that prevents nurses, midwives, and other health professionals from practising to their full potential in most parts of Canada. Other Guardian values—obedience, discipline, and respect for hierarchy—also hinder efficiency.

The health care system is intensely hierarchical. The typical hospital organization chart reveals layer upon layer of supervisory and management staff. Doctors give "orders" to nurses, who are expected to obey and carry them out. Nurses often have to twist themselves into knots trying to advise doctors about the right course for patients, all the while making the doctor think the ideas were his own.[7] There is some evidence that a strict hierarchical relationship and ensuing poor communication between doctors and other providers can compromise the quality of care provided.[8]

To break free of this paralysis, we need health care delivery organizations with strong Trader values. For their part, the provincial governments should maximize the positive aspects of their Guardian role by clarifying the goals of health care programs and by creating an environment that promotes innovation.

Reinventing Government's Role in Health Care

Recently a number of philosophy-of-government "star trekkers"—boldly going where no government has gone before—have called for redesigning the interface between the public and private sectors. Leading the current "away team" are Americans David Osborne and Ted Gaebler. Their book, *Re-inventing Government: How the Entrepreneurial Spirit is Transforming the Public Sector,*[9] takes a fresh look at how a government can create

---

* This does not, however, imply a for-profit system. In fact, some of the most successful entrepreneurs work in the not-for-profit sector.

an entrepreneurial environment at the level of service delivery. Since that seems be exactly what Canada's health care system needs, their advice is highly relevant to the reforms we propose.

One of Osborne and Gaebler's central points is that governments are too often tempted to "row" when they should really confine themselves to "steering." To Osborne and Gaebler, "steering" means setting priorities and monitoring their achievement within a democratic process (a Guardian activity). "Rowing" means organizing the production of a given range of goods and services (a Trader activity). Osborne and Gaebler are certainly not anti-government, nor are they particularly conservative in their views. In fact, some of their advice—for example, their recommendation for a comprehensive labour adjustment strategy—comes from the left wing of the political spectrum. But regardless of political stripe, all governments today realize that there are limits on what they can accomplish directly. There is a growing consensus that they need to focus more on policy direction, leaving program delivery to others.

What this means for health care is that provincial governments should set clear goals and monitor progress towards them, but let other agencies at arm's-length provide the services.

There are two major challenges to fulfilling these role assignments: constructing goals so that they really do steer health care services, and choosing rules that will maximize the Trader aspects of the delivery system.

Moving towards regionalization

One way to radically change our institutional arrangements is to switch from a model of health care funding based on institutions to one organized geographically by region. We talked about this briefly in Chapter 8, in our discussion of reforms in Saskatchewan and New Brunswick. This change would make it much easier to transfer resources from institutions to community care, and by doing so come much closer to matching real needs.[10]

Quebec set up a regional approach to health care delivery in the early 1970s when it first implemented public health insurance. Regionalization has been suggested by a number of Canadian government reports over the past decade, and it is being implemented to varying degrees in Prince Edward Island, Nova Scotia, New Brunswick, Saskatchewan, Alberta, and British

Columbia. Even Ontario plans to try it in its long-term-care reform. Various other countries, too, have regional approaches to planning, managing, or funding services, including Denmark, Finland, and the United Kingdom.[11] In fact, Lord Dawson of Penn proposed a regional organization of services for Britain as far back as the 1920s.[12]

One impediment to regionalization is the issue of accountability. The provinces are happy to pass along responsibility to the regions, but *not* authority. Provincial officials like to retain the power to micromanage the system when it suits them. That's because provincial politicians and bureaucrats always worry that if they relinquish authority, they will still be held responsible for any problems that occur. The prospect of tough questions from the Opposition in the legislature provides ample motivation for them to keep a tight grip on the reins of power. In fact, fear of political fallout is a key factor in understanding why provinces tend to keep the overall goals for the health care system very vague and why they continually interfere with local decision-making.* This clinging to power will always be a major factor influencing the development and implementation of regional funding.

In brief, reasons for favoring regionalization are as follows:

- Decisions will be made closer to the action. Mistakes will be discovered earlier and can be corrected without needing to wait for approval from some central authority—in this case, the province.
- It provides a basis for pooling resources and a mechanism for reallocation.
- It reduces complexity by limiting the number of stakeholders and establishments that have to be dealt with.
- It expands the chances for public participation.

---

* For example, it took the Ontario Ministry of Health four years to allow one southern Ontario community to shut four in-patient psychiatric beds and use the money for out-patient programming.

Steering the System: Performance Indicators for Health Care Delivery

Over the past five years or so, setting goals for health and the health care system has caught on with provincial governments. Ontario, New Brunswick, Nova Scotia, and Quebec have all published a set of provincial health goals,[13] and British Columbia and Saskatchewan are due to announce theirs in 1994.

The problem is that most of the health goals developed so far provide almost no direction when it comes to health care delivery. Most goals refer to traditional health status measures, such as life expectancy, illness rates, or death rates from specific diseases. These kinds of goals are important Guardian objectives related to protecting the public's health. However, formal health care services have only a tenuous relationship to many of these traditional indicators, such as the rate of low-birthweight infants* and death rates from cancer and heart disease.[14] As you'll remember from Chapter 3, major improvements in these measures usually result from changes in society's values and institutions and often require governmental Guardian activity (e.g. smoking bans, food and agriculture policies). Because formal health care services have relatively little impact on these health status goals, the goals provide little direction on how services should be organized and managed. And they are no more helpful when it comes to evaluating improvements in health care delivery. That's why provinces also need to set specific objectives that reflect what the health care system *ought* to accomplish. Developing "system-sensitive" health goals would provide clear direction to regions and local communities about specific programs to target for improvement. These same goals could then also function as performance indicators, allowing communities and regions to chart their progress. By establishing appropriate indicators for the health care system, the provincial government would be fulfilling its Guardian/steering role—in essence, setting out expectations.

---

* Prenatal care does have some impact on reducing low-birthweight rates, but this impact is dwarfed by social and economic influences such as the rate of teenage pregnancy, nutrition, education, smoking, family support, etc.

The kind of indicators we propose come in two varieties.[15] First are the population-based indicators, which relate to the performance of the health care system at a community level. Second are provider-based indicators, which relate directly to the performance of individual caregivers, such as hospitals, community health centres, and nursing homes.

Population-based indicators

Population-based indicators use the whole community (neighbourhood, city, province) as the basis for measurement. These indicators relate to the overall performance of the health care system rather than any specific component.

Some historical precedents might help you understand how these indicators can be used. For example, in the 1930s, New York City developed maternal mortality committees to investigate the deaths of women during pregnancy.[16] When a maternal death occurred, all the particulars of the case were presented to a committee of respected obstetricians. The committee focused on identifying and correcting flaws in the system—the failure of public health services, emergency services, obstetrical services, and so on—rather than singling out individual service providers for blame and punishment. Partly as a result of the committee's work, New York's maternal mortality rate fell dramatically, and policies implemented by the committee were swiftly picked up by other jurisdictions.

Another example comes from the investigation of airplane crashes and near misses. Investigators often go beyond the actual event itself to consider matters of airplane design, manufacture, maintenance, and operation. Again, the main focus is not to identify a single culprit, but to find and correct system and process flaws. For example, the investigation of the Dryden Air Ontario crash in the 1980s led to international policy changes requiring aircraft de-icing to prevent future tragedies.

In 1976, Dr. David Rutstein of Harvard suggested assessing the overall quality of health care by calculating the death rates from conditions that *should* be amenable to treatment by health services.[17] Subsequently, other investigators have modified the list of conditions and suggested further refinements.[18]

With this in mind, what does a population-based health care performance indicator look like? Examples include vaccine-preventable illness, amputation rates among diabetics, hospitalizations for people with chronic illness that should be controlled in the community (asthma, diabetes, heart disease), as well as deaths from cervical cancer, tuberculosis, acute respiratory infections, Hodgkins Disease, and hypertensive disease. A well-organized and effective health care system can have a major impact on these kinds of outcomes. Our enthusiasm for focusing on the broader determinants of health should not distract us from this important message. Measuring these indicators systematically would provide us with a good basis for identifying our system's strengths and weaknesses.

Provider-based health care performance indicators

Provider-based indicators relate to the performance of specific individuals or institutions measured against the caseload of the provider or facility. Procedural complication rates and death rates for individual surgeons or hospitals are an example. But this type of indicator could also be developed for primary care practices. These would look at patient outcome measures to determine, for example, whether there's been good control of hypertension and diabetes, how high the hospitalization rates are for persons with chronic illness, and also whether some key preventive care measures are being provided according to recommended schedules. For an example of the latter, the Canadian Task Force on the Periodic Health Exam makes recommendations for preventive care according to the age, sex, and health status of patients seen. An indicator to measure performance would calculate what percentage of patients who should have received a specific service actually received it.

How should indicators be selected?

Several criteria should guide the selection of a set of health care system performance indicators:

1. Indicators should relate to important health care problems.
2. There should be strong evidence linking system performance with the indicator.

3. Together, the indicators should span the spectrum of health care delivery, from preventive to curative, from primary to tertiary, and from cradle to grave.
4. Indicators should be relatively simple and inexpensive to measure reliably and validly.*
5. Indicators should be easily understood by the public as being relevant to health and helpful in choosing a caregiver, community service, hospital, or nursing home.
6. Indicators should measure both input (what was done) and outcome (how the patient fared as a result), with an emphasis on the latter. Indicators that measure structural variables, such as the availability of equipment or specific types of personnel, are not as relevant to system performance.
7. Indicators should include measures of patient satisfaction.

How does Canada measure up?

Over the past six years, Dr. Terry Montague of the University of Alberta Hospitals in Edmonton has shown how performance indicators can drive quality improvement. Since the 1970s, a host of new and potentially effective treatments for heart attack have emerged. Since the late 1980s, increasing international cooperation in large-scale clinical trials has allowed us to compare the effectiveness of many of these alternatives. However, the results of this research have not been incorporated uniformly into practice.[19]

When Dr. Montague arrived in Edmonton from Halifax in 1988, he wanted to create a network of physicians who managed patients with heart disease in western Canada. He visited doctors from Winnipeg to Vancouver to Yellowknife and back. Gradually, they became convinced that it would make a lot of sense if they all collected the same standard data on patients and got together regularly to review their performance. In 1993, Dr. Montague's network encompassed ten hospitals, and it's still growing.

---

* Reliable measurements are those that show little variation, while valid measurements are those that approximate the truth. A measurement might be very reliable without being valid (e.g. using a yardstick that is only thirty inches long), but in general the two run together.

In Edmonton, Dr. Montague used a key provider-based indicator—the death rate from heart attack—to motivate his hospital to improve quality of care. For example, data from 1987 showed that heart attack victims over seventy years of age had much higher death rates than younger patients. The hospital's poor performance on this indicator spurred Dr. Montague to look for an explanation. His subsequent investigation showed that older patients were much less likely to receive effective treatments. After appropriate feedback of this data to his colleagues, a greater proportion of older patients began getting the right drugs and their death rates fell by half—from 35 percent in 1987 to 19 percent in 1990.[20]

Like Dr. Bill McLeod, who spearheaded the drive to reduce the rate of inappropriate Caesarean sections in Windsor, Dr. Montague is really acting as a local opinion leader—encouraging others to use key health care performance indicators and to take action to address flaws in the system.

Until quite recently, Canada, along with the rest of the world, has ignored the potential of health care system performance indicators. Reforms to Britain's National Health Service were supposed to incorporate them, but so far they measure only inputs, not outcomes.[21] Even so-called clinical indicators measure structure (how many nurses? is there a fridge for medications? etc.) and process (admission rates, waiting times, etc.) rather than patient outcomes,[22] although Finland did use blood pressure measurements and diabetic control to assess their primary health care reforms. [23]

The real centre of action on health care performance indicators is in the United States. Since 1988, a group led by Dr. Albert Siu of the Rand Corporation has been working with a number of health care delivery organizations and insurance companies to develop system-sensitive quality of care indicators.[24] Together they set up the HMO Quality of Care Consortium in an attempt to spark competition on the basis of quality in the U.S. health care marketplace. Canada may have a different financing arrangement for health care, but we believe that the criteria for establishing indicators, and most of the indicators themselves, are readily transportable to this country.

In fact, the process has already begun:

- In 1991, Dr. Clyde Hertzman from the University of British Columbia authored a report for the British Columbia Royal Commission on Health Care and Costs. His analysis showed that death rates from treatable causes varied nearly threefold in different areas of the province.[25]
- In 1992, the Hospital Medical Records Institute (HMRI)* produced a report that, among other things, showed the variation across the country for a variety of procedures and services in fiscal year 1991–92.[26] For example, only 23 percent of women with breast cancer in St. John's, Newfoundland, have breast-conserving surgery, compared to 68 percent of women in Ottawa. The rate of births by Caesarean section varied from 13 percent in London, Ontario, to 25 percent in Victoria, British Columbia.

Changing the Structure of Primary Care

Once government has established its health care system goals, the responsibility for attaining them passes to the regions and communities, where health care delivery takes place. This raises several questions. How can the provincial government make sure that care providers and the organizations where they work behave like Traders? How can it be certain that innovative health care delivery systems will actually get created? We recommend two key tactics:

1. Give primary care centres the funding for primary health care (including primary social services and dental care) as well as for drugs, lab services, secondary, and some tertiary care.**

---

* The HMRI is being phased into the newly created Canadian Institute for Health Information.

** Primary care centres would receive funding for drugs and lab services that are relevant and appropriate to primary and secondary care. Resources for more sophisticated diagnostic tools and medications would be excluded.

2.   Foster competition between different publicly funded primary care centres based on quality of care and service.

To create a new delivery system, we think it is essential for the budgets of hospitals and community services to be linked. One way to integrate budgets would be to fund regional boards and allow them complete flexibility in deciding how much funding to pass along to different organizations at different levels within the system.

We favour a different option, however—one we think is more likely to result in the radical changes our delivery system needs. In this option, all the funding for primary, secondary, and even some tertiary care—as well as long-term care, drugs, and lab services—would be linked to patients (using a per-capita funding arrangement), and most of it would be under the direct control of primary care centres via patients who choose to receive their services there. Under these rules, primary care centres would pay for most other health services directly.

Britain recently made changes of this sort when it altered the funding rules for the National Health Service. In their reform, general practices with enough patients can qualify to become "fundholders." Fundholding practices are owned by the GP partners who receive capitation payments for primary care, drugs, x-rays, lab tests, and some elective specialty care.* The practices are somewhat protected because the National Health Service pays any costs beyond $10,000 per year for any individual patient. Fundholders can shift resources between budget categories but cannot use surpluses as profit. As a result, some income for specialists and hospitals now depends on how well they serve general practitioners and their patients.

And what a change this brought! Suddenly, the traditional medical hierarchy was turned on its head. GPs, who regularly complained about the great difficulty of arranging service from specialists and who were often left out of the communications

---

* Unfortunately, the capitation payments have not been adjusted for individual patient needs leading to complaints that they are too rich for practices with well-to-do healthy patients.

loop, now have specialists and hospitals courting them with offers of better service. For example, new specialty clinics held on-site at GPs' offices have begun to spring up, providing more convenience to patients and better continuity of care. Hospital clinics now fax test results and consultation reports to the GP, providing real-time communications relevant to the family doctors' plans to follow up their patients' conditions. These and other tangible improvements point to the unleashing of a new entrepreneurial spirit—brought about by a change in funding rules.

Here in Canada, some family doctors would like to adopt Britain's system of primary care. But we think that a model built exclusively on private practice GPs is too narrow. It doesn't give citizens or other health providers much of a chance to contribute to planning services.

Other people think our system should only fund non-profit, board-governed community health centres, but this is also problematic. Some community health centres are highly entrepreneurial and would likely thrive under the new funding rules. But others show much less Trader instinct and would probably display even less if there were no competing alternatives.

Competition in primary health care

What we offer instead is a hybrid model with an element of competition, at least in the vast majority of the country with sufficient population density to allow it.[27] In this model, each community would have at least one community health centre, but almost all would also have privately sponsored clinics. For example, there would be one community health centre for every 5,000 to 50,000 people. Depending on the community, several other community health centres and private clinics could also be in operation, but any primary care centre would have to satisfy provincial criteria for a licence, including:

- a demonstrated ability to deliver a full range of primary care services, including medical, nursing, social work, pharmaceutical, dental, psychological services, and other mandatory areas of professional practice;
- a clear strategy for meeting the system performance indicators set by the province;
- proof of ability to provide (directly or through contracts)

specialist care, laboratory services, hospital care, and nursing home services; and
- a willingness to abide by the provincial health care labour code.

Some rural and sparsely populated, remote communities would probably only need one primary care centre, and for them we suggest a community health centre.

Gaebler and Osborne make the point that when embarking upon publicly financed competition, it is often important to ensure that the public providers don't get "low-balled" out of existence. The term refers to the possibility that private contractors might initially provide good service at a good price but then quickly demand more money when there are no longer any public competitors left in the marketplace. That's one reason we recommend that there be at least one community health centre in each community—to ensure a "public" infrastructure and guarantee that the neediest patients always have a source of care.

In fact, in our model, CHCs would also be responsible for clinical occupational health services and community health promotion. The former would involve both preventive, diagnostic and treatment services for individuals, as well as consulting services to local industries and businesses. Despite the limitations of community health promotion presented in Chapter 3, we nevertheless believe that CHCs are in an ideal position to raise awareness in the local community about the broad determinants of health and to initiate action where appropriate. For example, Montreal's CLSC Notre Dame de Grâce proved to be a very effective advocate for a group of low-income tenants whose living arrangements were going to be massively disrupted by a large-scale redevelopment of their housing.[28] Toronto's South Riverdale Community Health Centre mobilized community action against lead pollution, culminating in the province's decision to remove and replace soil from a thousand households.[29]

In the system we propose, individuals would have to register and receive their care from a single primary care facility—except, of course, in emergencies or when they were away from home. People would have complete freedom to enroll with another centre whenever they wanted, but at any given point in time, they could be enrolled at only one centre.

Publicly financed competition in health care is already well established in some European countries. Drawing on experience there, policy analysts Richard Saltman and Casten von Otter identify the following criteria:

1. Public finance
2. Patient choice of primary care facility
3. Budgeting tied to market share.

All modes of primary care would rely primarily on public funding, although small amounts of funding would also come from workers compensation boards, insurance companies, etc. However, the total amount received by any centre would depend on the number of patients on the roster, and what kinds of illnesses and risks for illness they faced.

Probably the fairest way to allocate funds is to use a capitation payment, adjusted to reflect the need for care. As mentioned in Chapter 6, professors Stephen Birch and John Eyles and their colleagues at McMaster University have developed a formula for funding health care according to needs.[30] The McMaster group uses the standardized mortality ratio (SMR) for people aged zero to sixty-four to adjust per-capita funding for a region. The SMR is the death rate (adjusted for age and sex) in a particular community compared to the provincial average. Scotland uses this method to allocate hospital funds in their system.[31] Manitoba researcher Professor Noralou Roos and her colleagues recently suggested a socio-economic risk index to adjust per-capita payments.[32] Saskatchewan partly converted its districts to needs-based funding in 1994, and Alberta and British Columbia are also investigating the concept.

Mental health and public health inspection services would be exempt from this funding because we are concerned that without explicit protection these areas would always be underfunded.* And there are other reasons why these service areas logically fall

---

* This should not be misinterpreted to mean that a capitated mental health system is out of the question. On the contrary, all we are doing here is flagging the need to protect this mental health funding from primary and acute care poaching.

under the region's responsibility. For one thing, both types of services seem to align better with Guardian activities in that they are related to issues of public protection. Consumers of mental health services are particularly vulnerable to exploitation and would not necessarily be better served in a more competitive system.

As economist Robert Evans points out, it's impossible to push the balloon in one place without creating a bulge somewhere else. And our preferred model also creates some bulges—some practical problems to overcome. For example, capitated primary care centres would have an incentive to "cream skim"—each centre would be tempted to enroll the healthiest patients and shift responsibility for those needing heavy care to other facilities. Within a given region, you would still have a zero-sum game because the total payments for the region would be set by the province. But within a region the casemix from one centre to another could become quite unbalanced, and the connection between the funding level and patients' needs similarly ill-matched. One way to moderate the temptation to "cream skim" would be to make sure that each primary care centre received sufficient payments to care for the needs of its enrolled population.

There are a number of ways to handle this:

- Tailor the capitation amount to reflect the specific needs of each neighbourhood, using epidemiological and demographic information. That's how the United Kingdom funds its general practices—capitation payments there are adjusted using a factor called the Jarman index.[33]
- Use data specific to the actual patients seen by the centre (e.g. age, sex, chronic illness, and social factors) and prospectively adjust the capitation rate.
- Adjust capitation at the end of the year based on data about patient outcomes (e.g., the number of deaths,* number of hospitalizations classified as "unavoidable"). President Clinton's health reforms suggested some post-hoc adjustment process to make sure health plans with especially heavy-care patients were not penalized.

---

* In a population of 5,000, about 40 deaths per year would be expected.

None of these options is perfect, but choosing any of the above alternatives would be fairer than the system we have now. As it stands, per-capita health spending from one region to another varies enormously—often by more than 100 percent—and in many cases, high levels of spending do not correspond with high levels of need.

We recommend that the province establish baseline capitation payments for each region according to a needs-based adjustment factor (e.g. SMR for those aged zero to sixty-four years). Then this baseline payment could be adjusted for each patient within a region according to age, sex, chronic illness, and a socio-economic weighting factor. About 5 to 10 percent of the total would be held back for year-end bonuses to reward quality of care and service and to provide compensation to centres caring for very heavy-need patients. We suggest that the regional board be responsible for determining which centres should receive year-end adjustments and for allocating these resources according to provincially established rules.

Another difficulty is the fact that some patients would likely avoid enrolling in any primary care facility. As mentioned earlier, special arrangements would be needed to make sure that people with serious psychiatric problems had access to the care and services they need. People with AIDS and other terminal and near-terminal conditions might also need special arrangements or programs to meet their higher need for care.

Traders in Primary Care: Setting the Entrepreneurial Spirit Free

Traders can be found in all parts of the health care system, but they really stand out in primary care, where flexible, client-sensitive program planning can dramatically improve productivity.* Publicly financed competition at the primary care level would promote many innovative experiments in health care delivery. Health care represents one-tenth of our economy, but it's been

---

* Our use of the term productivity does not refer to how much servicing is done, but rather to the rate of successful outcomes per unit of cost.

stuck in the same production mode for decades. Competition could free the system to perform at its best.

The possible configurations are limitless. True, a group of doctors could qualify to become a primary care centre merely by employing some extra staff, like many doctors' offices now. But it would also be possible for someone like Marie-Louise Ansak, the social worker who founded On Lok, to establish the same kind of agency in Canada, because the capitation payment could be adjusted appropriately to cover the costs of serving high-needs groups, like the frail elderly.

Community groups and consumers could also set up and run primary care centres, or develop specific services offered on contract to primary care centres. Examples might include patient-run rehabilitation centres for psychiatric patients or self-help groups for heroin addicts. Coronary disease patients with experiences to share could be hired on contract by other primary care centres interested in offering their heart patients contact with a peer group. Companies with expertise in setting up self-help and mutual aid groups could sell their services directly to primary care centres.

We recommend that the province offer feasibility and start-up grants to community groups that want to establish primary care centres. Otherwise, doctors would have a significant advantage over other community sponsors by virtue of their existing practices and patients. We also recognize that consumer groups will need resources for capital from the province. It is somewhat less clear whether a private (doctor-sponsored) primary care centre with no community board should be eligible for provincial capital grants.

The system would also generate more use of research evidence about cost-effective alternatives. If massage and chiropractic turned out to be more effective than drugs and surgery for many musculoskeletal problems, they would likely be offered as the first approach to the problem. If Dean Ornish's lifestyle program turned out to be more cost-effective for coronary patients than drugs or surgery, these services could be offered routinely. As centres searched for better ways to serve their clients, there would be a surge in demand for health services research, and especially for evidence related to outcomes. Knowing and doing what works best would be a critical competitive factor.

Using incentives effectively: lessons about what not to do from Ontario

Ontario has ninety family practice centres called health service organizations (HSOs), which are funded by capitation. However, this program was flawed from the start, not by the principle of capitation payment, but by poor planning and management.

For example, the program didn't have appropriate rules for creating and managing the patient roster. Some doctors registered patients who weren't really theirs; some patients on the roster were long dead. Another problem was that HSO physicians were allowed to bill fee-for-service for transient patients, which provided an incentive for doctors to put low-needs patients on the roster but continue to bill fee-for-service for frequent users. HSOs used to receive a bonus if their patients used hospitals less than the county average. The problem was that there were no controls to make sure that the HSO's patients actually matched the county's in terms of average need for care. In fact, there was good reason to believe that, because of "cream skimming," the average HSO patient was considerably healthier than the average county patient. Formal studies on HSOs showed that they didn't necessarily engage in more appropriate preventive care than fee-for-service practitioners,[34] and that their hospitalization rates were in fact similar to matched patients from fee-for-service practices.*[35]

In the late 1980s the Ontario Ministry of Health grew concerned about these and other problems with the program and halted its expansion in 1991.[36]

There are lessons here for our reform proposals. For one thing, to avoid the problem of Ontario's HSOs, publicly financed competition among primary care centres would also have to set some income restrictions for family doctors and other staff. Otherwise there could be too much incentive to underservice and, in the case of private centres, pocket surplus funds as profit. We suggest a schedule of salary ranges for doctors, nurses, and other workers, with the opportunity for bonuses if certain targets are met. There should also be limits on the amount of surplus that can be

---

* Of course, some HSOs, like the Sault Ste. Marie Group Health Centre, are spectacular successes and should not be tarred with the same brush.

carried over from year to year. These measures would force primary care centres to plow their revenues into services.

Patients can be effective consumers at the primary care level

There's little doubt that more and more consumers are demanding better-quality care and service. Publicly financed competition gives citizens the opportunity to make their voices heard in the political process while also allowing their choice of provider to affect the development of services.[37]

Some readers might think we've contradicted ourselves because we argued earlier that patients have trouble being informed consumers of health services. The catch is that, while it's extremely difficult for patients to be knowledgeable consumers of highly technical aspects of health care, we think that they could make good decisions about which primary care centre to join. Here's why.

The average Canadian sees a GP about four times a year. But people with high health care needs—like the frail elderly, young women, and children—could easily make a dozen or more visits to the doctor in a single year. This level of contact allows patients to assess how user-friendly their primary care centre is. Do they have to wait hours to see a caregiver? Are they put on hold for twenty minutes when they call for advice? Is the food in the seniors' day centre unpalatable? Are their homemakers always late? Do they have to wait months to see a specialist?

Most patients—especially frequent users—could answer these questions right now; some doctors and community health centres already attract patients because they pay more attention to consumer preferences. But what would happen if the centre's viability depended on these kinds of factors? What would happen if the incomes for doctors, nurses, and indeed all staff were directly dependent on being able to attract and retain patients' loyalty? We predict that the quality of service would be even better. According to policy analysts Saltman and von Otter, only a few patients actually have to switch providers before a new atmosphere of consumer awareness takes hold.

However, primary care centres would also compete on the basis of quality of care, not just quality of service. Every year the province would release "report cards" for each region's hospitals and nursing homes and primary care centres, noting their performance according to provincially selected performance indicators. Consumers could use these to make their choices. It would be clear at a glance which centres were more likely to keep patients healthy and out of hospital.

Having publicly available data on quality of care would help stem a centre's temptation to focus only on the cosmetic aspects of care. If a primary care centre spent too much money on fancy waiting room furniture, or offered housecalls to people with the sniffles, it would risk not having enough to pay for more useful services—and this could cause the centre to do badly on its performance indicators. A centre that spent most of its time on care for healthy people with minor illnesses—as too many family doctors now do—wouldn't have enough left over to take proper care of those who really needed attention. Many of these people would end up in hospital, and the primary care centre would have to pay for this costly institutional care.

All in all, we think public competition in primary care would have a salutary effect on the system. Many family doctors, nurses, administrators, and other health workers already demonstrate a degree of entrepreneurism—and many express frustration at existing funding rules and perverse regulations that limit their creativity and desire to offer better care and service. Let's unleash them from these chains.

Regional Responsibilities

Our reform proposal would put regions in charge of hospitals and some tertiary care services. Regions would also have responsibility for mental health, communicable disease control, environmental health services (including public health inspection services), and the effective coordination of emergency and ambulance systems. The size of a given region would be determined by the size of the population and its need for service, rather than arbitrary lines on maps. In general, a region would serve between 30,000 and 300,000 people. People would be able to get most of their needs for secondary care health services within their own region—including obstetrics, pediatrics, internal medicine, psychiatry, and general surgery. They would also be able to receive the more common sub-specialty services such as ophthalmology, orthopedics, and cardiology. Health care performance indicators set by the province would guide the development and improvement of secondary care programs.

For example, suppose a region's health status information revealed a much lower than average death rate from heart disease and a population with lower levels of smoking, dietary fat, and other identifiable risk factors. But then suppose the health care system's performance indicators revealed a higher than average death rate from heart attack in the hospital. This regional scenario would prompt an investigation (along the lines of Dr. Terry Montague's program in Edmonton) to look at the whole picture and try to focus on identifying system flaws—a kind of diagnostic journey to find the relevant causes and correct them.

A first step would be to rule out the chance that the finding is just a statistical artifact. For example, maybe more patients in this region get transported to hospital and die there as opposed to being declared dead at home. This could be investigated by looking at all heart attack deaths in the region, wherever they occur. Or perhaps heart attack patients in the region delay seeking medical attention. Maybe there are problems with the region's emergency response system. Perhaps the hospital emergency department staff are slower recognizing and treating new heart attack patients. Perhaps the coronary care unit doctors aren't using the right drugs, or are not using them correctly. A systematic, data-driven investigation could help answer these questions and provide the basis for taking corrective action.

Choosing another example, suppose a region's Caesarean section rate is 50 percent higher than the provincial average. Suppose further that the data show that the rate at which women are offered the chance to try a vaginal birth after a previous Caesarean section is one-quarter of the provincial average. This information would be more than enough for regional council members to start asking questions and pushing administrators and clinicians to investigate and take action. The key question for board members is "Why?" Why the variation? How can we reduce it by moving in the right direction? Once again, the focus wouldn't necessarily be punitive, but this kind of information clearly empowers consumers to demand accountability from service providers.

Regional secondary care facilities

Our arguments favouring competition in primary care don't apply to secondary care. That's because there are many potential efficiencies competition could produce at the primary care level, but competition among secondary care providers would, in fact, create more waste and inefficiency. For example, most communities and regions with between 100,000 and 200,000 people need only one acute-care hospital, but many areas of Canada with this many people are already served by two hospitals or even more. Having hospitals compete with one another is extremely wasteful.

Regional hospitals and long-term-care facilities should be funded from primary care centres. If a person has to have his leg amputated because of poor diabetic control, then the hospital will be paid for that case by the patient's primary care centre. As much as possible, the price charged should be based on the actual cost of services provided, as opposed to case-mix or per diem funding. This would ensure that the payment reflected the resources actually used. It would also supply a powerful incentive to primary care centres to keep patients out of hospital and get hospital patients out as soon as possible. New computer costing systems should make this task fairly easy and inexpensive.

In this system GPs would be responsible for admitting and discharging most of their own patients. But if specialists were responsible and a primary care centre was unhappy with the service of a particular hospital, it could send elective patients to a neighbouring region's hospital. The loss of regional funds would be a powerful incentive for the regional board to take remedial action at their local hospital.

By and large, the proposed system would not require human resources planning for the first level of specialists. And it doesn't particularly matter to the system's integrity how they are paid, whether on fee-for-service, salary, retainer, contract, or some combination arrived at through negotiation with the primary care centre.

We don't want to give the impression here that we've dotted all the "i"s and crossed all the "t"s. Certainly, we admit that there are a number of challenges inherent in this model. One is our recommendation to guarantee employment security to workers—this will be a preoccupation for unions and managers alike. Another is the fact that regions will have an incentive to off-load patients to tertiary care, and therefore to provincial responsibility.

The Governance of the New System

For two decades, many reports and commissions from across the country have said that we need more democracy in the way we govern our health care institutions. We agree. More citizen participation and more opportunity for patients to influence the delivery of services could lead to better care.

We also recognize that initiatives to increase citizen participation can turn out very badly. For example, Quebec's most recent reforms require that the boards of all the province's health establishments—hospitals, nursing homes, *centres locaux des services communautaires* (CLSCs), etc.—be elected.* Unfortunately, the government allocated almost no resources to support the development of this new democracy. The new law also allowed all residents of Quebec to vote anywhere in the province, regardless of where they lived. As a result, in the first elections, held in the fall of 1992, busloads of people were driven around Montreal to vote for boards in up to twenty different establishments. Many voters were electing people they didn't know, in agencies they didn't use. There weren't even any age limits for voting! The minister's office spent a frantic time phoning agencies the day before balloting, warning them not to let babies vote! Terry Kaufman, the executive director of CLSC Notre Dame de Grâce in Montreal, says many of these problems occurred because citizen participation was merely an add-on to the reform process. He worries that it was done so badly that it could discredit the entire reform process.

We also need to consider the fact that local citizen boards are just as capable of making bad decisions as good ones, and that the mere presence of citizen boards does not guarantee accountability. This is a sobering thought for those who are uncritically gung-ho on democracy! That's why it's so crucial that board selection processes are carefully designed to attract good people. Also, Saskatchewan's Steven Lewis and Lawrie McFarlane both stressed that board size be kept as small as possible (about six members) to

---

* The actual rules are very complicated. Some of the directors' seats are open to public election every year. Others are reserved for representatives from various "electoral colleges" representing assorted professional groups.

avoid factions and promote group cohesion. "Don't discount
the impact an influential leader can have," says Saul Panofsky,
executive director of of CLSC St. Louis du Parc in Montreal. All
three say board credibility is critical and that having board members who are trusted by the community makes change much easier. "You can learn the details of health care fairly fast, but
credibility and stature take years to develop," says Lewis. And all
three acknowledged the need for provinces to make a serious
investment in appropriate board development. Volunteer board
members need help to do a good job. If they get that support,
they can be outstandingly effective.

   In essence, we are looking at two types of boards: one would
govern the community health centres; the other would operate
at the regional level to govern public health, emergency services, mental health, and the region's facilities for acute secondary care, long-term care, and some tertiary care. What
follows is a series of principles we propose for governing the
new system of community health centres, some of which are
already in place:

1. More than half of the board should be elected by the
    centre's users, with three-year terms staggered so that
    one-third of board seats are up for election every year.
2. Some board seats should be reserved for members
    appointed by local municipal councils and the province.
3. The board should be able to appoint additional mem-
    bers to make up for any areas of deficiency they per-
    ceive after elections and appointments.
4. Staff should be prohibited from running for board
    membership but should have access to board meet-
    ings as non-voting observers.
5. The board should focus on policy and delegate the
    management role to staff.[38]

We also think private primary care centres—those sponsored by
family doctors or other professionals—should also incorporate
patient/citizen input in their program planning and should be
required to demonstrate how they intend to accomplish this as a
condition for licensing. Many health care professionals (even
some working in community health centres) would prefer to

limit community input to token involvement, but others know there's a lot to be gained from actively seeking advice and comments from patients and the broader community. This input can, for example, provide:

- structured feedback about existing services and programs;
- assistance with planning new programs;
- help to broaden the impact of health promotion and disease prevention; and
- one of many small steps needed to facilitate a sense of community cohesion.

Regional governance

When it comes to regional governance, we are recommending that individual boards for facilities in the region be replaced with a regional board. Since primary care facilities will be responsible for funding regional secondary care, it makes sense for the regional board to be mainly composed of representatives from these primary care centres.

1. More than half of the board should be appointed by primary care facilities (including community health centres and private clinics), with three-year terms staggered so one-third of these board seats are selected every year.
2. Some board members should be appointed by regional/county councils* and the province.
3. Some board members should be elected at large during municipal elections.
4. The board should be allowed to appoint additional members to make up for areas of deficiency they perceive after elections and appointments.

We recommend that the regional board take overall responsibility for all the institutions within its area. This would mean dissolving

---

* Of course the models of regional or county government vary considerably across the country.

existing institutional boards (as has already happened in New Brunswick and in Saskatchewan). The bulk of existing administrative personnel from hospitals should be seconded to staff the regional level. Some hospital and facility administrators could also move to the primary care centres. A few would remain in the institutions as operational managers.

Dissolving hospital boards and dispersing administrators are key political tactics to facilitate regionalization. Too many managers and too many boards will perpetuate a focus on concerns within the four walls of an individual facility and will make it harder to deal with system-wide issues. The provincial Ministries of Health could deal with Catholic hospitals the way Saskatoon did: St. Paul's Hospital in Saskatoon kept its own board and retains its religious identity, but major program planning decisions now take place at the regional level. We do not make these recommendations because we think hospital boards have been doing a bad job, but rather because they've been doing too good a job for their respective insitutions, to the detriment of the total system.

Tertiary Care: The Province's Responsibility

We could complete the symmetry of our proposal for reforming the system by allowing regions to fund tertiary care, thus allowing this part of the system to function as a quasi-market also. In fact, this was discussed in the late 1980s, as Quebec was putting together its most recent reform package. The idea was attractive to many at the primary and secondary care levels for the same reasons that primary care centres would like to fund secondary care. Money is power, and holding the purse would force tertiary care facilities to be more responsive to other levels within the system. Against the idea, however, is the fact that the province would still bear the ultimate political responsibility for any screw-ups. What's more, larger provinces share a pressing need to coordinate the overall development of tertiary care.

There's yet another important consideration arguing against regional funding for tertiary care. There's a highly competitive international market for certain types of specialists. It's a bit like the National Hockey League, where Canadian teams have to compete with American teams for free agents. For example, in the United States, cardiac surgeons and neurosurgeons make fantastic amounts of money. If provinces want to cover these specialty areas—and they certainly do—they must be prepared to pay dearly for certain doctors. However, these decisions should be made within overall provincial priorities and with full consideration of the political implications.

We suggest that provinces establish a mechanism for joint governance over tertiary care facilities with input from communities, regions, and university training programs for health professionals (which are usually based in tertiary care facilities). Again, we see the key to success being the establishment of appropriate indicators that would drive the development of health care programs. If one area of a province had a particularly high rate of low-birthweight babies, the province should be able to fund either better social interventions for pregnant women or improved neonatal intensive care. We would hope that the ultimate decision would depend on which alternative has the best chance of improving the indicator. However, other political factors would also affect the decision, which is why we recommend the provinces retain the responsibility.

Provincial Health Councils: The System's IQ

Over the years, various bodies have been set up to advise Ministries of Health. For example, the Ontario Council of Health was established in 1966, and in 1972 it was given statutory recognition in the Ontario Ministry of Health Act. Over the years, this agency conducted research, for example, on community health centres and the use of nurse-practitioners. In the early 1980s, Ontario's activist Health Minister Larry Grossman turned the Health Council into a much more public body, using it to hold forums on health policy reform. Unfortunately, the council rattled too many officials within the Ministry of Health. When the council lost its political cover (Mr. Grossman was promoted to Treasury), it was killed off.

In 1987, the Ontario Health Review Panel, chaired by Dr. John Evans, recommended a new Provincial Health Council, and later that year Premier David Peterson set it up. In 1989, the Premier's Council on Health Strategy was working in five areas, one of which was developing strategies for health status and health care. Various reports were released, including several on health goals for the province. When Bob Rae's NDP government took office, it was renamed and reconfigured as the Ontario Premier's Council on Health, Well-Being, and Social Justice. More recently, government merged this council with the Premier's Council on the Economy. Since then it has pretty much faded from view and policy-makers' attention.*

New Brunswick appointed its Premier's Council in 1989, but it had a time limit on its mandate and it was dissolved early in 1991 after suggesting health goals for the province. Nova Scotia appointed its Provincial Council on Health in 1991. With strong leadership from its executive director, Mary Jane Hampton, and a small staff, it has released health goals for the province and conducted consultations on health policy reform with thousands of people in dozens of communities. It has also been something of a thorn in the side of the Ministry of Health in its role as a public watchdog on the government's health reform agenda.

Late in 1993, Saskatchewan appointed its provincial Council on Health with a mandate to advise on public policies that affect health. British Columbia intends to appoint a provincial health council in 1994.

Although the idea behind these provincial councils of health is admirable, their track record so far shows limited success. We suggest that provincial health councils should have three main purposes: measuring health status, monitoring and publicizing health system performance and supporting quality improvement throughout the system. The provincial councils would be responsible for facilitating and supporting the work of opinion leaders like Dr. Terry Montague, as well as his counterparts in other professional disciplines.

Finding the right roles for provinces, regions, and communities

No one experienced with horses would recommend a standardbred for a jumping competition or a thoroughbred for the plough. In the same way, it's important to select appropriate

---

* A recent report they released on "patient abuse" of the system and the role of user fees did, however, capture significant media attention.

roles for each level of governance within our reformed health care system. Table 9.1 outlines the roles we see for the province, regions, and communities. We have tried carefully to partition the Guardians from the Traders. The provincial Ministry of Health must be a guardian of the public, but we see the provincial health councils as mainly having Trader responsibilities. They should stay away, as much as possible, from any disciplinary or fiscal responsibilities.

We hope this introduction to a reformed health care system will provoke some serious thought. If you want to play a new game, you have to be prepared to change the rules. And that's what we've done here—a major shake-up in how health care is funded and organized. We believe the approach we've taken is consistent with Canadian values concerning health—equity, quality of care, informed choice, accountability, efficiency, and, most importantly, citizen participation. More emphasis on this last value could be just the shot of medicine our flagging democratic tradition needs. To quote John Stuart Mill: "The most important point of excellence which any form of government can possess is to promote the virtue and intelligence of the people themselves."[39]

Table 9.1

NEW ROLES FOR HEALTH CARE

Provincial Health Council

Measures the health status of the population.

Sets health care system performance indicators with public input.

Measures the performance of the health care system.

Publishes performance scores for primary care centres and institutions.

Facilitates continuous improvement in the quality of clinical care by:

- Acting as a clearing house for relevant research evidence.
- Supporting the work of local opinion leaders.

Ministry of Health

Budgeting:

- Sets an overall budget for health care.
- Sets a needs-based capitation funding formula for regions and for primary care centres.
- Sets specific budgets for: regional mental health; regional public health inspection; regional administration; tertiary care.

Planning and Coordination:

- Plans and coordinates tertiary care.
- Plans and coordinates inter-regional and interprovincial and federal/provincial/territorial policies.

Financial Accountability and Quality Assurance:

- Assesses performance of regions and primary care centres.
- Sets sanctions and retains the right to take over the administration of any health care delivery agency.
- Sets the laws for professional licensing.
- Sets the conditions for licensing and grants licences to primary care centres.

Regional Health Authority

Governance:

- Is responsible for the region's health care facilities and some tertiary care.

Planning, Coordination, and Management:

- Is responsible for mental health services in the region.
- Is responsible for the region's communicable disease control and environmental health services, including public health inspection services.
- Is responsible for emergency services in the region.

Budgeting:

- Makes year-end adjustments to primary care centres' budgets.
- Makes year-end adjustments to institutional budgets.

Health Facilities within a Region (acute, long-term care, and rehabilitation)

- Are responsible for day-to-day operational management and delivery of services.
- Are responsible for collecting and supplying performance data.

Primary Care Centres

- Are responsible for operational planning, management, and delivery of services.
- Have twenty-four-hour responsibility for patients.

CHCs

- Have the same resposibilities as all primary care centres but in addition are responsible for:
  - clinical occupational health;
  - community health promotion.

Chapter 10

Changing the Health System's Lineup: A New Game Plan

IMAGINE WHAT WOULD HAPPEN if Canada's Olympic hockey team had a superstar offence but no defence at all. We might score plenty of goals, but we'd be certain to lose most games. That's more or less what we've done in our health care system. Acute care is the "star" and gets most of the resources. Meanwhile, primary care, our first line of defence, is in such a terrible state of disarray that it's been benched for lack of coordination. This is holding back the overall performance of the entire system.

You already know that innovative approaches to primary care can improve health and reduce the need for specialist and institutional care.[1] Most of these innovations are incompatible with a system based on solo practice, fee-for-service doctors. Even the Canadian College of Family Physicians makes the claim that fee-for-service actually penalizes family physicians who are trying to do a good job. That's why they want to see more experimentation with salary and capitation funding for primary care.[2]

We believe capitation is the most appropriate means of funding because it makes a very direct link between the centre's revenues and its ability to attract and retain patients. Centres that fail to please patients will lose income. Capitation has the added advantage of giving centres enormous flexibility to innovate and make changes to accommodate patients' needs. This freedom means centres can spend their resources where it makes the most sense. Those that are the most entrepreneurial will be the most successful.

The Scope of Primary Care

Except for emergency care, most people make their first contact with the system when they see their family doctor. The physician hears about the person's problem, undertakes what's needed to make a proper diagnosis, and makes recommendations for therapy. The whole process is highly individualized and private—as it should be. The main focus is whatever problem the patient has brought to the doctor's attention.

But the visit is also an opportunity to explore other issues. What should happen when patients visit their primary care provider is sometimes called the "quartet of the consultation":

1. Management of the presenting problem.
2. Surveillance of chronic illness.
3. Opportunistic health promotion.
4. Education about the appropriate use of services.

We've discussed the importance of a move to non-fee-for-service payment and how a more meaningful involvement by patients and community members in the governance of health care institutions can benefit everyone. Here are more key features of effective and efficient primary care:

1. A focus on "whole population" primary care.
2. Seeking and showing respect for patient choice.
3. Collaborative practice between family doctors and primary care nurses.
4. Integration of primary care with secondary and some tertiary care.
5. Integration of primary care with community and social services.

"Whole Population" Primary Care

Dr. Julian Tudor Hart began general practice in Glyncorrwg in the Afan Valley in Wales in 1961. Over the next three decades, the two thousand or so inhabitants of the area faced serious problems following the mass closure of coal mines. Male unemployment ballooned from 8 percent in the mid-1960s to 40 percent by the 1980s. Glyncorrwg's overall social and economic status stood among the lowest 5 percent of wards in Wales.

During the 1960s, Dr. Hart and his staff used a "whole population" approach in delivering primary care. For example, they screened almost everyone in the community for high blood pressure. They also systematically identified people with diabetes, asthma, and alcoholism and offered them specific programs aimed at enhancing their health and teaching them how to manage their own illnesses. At the same time, Dr. Hart made extra efforts to convince his patients to reduce their risks of illness, advising them, for example, to quit smoking, reduce fat and salt intake, lose weight, and get more exercise.

The results of Dr. Hart's work were striking. Within thirteen years, over half the hypertensives had well-controlled blood pressures and 40 percent had fair control.[3] The proportion of diabetics or hypertensives who smoked fell by two-thirds. At least partly as a result of excellent primary care, the 1980s death rate among people under sixty-five in Glyncorrwg was 40 percent lower than that of a neighbouring village.[4]

Other examples of highly effective "whole population" primary care include the Community Oriented Primary Care program popularized by Dr. Sydney Kark,[5] and the nurse-led primary health care developed by the Victorian Order of Nurses and amply demonstrated by outpost nurses in Canada's north over the past century.[6]

Capitation funding makes it much easier to provide "whole population" primary health care, for two reasons. First, it encourages providers to find innovative and efficient ways to deal with community health problems. Second, it provides the budgetary flexibility to actually change how things are done.

A focus on "whole population" primary care is logically linked to key health system performance indicators. For example, is the centre doing a good job for people with high blood pressure, diabetes, and other chronic conditions? How many are hospitalized for flare-ups that should have been caught and treated at an earlier stage? What about the community's rate for invasive cervical cancer and other preventable conditions—how do these measures compare with neighbouring communities? Centres that perform well should be able to demonstrate lower community death rates for people under sixty-five. Dr. Hart's research shows that excellent primary care can be a life-saver.

Using Patient Choice to Change the System

Our proposed system will rely enormously on patient choice to drive the planning and delivery of care. Capitation funding will ensure that dollars follow patients. Except in the areas of mental health, public health services, and most tertiary care services, funding will not be attached to specific programs.

In today's system, patients don't have much choice about the care they receive. If they had more opportunity to express their preferences, the system would change dramatically. There's evidence, for example, that informed consumer choice would lead to lower rates of elective surgery and far less intensive care for patients with terminal illnesses. This would cut the need for doctors' services, hospital beds, and nursing homes, but it would also greatly expand the demand for community services and home care.

A new way of death

From the perspective of other cultures and other societies, North Americans have a highly unnatural view of death. In fact, how we care for terminal patients has helped transform health care from the cottage industry it used to be into a mega-enterprise representing 10 percent of our gross domestic product.

In any given year, between one-quarter and one-third of the system's budget is spent on patients who die.[7]

- Most people die in an acute-care hospital and often receive aggressive medical care aimed at postponing death.
- Not all, but certainly some of the care dying patients receive is not wanted by the patients themselves.
- Many people would prefer to die in their own homes or in homelike settings—provided they have good pain and symptom control and can count on help for family caregivers.

Many older people find it curious that governments spend so much on institutional care and so little on measures that would help them retain their independence in the community. Even though recent reforms in some provinces have expanded community care options, many older people and their families still have trouble finding publicly financed programs to meet their needs. In many parts of the country, home care, respite services, and day centre programs for the frail elderly are in very short supply. In contrast, there seems no limit when it comes to acute care. Thousands of dollars are spent on invasive services for terminal patients—machines that feed them, breathe for them, and eliminate their body wastes, or drugs and surgeries that only prolong the dying process.

Lately, however, a rising tide of consumerism has been helping to change this dynamic. Many seniors' organizations across North America are demanding the right to determine in advance what kinds of limits—if any—they want on their care in the event of a terminal or acute illness. Sometimes this is called an "advance directive," "living will," or "health wish."

Dr. Willie Malloy is a geriatrician at Ontario's McMaster University. He worked with the staff of Idlewyld Manor, a long-term care facility for one hundred elderly women, to introduce the concept of advance directives. The women were given information and encouraged to spell out their treatment preferences before they developed an acute illness. For example, staff asked the residents if they wanted cardiopulmonary resuscitation (CPR) if their heart stopped or if they stopped breathing. The women were also asked to specify the intensity of treatment they'd choose for reversible and for irreversible conditions.* Nearly 80 percent of the residents completed the directive and, among this group, 88 percent refused to have CPR.

In the year before the directive was used, there were nine deaths among Idlewyld Manor residents—eight occurred in hospital and one in the Manor. In the second year after the Manor began using the advance directive, there were eight deaths—seven within Idlewyld and one in hospital.[8] In that

---

* Intensity was defined in four levels: supportive care, limited care, maximum care, and intensive care.

year, Manor residents also used 50 percent fewer hospital days compared to the year prior to using the directive.

Obviously, great care must be taken to spell out the process for introducing and responding to advance directives in order to limit the potential for abuse. This can, however, be accomplished with appropriate legal, ethical, and religious monitoring. Above all, the process should support patients' decisions even when they run counter to prevailing wisdom. For example, patients who review the options and still want "everything done in every circumstance" should, as much as possible, have their wishes respected. Experience to date, however, suggests that people opt overwhelmingly for less invasive care, not more. Most consumers put a high premium on personal comfort and consistently indicate a preference for "high touch" over "high tech" services.

Overall, we believe that widespread use of advance directives would vastly improve the quality of care our system delivers. Besides, invasive medical intervention often interferes with the more spiritual aspects of death and dying. Encouraging terminal patients to choose their version of a "good death" could inject some badly needed humanity into the dying process.

Honouring informed choice is the primary reason we advocate advance directives. However, we also know that using them would produce major savings in acute care. These freed-up resources could be spent on acute care for people who really need and want it. Or they could be used to provide care that would actually improve the quality of life for older and terminal patients. Using living wills and advance directives would allow us to shift the focus of health care to living life instead of prolonging death.

Doctors and Nurses Working Together

Our proposed system relies heavily on nurses working as fully functioning members of the health care team. For this to happen, however, the relationships between nurses and other health professionals—especially doctors—need improvement.

In 1967, American psychiatrist Dr. Leonard Stein wrote a provocative article describing how doctors and nurses interacted. He called it "The doctor-nurse game."[9] The "game" involved elaborate strategies nurses had to use to get doctors to do the right things for patients. The big challenge for the nurse was to find a way to advise the doctor that allowed the physician to think the recommendation was his idea.

In 1990, Stein and some physician colleagues revisited the topic and found that a number of social changes had occurred in the intervening years. There were more female doctors, for example, and more appreciation of physicians' fallibility. Nursing itself had also changed. Educational standards were higher. The old-fashioned "handmaiden" role had been soundly rejected as nursing increasingly became recognized as a separate, valuable, and autonomous profession. As much as things had improved, however, the authors noted that "in many places, [the game] still functions essentially as described."[10]

Marianne Cheetham has been a nurse-practitioner at Toronto's South Riverdale Community Health Centre since 1981. Until 1982, the centre's doctors and one nurse-practitioner worked as autonomous, independent caregivers. That year, however, South Riverdale's board decided to set up a "collaborative practice" model based on teams, each one staffed by a doctor and a nurse-practitioner. The idea was to create more interaction, more synergy between the two professions, with the skills and knowledge from each influencing the care provided.[11]

Ever since, patients have been able to choose one of three teams to manage their care. Within the team, who does what depends on who is the most appropriate caregiver for a specific visit. At South Riverdale, Ms. Cheetham and the other primary health care nurses are responsible for most "well person" care, including prenatal care, well-baby visits, and routine physical examinations. The nurse is also the most likely professional to follow up on patients with chronic illnesses, although this varies somewhat from team to team. This division of labour allows doctors to focus on what they know best—the diagnosis and treatment of illness.

Ms. Cheetham thinks patients benefit from having two practitioners instead of one. And practitioners benefit, too, from being able to share the stress and pressure of delivering high-quality human services.

Depending on the size of the practice and the population's needs, a single physician-nurse team could handle most primary care for between 1,200 and 2,000 patients. Most parts of the country have a high enough population density to make it efficient for three or four teams to operate out of a single centre. This concentration of resources would also make it possible for the centre to hire other types of staff—social workers, midwives, home care workers (including RNs, RPNs, and homemakers), mental health workers,* chiropodists. Pooling staff also makes for more efficient administration and better after-hours service— South Riverdale is open four evenings a week and on Saturday mornings, too. And the doctors there, and at a number of CHCs, take their own night calls and feel strongly about doing so.

Patty Sullivan, the executive director of Klinic, a Winnipeg community health centre, cautions against limiting team membership to just doctors and nurses, arguing that this could de-emphasize the social and psychological aspects of care. We agree that there is a need to "de-medicalize" health services. Social workers should be included on some primary care teams, once again depending on the needs of the population served. In some centres, it might be more appropriate for social workers and other psychological counsellors to work as consultants to the team.

However, if we adopt this model, what we face is a staffing problem. There are almost a quarter of a million RNs in Canada but very few in primary care centres. Most nurses work in acute-care hospitals, where they are at high risk for lay-offs as hospital beds are cut and middle management jobs vanish. We also have 6,000 RNs working in physicians' offices, 7,000 working in home care, and almost 10,000 public health nurses.[12] Home care nursing in most parts of the country is expanding, but, except in Quebec, it has few formal links with other primary care services.**

Meanwhile, over the past twenty years, the role of public health nursing in our system has become blurred. At the start of this century, community physicians were scarce and too expensive for poor and working-class people. At the same time, a middle-class

---

* In our model, funding for the mental health worker would come from the region.

** Some home care nursing is administered by public health departments (e.g. in some parts of Ontario and Alberta) but, even in these locations there is little coordination with other primary care services.

movement attempting to eliminate poverty by educating women in the "domestic sciences" was sweeping North America.[13] Community nursing tackled both issues. Public health and Victorian Order nurses were highly visible as they moved through the community treating illness, administering vaccinations, and teaching basic child care skills and the fundamentals of hygiene. With more modern times, authoritarian methods that tended to patronize or teach down to people were replaced by new approaches that recognized the importance to health of an individual's self-esteem, sense of autonomy, and network of friends and family. But today many public health nurses are in a quandary over demands in some jurisdictions that they become community organizers or health promotion consultants.[14]

We think it would make a lot of sense to relocate these public health nurses to primary care centres. Some could easily retrain to function as primary care nurses on teams like those developed at the South Riverdale Community Health Centre. Others could continue providing home nursing, but with a key difference: they would be part of an integrated team of health and social service caregivers. Still others could continue their public health mission by working with small groups on a range of health-promotion and disease-prevention objectives.

Integration of Primary Care with Secondary and Some Tertiary Care

Transition is the critical point in a basketball game. When the ball changes hands, how fast the team in possession moves to the offence and the other team moves to defence often determines who wins. It is also a crucial part of health care. Every time a patient is transferred from one practitioner or facility to another, there are chances for disaster.

When a patient arrives at a hospital's emergency department, usually there is very little information that accompanies him. Staff in the emergency department have to take the patient's history, without any background on the person's medical or social circumstances. Sometimes this might not matter much— background information wouldn't change the recommended therapy for an otherwise healthy person with a broken leg, for example. But in many circumstances, background information can be crucial. Hospitals can be hazardous places—especially when no one really knows you—medically, psychologically, and socially.

Problems occur when it's time to return home, too. Hospital discharge planning is still very uneven.[15] All too often the patient is sent home before community nurses can be mobilized and without any contact with the family doctor. Now, with more patients leaving "sicker and quicker," discharge planning is more important to the well-being of the patient than ever.

Heaps of health care reports call for a seamless spectrum of services such that patients can move effortlessly through the system. One success story is the palliative care service at Montreal's Royal Victoria Hospital. Pioneered by Dr. Balfour Mount in the mid-1970s, the program began as an in-patient service, but it soon became apparent that many terminally ill people wanted to stay home as long as possible. The staff responded by setting up their own home care teams of nurses and doctors, who also coordinated services from homemakers and community nurses.

By the late 1980s, however, home care in Quebec was a CLSC service, so today, the CLSCs handle most of the Royal Vic's palliative care patients. CLSC nurses and homemakers know the palliative care staff are always available for consultation; this direct link means patients and their families are always dealing with someone who knows their case. Patients know they can access the palliative in-patient unit when community care is no longer possible or desirable. As it happens, many patients use the in-patient unit only briefly, preferring to return home once symptom control has been re-established.

To forge better links between service levels and enhance the development of a seamless system, it makes sense to consolidate funding for secondary and some tertiary care at the primary care level.

Integration of Primary Care with Community Social Services

Noting the connection between social well-being and health status, many reports recommend integrating primary health care with social services at the delivery level. Most parts of the country have ignored this advice. In most provinces, health and social services are delivered by separate agencies and funded by separate ministries. Even our federal government has split the former department of health and welfare into separate entities.

We believe, however, that the best way to ensure effective coordination is to insist on integration at the delivery level by putting primary health and social services under one budget.

That's what Quebec has done through its CLSC network. Each CLSC offers a range of social services along with primary health care and home care. Quebec's most recent reforms extended this direction by transferring about four hundred social workers from a host of different agencies to the CLSCs. Terry Kaufman, the executive director of the Notre Dame de Grâce CLSC in Montreal, says people in Quebec have now come to think of the CLSC as "one-stop shopping" for primary health care and social services. It's startlingly efficient—and humane—for people seeking formal care to know they can go to their local CLSC and let the staff help them in develop a care plan instead of searching throughout the city for what they need. A family coping with a schizophrenic son and a mother with breast cancer has enough problems without having to plan its own care unassisted.

People living outside Quebec aren't so lucky. In cities like Winnipeg and Ottawa, for example, we find hundreds of tiny social service agencies—and literally thousands in Metropolitan Toronto—each with its own board and administration. We have no quibble with their sincerity or with their ingenuity in being able to stretch slim budgets to do a good job. Most of these agencies attract loyal support from volunteers and many have become quite effective advocates for their clients. However, like hospitals, these independent, small, non-profit agencies also suffer from built-in incentives for non-cooperation. Their tendency to disregard duplication and fiercely guard their own autonomy has produced both gaps and overlaps in services.

That's why mental health patients and their families in Saskatoon lobbied the Saskatoon District Health Board to assume responsibility for coordinating and rationalizing mental health services. Former health board president Lawrie McFarlane (now British Columbia's deputy minister of health) said, "In Saskatoon alone, there are more than fifty agencies delivering mental health services. Finding your way through the system is a nightmare. We heard tales about patients finding out in the grocery store about a therapy they needed that they couldn't find out about any other way."

A similar situation arose in Windsor, Ontario. The District Health Council's steering committee wants to completely reconfigure its health and health-related social services system. They are making plans to close hospitals and, at the same time, develop an expanded, but more rational, community service system. At the outset, they assumed they'd only have to deal with about 70 local agencies. But as the consultation process progressed, it turned out that there were really about 230 organizations delivering health and health-related social services in the community! In 1994, the project's implementation group will be developing a plan for consolidating community service delivery. In return for a net new investment of $22 million, these separate agencies will be expected to amalgamate into about thirty organizations.[16]

Our proposed system will provide incentives for cost-effective delivery in both community and institutional settings. Overall, this means the number of boards and administrative staff will decline as services are consolidated.

Timing is a key factor in making the shift to community care work. Lawrie McFarlane cautions against thinking you can make cuts to the hospital system without developing community care first: "If you cut services or programs in hospitals and then try to build something in the community—you'll be doing it under pressure and probably badly. So do the community side first—get it up and running and appreciated."

By consolidating funding at the primary care level, we solve this timing problem. Expansion of services will occur at the community level first. The impact on secondary services will be felt quickly, but only *after* this key funding shift has occurred.

A Health Human Resource Strategy that Works

Now that we've outlined our proposal for a new system, it is time to look at some of the changes that will be necessary to make it work effectively.

You'll remember from Chapter 6 that health human resource planning has mainly been absent in our system, with disastrous consequences for caregivers and the public. We propose a major revamping of health human resources based on the following three principles:

1. The numbers of health professionals trained should correspond to the population's need for care as determined by the burden of illness and the most cost-effective ways to diagnose and treat these problems. We recommend a zero-sum process like the one used by the U.S. Graduate Medical Education National Advisory Committee (GMENAC), described in more detail in Chapter 6.
2. Training for health and social service professionals should prepare them to be lifelong learners. Health care information changes quickly. All health professionals must be able to learn on the job and need to know how to use new information technology to access data to make the best recommendations for patient care.
3. In addition to technical skills, training should equip all students to work well on teams. Too many of our present-day teams are positively dysfunctional, loose affiliations rather than high-functioning, mutually supportive groups. New workplaces that support cohesive teamwork can help, but training different health professionals together, rather than in isolation from one another, would be a key step in setting the stage for better teamwork.

Dr. Tyrone Turner, now chief of psychiatry at Toronto's Doctors' Hospital, recalls how the two years he spent working as an attendant at a psychiatric hospital ultimately led him to choose a medical career in psychiatry. He says the hands-on work he did at the Whitby Hospital nearly thirty years ago was a profoundly "grounding" experience, one that still inspires him to keep on fighting for better services for people with serious mental illness, even when it means he has to sit through interminable, often very frustrating meetings.

For many years, the palliative care service at Montreal's Royal Victoria Hospital has provided postgraduate training for students from many different disciplines, including medicine. For the first week, regardless of the student's field of study or prior training, he assists the nurse by making beds and helping patients with bathing, toileting, and other aspects of personal care. This rejigging of the traditional hierarchy is deliberate. Staff know that having students assist nurses in providing basic, hands-on care fosters a profound sense of humility—a good grounding that sets the stage for later training appropriate to the professional's particular discipline.

We think providing hands-on care should be part of the early training for all people who want to work as health care providers— including physicians, nurses, physiotherapists, occupational thera-pists, and midwives.*

In addition, we think all health professionals should do more of their training together. Interdisciplinary programs should be the rule for early training where the course work that has to be covered is essentially the same. Profession-specific training would come after this basic beginner's program, but teamwork would continue to be an integral part of even the more advanced stages of clinical training.

This kind of change would also facilitate opportunities for "clinical laddering"—allowing people to exit and then re-enter training for a new discipline without having to start their course work all over again.

Changing how health professionals learn will no doubt take considerable time to implement. However, two aspects need immediate attention: we need to make further cuts to medical school enrollment, and we have to retailor nursing education to support the necessary shift to community care—especially primary care.

Radical surgery: sometimes the kindest cut

The 10 percent cuts in undergraduate medical school enrollment imposed in 1993 are not sufficient to deal with our surplus of doc-tors. In fact, if applied across the board, further cuts could under-mine the continued viability of medical education altogether.

---

* Consideration could also be given to applying this training model to den-tists, dental hygienists, pharmacists, optometrists, chiropractors, massage therapists, naturopaths, and others.

That's why Canada has to close at least one medical school. We recommend this rather than continued across-the-board cuts for the same reason we recommend closing some hospitals. First, reducing the budgets of all hospitals equally doesn't discriminate between efficient and inefficient ones—it's really quite unfair. It also doesn't save much money. The hospital still has to support its infrastructure and maintain all services— although at a reduced level.

The same applies to medical education. Federal transfer cutbacks and dwindling provincial capacity to support medical schools are making it very difficult for them to maintain a high level of quality. The cuts are hurting strong and weak schools alike. Closing the weakest one(s) would protect the continued viability of the rest.

However, we think some schools should be protected from outright closure. For example, eliminating the schools in Saskatchewan and Newfoundland would hurt the delivery of specialty services in those provinces. But why does Montreal need to have two schools—McGill and l'Université de Montréal? Why does Alberta need two (the University of Alberta in Edmonton and the University of Calgary) when British Columbia, with 50 percent more people, gets by with just one?

And some people ask whether Ontario really needs five medical schools.* If the province believes it does, it should at least consider moving one to northern Ontario, to Sudbury, for example, and making this new location the hub of a multicampus school for all of northern Canada.

Renewing nursing education

There are almost no full-time job openings for graduating nurses. Most are leaving the country to find work, while a few are cobbling together several part-time or casual jobs into full-time employment. This situation would change dramatically if Canada's health care system moved in the directions we're suggesting. In fact, we'd predict an increased demand for nurses at

---

* Ontario's medical schools are located in Toronto, Ottawa, Hamilton, London, and Kingston.

all levels of training, from registered practical nurse to clinical nurse specialist, although primary care nurses would be the most sought-after.

To accommodate the new system, however, nursing schools would have to shift their priorities by:

- training far more of their students to work in community settings;
- providing skills that support collaborative primary care practice;
- offering retraining to nurses losing their acute care jobs; and
- instituting "clinical laddering" so that nurses could easily take advanced training within nursing or pursue training for another health profession altogether without having to start over.

Easing Labour's Pains

There's no way around it. Our proposed reform has major implications for organized labour in our system. Staffing levels per bed in hospitals and long-term-care institutions will have to increase to cope with higher levels of acuity. And many new employment opportunities will be created in the community sector, jobs that should offer greater worker autonomy and higher job satisfaction overall. Nevertheless, it appears that the net impact of our proposed health reform will be an overall reduction in the numbers of people employed in the sector.

Already, thousands of health care workers have lost their jobs—mostly in acute care, as provinces have cut back hospital budgets. Working conditions for those still employed in these institutions have deteriorated. "It's just brutal here," said Lawrie McFarlane, when he was still president of the Saskatoon District Health Board, referring to the impact on unions. How can you expect them to be real supporters of reform, he asked, when employers "are firing staff left, right, and centre"? To Steven Lewis, who heads Saskatchewan's Health Services Utilization and Research Committee, the province's (initial) failure to develop an effective labour adjustment strategy was a big oversight:* "We know that probably we don't need as many health care workers, and that many certainly need to be redistributed to community care. But a civilized society doesn't just toss workers onto the slag heap because we don't need them doing the same things any more. It acts progressively to create opportunities for new work in new areas."

Organized labour in this country has been a major force behind many progressive social changes, including Medicare itself. In fact, the United Steelworkers Union pioneered prepaid medical care in Sault Ste. Marie, before Canada even had public insurance for physician care. Canadian unions were also highly visible supporters of the Canada Health Act. All the same, we can predict that health sector unions will oppose any health reform proposal that does not offer a "sane and humane" labour adjustment strategy.

There's a very strong connection between unemployment and illness. Losing a job is a very serious health risk. The health care system ought be acting on this knowledge by offering its workers iron-clad employment security. This single measure would take much of the sting out of health reform. Worker anxiety would decrease, and unions could, in good conscience, actively support the many progressive aspects of real reform.

Offering employment security is not in any way incompatible with our prediction that, overall, the number of jobs in health care might decline. The annual attrition rate in our system is between 4 and 10 percent. People leave the system voluntarily all the time when they move away, die, retire, or find other jobs. This level of attrition provides more than enough leeway to shrink the system without threatening existing employees.

However, there is a quid pro quo for job security. In return, unions will be asked to be more flexible, allowing, for example, current job descriptions to change and the relocation of jobs from one site to another. If a patient's blood pressure needs to be

---

* In fact, in 1993 Saskatchewan addressed this failing by proposing a model for a labour adjustment strategy. However, the province did not require the districts to follow the provincial strategy. Reports from Saskatchewan's health care unions say the program is working better in some communities than in others.

taken, it should be done by any available hands-on worker who knows how to do it. If a light bulb needs changing in someone's house, it should be done by whoever is there. A person's job might shift from the hospital to the community. Without this kind of "who does what where" flexibility, innovation flops, efficiency is out the window, and we're back to the beginning of the book, debating whether we can afford Medicare.

Protecting workers' rights is the unions' responsibility. However, shifting the location of jobs from institutions to community settings poses some thorny problems for organized labour. For example:

- People working in the community typically earn less than those employed in hospitals. Wage parity between the two sectors is therefore an essential precondition to successfully shifting jobs from one sector to another.
- The new system must ensure the portability of wages and benefits and system-wide recognition of seniority to facilitate the shift. Anything less than this will create insurmountable barriers to staffing.
- Many different unions represent health care workers, but organized labour has its greatest presence in institutions. A great deal of organizing work needs to be done to extend union membership throughout the system.

Furthermore, while collective bargaining is a key union function, it is also an expensive and very time-consuming process, made even more so in those cases where it is decentralized at the local establishment level. We think central bargaining for basic wages and benefits for all health care workers—sometimes called "sectoral bargaining"—would be much more efficient. Models for central bargaining in health care have already been implemented in Quebec and, more recently, in British Columbia. The rest of the country needs to catch up.

Deregulation of Health Care

The regulations that tightly limit health care workers also need to change. Many of these restrictions serve to protect the private

interests of doctors and dentists much more than the public's
health. Many conflict directly with current evidence about the
type of professional competent to provide various services. In
many provinces, the result is that midwives, dental hygienists,
and practical nurses are confined to narrow job descriptions
that ignore their real training and skills. Our proposed system
will need to make sure these workers are free to perform to their
full potential.

Accordingly, we think the provinces should review current
laws and regulations governing health professionals and make
the changes needed to facilitate innovative health programs in the
regions and communities. Ontario may have a model worth following in their recently proclaimed Regulated Health Professions
Act.* However, it's still too early to judge whether this new
approach to regulation will actually serve its intended purpose.

Organization and Staffing of Provincial Health Ministries and the Regions

In our proposed system, Ministries of Health in each province
would concentrate on setting policy and evaluating outcomes, as
we outlined in Table 9.1. This new job description has major
implications for how the ministries themselves are organized and
staffed. For example, the typical Ministry of Health organization
chart mirrors the kind of fragmentation seen in the system itself.
There's a branch or division responsible for institutions, another
responsible for physician payment, another for the drug program,
another for public health, and so on, each with its own separate
staff and budget. More than anything else, this structure reflects
the power of dominant interest groups within our system.

Our proposed reforms will make these "functional chimneys" irrelevant, obsolete. Instead, ministries will need a new
organizational structure capable of evaluating regional and

---

* Ontario's approach involved identifying thirteen "controlled acts" deemed
to pose some risk to the public's health if provided by an unregulated worker.
The legislation spells out which health professions have the right to provide
all or some of these acts. (Only doctors have the right to perform all thirteen.)

province-wide performance. This means being able to address the system as a whole, rather than the bits and pieces that comprise it. In provinces experimenting with regionalization, this is already starting to happen. Saskatchewan, for example, now has a computer information system capable of tracking costs and quality throughout the province and making district-to-district comparisons quickly and easily.

Overall, Ministries of Health will probably need fewer staff, not more. On the other hand, they will require far more personnel with expertise in the evaluative sciences, including epidemiology, health economics, program evaluation, and information systems.

By contrast, operational planning and management of the system will become a regional and community responsibility. Both levels will need personnel skilled in community development and group animation. And both will need staff with substantial administrative and technical expertise—including people with strong backgrounds in the evaluative sciences. Where will these people come from? A major source for administrative and technical personnel could be the hospital sector. Larger hospitals have lots of administrative and planning staff. In the new system we propose, most of these positions would be reallocated to the regional and community level.

This, in fact, is precisely what happened in New Brunswick when it regionalized its hospital system. A number of hospital CEOs relocated to take senior positions at the regional level. Marcelle Fafard-Godbout used to be the CEO of Grand Falls Hospital—a small facility with fewer than two hundred employees. Today, she is responsible for patient care and nursing services for an entire region. Of course it's one of the province's smaller regions, she's quick to point out, involving some 300 beds and about 500 staff: "What counts, I guess, is a positive attitude about the future—I see my new job as a new opportunity, a new direction."

A Comprehensive Research Strategy for Health Care

Jonathan Lomas, a professor at McMaster University, says it's been hard for health service researchers to identify the audience for their work.[17] This is changing, however. Driven by economic constraints, governments are beginning to make use of information from health services research to justify downsizing and rationalizing our over-built acute-care hospital sector, for example. Research information relevant to clinicians is also having an impact on changing practitioner behaviour; we've seen how local opinion leaders can reduce inappropriate Caesarean sections and improve survival rates for heart attack.

Almost certainly, our proposed system will create an enormous demand for clinical research and program evaluation. The incentives to create this demand are built in. For example, in our reformed system, a primary care centre that manages to reduce its hospital use by as little as 5 percent could produce enough savings to hire a dietician and a physical education consultant. Offering these services would give the centre a significant advantage over competitors and would no doubt attract new patients and more income.

This means, of course, that primary care centres would have to figure out how they could reduce hospital care without risking their patients' health. Soon, these centres would be scrambling for new health services research. Finding the funds to support this new demand for research might involve joining forces with other centres, or perhaps using the provincial primary care association to tap the Ministries of Health, the federal government, or other granting agencies.

Unfortunately, money for research on quality of care or to develop practice guidelines is hard to come by. The need is widely acknowledged, but medical associations and licensing/regulatory agencies claim they just don't have the resources. Governments too have slashed research budgets and have very little manoeuvring room to restore them in the current economic climate.

So we'd like to propose another promising candidate to supply new research funding—one that's fairly bursting at the seams with ready cash. Our nominee is the Canadian Medical Protective Association (CMPA), a physician-owned, non-profit malpractice insurance company. Nearly all of Canada's doctors belong to it. The objectives of the organization are perfectly suited to funding health services research—at least as it pertains to medical practice, as the following excerpt from their 1988 annual report reveals: "As was enunciated in the act of the Canadian Parliament incorporating the Canadian Medical Protective

Association in 1913, an important objective of the Association has always been 'to promote and support all measures likely to improve the practice of medicine.'"

Until 1983, all doctors in Canada, regardless of specialty or risk of lawsuit, paid the same low fee for malpractice insurance—about $500 a year. However, in the early 1980s, the CMPA predicted that Canada was going to witness a rapid escalation in litigation, as had already happened in the United States. To prepare for this onslaught, the CMPA hiked fees dramatically and began to charge doctors differently according to their risk of being sued. By 1994, an anaesthetist or obstetrician (both in the highest risk category) was paying $17,000 for malpractice insurance. Even family doctors who did no obstetrics or emergency work were paying $1,500.

But the malpractice crisis predicted by the CMPA never materialized. According to their own annual reports, the rate of legal actions commenced barely grew at all. The rate of judgments in favour of patients has also remained stable, with doctors winning between 70 and 80 percent of all cases that go to trial.

What did grow, however—and very impressively, too—was the CMPA's reserve fund for claims. From a base of $24.5 million in 1983, the fund had ballooned to $614 million by the end of 1992! And it's still growing at the rate of about $100 million a year; membership fees in 1992 were running at 70 percent above total expenses.*

In fact, today the CMPA has so much money that it has begun to cover legal costs of doctors involved in "billing disputes" with provincial health insurance plans—a move provincial governments dislike intensely, because government itself pays a substantial proportion of physician malpractice fees as part of their negotiated agreements with medical associations.

We think that the CMPA is a perfect choice for injecting badly needed cash into research aimed at improving the quality of medical care. Creating a Quality Care Research Foundation

---

* In fairness, CMPA's costs grew too. Spending on awards, settlements, legal services, and expert witnesses increased from $24 million in 1985 to $74 million. But this was more than offset by the enormous increase in revenues flowing to the organization.

would serve at least two of the CMPA's key purposes: it would reduce the likelihood of malpractice suits, and it would provide evidence useful in defending practitioners named in a lawsuit. Using just the investment interest on the reserve fund could easily produce $40 million every year to support clinical research, guideline development, and quality assurance programming. This idea was, in fact, proposed at a recent meeting of the Conference of Deputy Ministers of Health, but, according to Michael Decter, Ontario's former deputy minister of health, the CMPA failed to respond, except to acknowledge receipt of the Conference's letter.

Promoting non-traditional approaches to health care

The research agenda for health services, however, should not be limited to medical care alone. We are already finding out that competing alternatives have much to offer:

- As already discussed, Dr. Dean Ornish, a cardiologist from San Francisco, has shown how a strict low-fat vegetarian diet, combined with moderate exercise and other techniques to reduce stress, can melt away fatty plaque in patients' coronary arteries.[18]
- Within a short period of time, a low-fat diet can also control angina pains without additional medication.[19]
- Physical exercise and weight loss have been shown to prevent adult-onset diabetes.[20]
- A recent review of chiropractic shows it is more cost-effective in treating most acute low back pain than traditional medical therapies.[21]
- Nursing interventions aimed at reducing stress in certain heart attack patients can reduce their risk of a second heart attack.[22]

This list is far from complete, of course. But it would be even longer if more research funding were available to evaluate non-medical remedies. We could then talk about the relative merits of services from naturopathy, homeopathy, Chinese medicine, and a host of other competitors for the health care dollar. This research will never be done, however, as long as our system views drugs and surgery as the only legitimate therapies for disease.

For example, some heart patients swear chelation therapy helps them, but there's never been a properly designed randomized controlled study on its effectiveness.* Chelation therapy for a single patient can cost thousands of dollars, but of course if it really worked it could save the system tens of thousands of dollars in drug and surgical costs.

That's why it's so important to evaluate these alternatives properly. Those that work should be available through our publicly funded system. Those that don't work shouldn't be eligible for public funding, or private spending, either. Who wants to pay for a service that doesn't work? In fact, we think that providers who offer services proven to be ineffective should be liable for professional and, if necessary, legal sanctions.

During the 1930s, there were frequent demonstrations in Britain supporting the creation of the National Health Service. At many, Dr. Archie Cochrane, the famous epidemiologist, could be seen standing off to one side, away from the crowds, holding a placard with this simple message: "All Effective Care Should Be Free."

What more is there to say?

---

* Chelation therapy involves the intravenous injection of a drug (EDTA) in an attempt to dissolve plaque. It is a popular but unproven and potentially dangerous therapy.

Chapter 11

Getting from Here to There: Strategies for Success

IN THE EARLY 1970s, associate deputy health minister Dr. Ted Tulchinsky proposed a comprehensive reform of Manitoba's health care system. In retrospect, the plan he proposed was twenty years ahead of its time.[1] It made sense scientifically and managerially, calling for a larger and stronger primary care sector and a regional system for planning and management. But Dr. Tulchinsky's plan never really got off the ground because it lacked a comprehensive political strategy for winning support.

Health Minister Frank Miller ran into a similar problem in 1975 when he tried to rationalize hospital services in Ontario. Hospitals organized a series of highly emotional protests, and finally, the strain led to a heart attack for Mr. Miller, which effectively sidelined both him and his policies.*

The power of governments to legislate change—to impose reform from above—may appear limitless to those not directly involved in public service. But governments need allies to make substantial changes. To succeed with major reforms, politicians need public support.

Former health minister Monique Bégin admits that when she was just a rookie in Prime Minister Pierre Trudeau's cabinet she didn't really understand this. "I thought a good idea would just sell itself," she says. But Allen MacEachen, a cabinet colleague, set her

---

* Mr. Miller did recover enough to be an active minister in Bill Davis's government and, later, premier for a short period in 1985.

straight when he asked pointedly, "Where's the political demand for your proposals, Monique?" For Bégin, this was a turning point, and she began to understand that "politics is a balance of forces ... it's strategy that makes you a winner or a loser."[2]

And Bégin proved to be an outstanding political strategist. During the period leading up to the passage of the Canada Health Act—the law that permits Ottawa to penalize provinces allowing extra-billing or user fees—she and her staff worked tirelessly with national and provincial health coalitions to garner public support for the proposed law. She commissioned an opinion poll to demonstrate to her cabinet colleagues that she had grass-roots support. After winning their approval, her department published a white paper, *Preserving Universal Medicare*,[3] and distributed it strategically, so that requests for additional copies soon flooded the department. She tackled opposition from medical associations and most of the provinces by hosting a series of community forums that gave the "repressed structural interests"—especially nurses and consumers—a real voice in the debate. It paid off. The House of Commons unanimously passed this landmark legislation in 1984.

In *Medicare: Canada's Right to Health*, her book documenting this turbulent period, Bégin concludes: "Only the public can change the orientation of the health care system. If the public does not make demands, no politician, man or woman, can make the changes we need."[4]

Prussian statesman Otto von Bismarck said something similar back in 1867, when he declared that "politics is the art of the possible." Public demand is what makes policy change possible—especially if the change is dramatic and sweeping.

Covering the Bases

To succeed, a reform strategy has to cover all the bases: it must be based on accurate information and careful analysis; it must be managerially sound; and it has to resonate with the public's beliefs and values. Reforms often fail because one or more of these essential elements is ignored. For example, scientific knowledge from epidemiology doesn't readily translate into an implementable policy; merely knowing the evidence on treatment variations and inappropriate care does not tell us *how* to improve in ways that make managerial sense and are politically acceptable. Relying on management expertise alone can produce reforms that are politically damaging or scientifically off base. Politically popular reforms that reject scientific evidence and management considerations will probably produce systems that don't work.

Take, for example, the joint management committees in Ontario, Alberta, British Columbia, Manitoba, Newfoundland, and Nova Scotia established between the Ministries of Health and the provinces' medical associations. This kind of liaison might seem sensible from a managerial point of view; a joint management committee (JMC) provides a forum for physicians and government to deal with the many issues they face in common. Politically, however, they're a disaster. For example, most of these agreements allow the provincial medical associations to veto transferring money out of the fee-for-service pool to pay doctors on a different basis. With JMCs holding the balance of power, decisions are made behind closed doors. The public doesn't get access to information that would help change key beliefs. Other health care providers are also out in the cold—essentially "non-players" in the health reform debate.

Often, when the less powerful forces in our system try to participate in debate, the dominant interest groups slap them down. In 1993 the Ontario Nurses' Association (ONA)—the province's largest nurses' union—put together a well-written pamphlet that advocated, among other things, a stronger system of community-based care and a broader role for nurses. The pamphlet was designed as a newspaper insert and in November some 800,000 households in Ontario got a copy with their Saturday paper. The pamphlet also had an interactive component: a mail-in questionnaire. Ina Caissey, the ONA's president, was delighted with the response: "Thousands sent back their forms, often with a letter outlining their concerns in more detail. Many, many people indicated their desire to get involved."

Many health professionals—including some doctors—reacted favourably too. "It grabbed my attention," said Dr. Phil Berger, the chief of family medicine at Toronto's Wellesley Hospital.[5] Dr. Gordon Dickie, president of the Ontario College of Family Physicians, said he saw little in the document he could disagree with, although he wished the nurses' union had put more emphasis on health professionals working together. But the Ontario Medical Association blew a gasket. ONA's analysis criticized the drug industry, hospitals, and doctors, according to OMA president Tom Dickson, who said, "Insulting the other people who work with you on a daily basis is not the way to constructively reform a health care system." He characterized much of the material in the document as "judgmental, inflammatory, malicious and wildly inaccurate."[6] So far, the nurses' union has made no public response to this stinging rebuke. "I'm not sure we want to draw attention to the OMA's reaction," said Caissey. "We know the public's on our side."

Find the Winners and You'll Have Allies

The example above provides some clues about who stands to gain from health reform—and conversely, who is determined that it won't happen. Identifying the potential winners early on and devising ways to give them a real voice in the policy debate is central to the political strategy we outline in this chapter.

We've already described what we would like to see happen to the health care system in Canada. Let's now go ahead and ask this question: if we implemented our reforms—changed the funding rules, gave most of the system's resources to primary care centres, activated competition among them, and transferred management and operational responsibilities to the community and regional levels—who would win?

Winner Number 1: consumers and family members

We know that anticipatory primary care can catch problems early and forestall serious illness—when this strategy is applied systematically using a "whole population" approach, the community's overall health can improve substantially. To the extent that we make this clear to the public, people will support a reorganized and stronger primary care sector.

Consumer choice will also drive publicly financed competition in primary care. Provinces will issue public reports on the performance of regions, primary care centres, individual hospitals, and long-term-care facilities. This information, with relevant indicators (e.g. success of diabetic control, rates of surgical wound infections, bed sores, etc.), will help consumers choose where to get their care. Advertising restrictions will have to be softened to permit centres to publicize their programs, letting the public know, for example, whether dental care, a massage therapist, or a dietician is available on site. And consumers will also give direct feedback through routine surveys about their satisfaction with care and service. The results will help guide service improvements and, when published, will provide consumers with an added source of information about where to get care.[7]

As partners in managing their own care, patients and their families have a lot to gain from these reforms. For one thing, the new system will have an enormous incentive to help patients become truly informed about their conditions. It will also reinforce the right of patients to exercise their own preferences in choosing among diagnostic and treatment alternatives. The right of an informed patient to refuse treatment, even when this choice runs counter to professional advice, will be respected. Timely access to necessary and desired care will be guaranteed because the dollars to pay for primary, secondary, and some tertiary care will follow the patient throughout the system. And the implementation of priorization programs for waiting lists will ensure that everyone gets the high-tech services they need when they need them.

Health promotion and disease prevention services will be coordinated at the community level, and a more comprehensive range of health and social services will be offered locally. Even when patients need hospital treatment or care in a long-term-care facility, their connection to the primary care centre will always be maintained. This revamped system of primary care will bridge the gaps of poor coordination and service fragmentation.

Timely help for consumers will be only a telephone call away. Anxious parents, worried seniors, and concerned family members will be able to get speedy advice from specially trained nurses about how and when to use the health care system. The Toronto Hospital for Sick Children already has such a service in place for parents. Rachel MacLeod, a Toronto resident and mother of two young children, sees the service as "necessary and even essential, especially when it's four in the morning and you're all freaked out. When my daughter was going into her third day of fever, I looked through all the books I had at home with medical information to see how long we should wait before calling a physician, but I couldn't find any advice." Sometimes, she says, parents are very uncertain about how serious the illness is. "When the nurse answers the phone you get to talk to someone knowledgeable. You're already upset when you feel your child is really sick—just being able to talk to the nurse is very reassuring. With good information you can make a good decision about what action to take."

Consumers will also play an active role in governing the system, through community health centre boards and regional councils. Appropriate training and other support for board members will help consumers participate on an equal footing in decision-making. It's true that the boards of many individual agencies and hospitals will disappear, but overall, consumers will have a much better chance to really influence service delivery.

Opportunities for volunteer work will also expand as primary care centres search for ways to serve patients and clients better. Volunteer programs for friendly visiting, peer counselling, self-help, and so on could vastly enhance a centre's ability to reach out to people who need extra support. Centres will have an incentive to make sure volunteers have access to training and other supports to take on these important tasks.*

Winner Number 2: nurses

Nurses have a lot to gain from meaningful health care reform, and a lot to lose if it doesn't happen. For example, if our reforms are implemented, job prospects for nurses in primary care will explode. Under our proposed system, the number of nurses working in community settings of all types will more than double.[8]

New demands for efficiency and better treatment outcomes will foster more team-based, collaborative practice among nurses, doctors, and other health professionals. With capitation funding in place, it will make economic sense for nurses to take on substantial responsibility for primary care, and certainly the scientific evidence supports their doing so. We expect that the RN will look after the needs of healthy people in the practice

---

* The intention here of identifying a role for volunteers in service delivery is not to replace paid staff, but to underscore the idea that volunteers will continue to be important in human services.

and, in most cases, will keep tabs on those with chronic conditions, alerting the doctor to step in when problems arise.

Nurses will also play a key educational role in teaching patients how to manage specific conditions, which signs and symptoms should trigger an office appointment or an emergency room visit, and which ones are safe to handle on their own. "Call-a-nurse" programs, like the one at the Hospital for Sick Children, are already set for province-wide implementation in Quebec and are in use across the United States; their more extensive development will create even more job opportunities for nurses.

New nursing jobs in primary care centres will also open up for public health nurses, who will be working with individuals and groups on everything from family planning to quitting smoking, from the care and feeding of newborns to medication awareness. And although we favour physician-nurse teams for providing clinical primary care, experiments with clinics run entirely by public health nurses in Newfoundland might show this model to be a cost-effective alternative—especially in rural and remote areas having trouble attracting physicians.[9]

What about hospital work? That, too, will become more rewarding. Hospitalized patients will be more acutely ill and will need a greater degree of skilled nursing. Informed choice and patient demand will increase the supply of "high touch" care. Both will force a richer staffing complement for every remaining bed in the hospital. Although not all of these new positions will necessarily go to RNs, some definitely will. In addition, new opportunities for nurses to substitute for certain medical specialties will be created as hospitals try to satisfy demands from primary care centres for cost-effective, high-quality care, and as postgraduate physician training positions (cheap medical labour) are cut in some areas. As in other modern organizations, hospitals will have new incentives to flatten the hierarchy and promote real collaborative teamwork.

Hospitals will be under pressure from primary care centres to release patients as soon as they can be well cared for in the community. This will substantially increase the demand for home nursing care, as well. These nurses might work for primary health care centres or nurse-run collectives that would contract with various primary care centres.

Winner Number 3: other health care and social service professionals

As the entire system becomes more patient-driven, community jobs for other health care and social service workers will also expand. As just one example, the demand for timely discharge planning in hospitals will create new, higher-status jobs for nurses and social workers. Both will be needed on quick response teams working in every hospital emergency department, helping patients avoid unnecessary hospitalizations by arranging care closer to home.

Primary care centres and hospitals will both have an incentive to use the most cost-effective care-provider to match their patients' needs. Many service areas will experience a change in staffing patterns as a consequence. Who will perform foot care—RNs, practical nurses, chiropodists, or podiatrists? Who will provide home nursing—RNs or practical nurses? Who will deliver physiotherapy—or should we use chiropractic? Should the doctor do the counselling, or the nurse, or the social worker? Should we hire a psychologist or refer to an outside psychiatrist? Regions and primary care centres that get the right answers to these questions will quickly achieve a comprehensive human resources plan, based on quality of care, patient satisfaction, and economic considerations.

Overall, the new health care system will offer more opportunity for many health and social services workers to demonstrate their skills and earn recognition for their efforts.

Winner Number 4: primary care centres

He who pays the piper calls the tune. Because primary care centres will control most of the health care budget, they'll be in a strong position to negotiate for better service from specialists and hospitals. They will also be able to expand greatly the range of services they themselves offer. Capitation funding provides ample flexibility to accomplish this.

And because the per-patient funding will be adjusted according to the individual rostered patient's need for care, centres serving the most disadvantaged areas could easily receive two to three times more funding than centres operating in wealthier and healthier communities. For existing community health centres, many of which operate in high-needs areas, these enhanced resources will make it possible to provide more services.

Health system performance indicators will show how effectively each centre has been able to promote health and prevent disease. Publication of results and word of mouth will reward successful centres, thus attracting more patients—and more revenue.

Winner Number 5: good doctors

The new system promises great rewards for good family physicians—particularly those trying hard to serve high-risk patients well. Many of the best primary care doctors today can work sixty-plus hours every week and earn less than a plumber who puts in fifty.[10] That's not fair—particularly when they see colleagues dealing with a high volume of "easy" patients who are able to take home twice as much as the Prime Minister!

Under our proposal, doctors who want to work like nurses and social workers will probably be out of a job, but many of this country's better family doctors will actually make *more* money after reform, in most parts of the country netting at least $100,000 for a forty-hour week. Those wanting to work longer hours, perform obstetrics, work in emergency departments, or look after patients with heavier needs could net up to $150,000, or more.[11] Ultimately, we recommend that a pay scale be set by negotiation between the association representing family doctors and the province. However, the settlement should leave some flexibility for negotiation between individual centres and their doctors.

Good family doctors would also be able to practise medicine at an unparalleled level of quality. The strains and pressures of work will lessen too, through collaborative practice with nurses and other health professionals and the ready on-site availability of other primary care doctors.

Rural doctors will see dramatic improvement in their quality of life. They will be able to share the load for after-hours and emergency services with others and be paid for the hours they actually work.

Academic doctors won't have to jam patients through their offices in order to generate enough fee-for-service billings to support their teaching and research activities. Dr. David Sackett, professor of internal medicine at McMaster University, recently complained that he and his colleagues were being forced to practise high-volume medicine just to keep their faculty afloat.[12]

In 1993, the chiefs of the five Ontario university family medicine departments said they'd love to see fee-for-service junked in favour of a capitated system. Dr. John Forster, an outspoken advocate of this approach, is the chief of family medicine at Ottawa University. Twenty years ago, he left England. Now he wonders if he made the right choice as he sees his British colleagues increasing their income and prestige under the new reforms to the National Health Service that put primary care in the system's driver's seat by creating fundholding practices. In fact, fee-for-service for clinical instructors in Canada's medical schools could one day be as outdated as bleeding and cupping. In 1993, Queen's University made a landmark agreement with the Ontario government that eliminated fee-for-service payment entirely in that institution.

The demand for scientific evaluation of alternative diagnostic interventions and therapies will also increase. And of course, if the Canadian Medical Protective Association agrees to establish a Quality of Care Research Foundation funded by the interest earned on their growing reserve fund for claims (as recommended in Chapter 10), the money to support this research would be there—to the tune of $40 million or more every year.

Winner Number 6: public health

In the nineteenth and early twentieth centuries, health policy was public health policy, almost completely concerned with preventing the spread of infectious disease. But then came undreamed-of advances in scientific medicine and changes in public attitudes, which left public health departments resigned to a less relevant role. Now is the time for the public health ideology to once again permeate the entire system. Relocating public health nurses to primary care centres would energize a much-esteemed Canadian profession.

In a similar fashion, public health epidemiology—monitoring the health status of the population and tracking the spread of diseases and risk factors—would be revitalized as scientists skilled in epidemiology and biostatistics joined with their clinical colleagues to form the central nervous system of the new health services. Having a real role in assisting regions and primary care centres to achieve better and better performance would be just the tonic these epidemiologists, data analysts, and evaluators need. They've been on the sidelines too long.

Finally, new mandates for provincial and regional health officers would enhance the prestige of these archetypical guardians of the public's health. The new job description for British Columbia's provincial health officer gives the position a much higher public profile and could be a template for other provinces. Not unlike the U.S. Surgeon General, British Columbia's provincial health officer is expected to issue a health status report every year and to speak out publicly on issues affecting the province's health.[13]

Winner Number 7: health service researchers

The search for better and more cost-effective ways to produce good health outcomes and higher patient satisfaction will produce a phenomenal demand for new health services research.

It's already happening in Saskatchewan. The province's new Health Services Utilization and Research Commission (HSURC) has been conducting extremely relevant research to guide system planning. According to executive director Steven Lewis, its mandate is "to produce evidence that leads to action."

In 1993, the commission published a study aimed at finding out how sick the people in Saskatchewan's hospitals really were. The results showed that about half the people in hospital could have had their needs met more appropriately in other, less costly settings.[14] "It's hard to believe that such a study had never been done before, but there you are," says Lewis. Dr. Stewart McMillan, who chairs the commission, said many of the patients now taking up expensive beds would be better off in home-care or out-patient programs.[15]

Lewis believes that studies like this one can be powerful tools for change: "Research evidence can be transformed into policy advice—it can tell us what direction we need to go in. And when we use it and start moving in the right direction—the major shifts that need to occur start to happen." In fact, Lewis is convinced that any movement—even a small one—is positive, provided it's in the right direction.

With Saskatchewan's district boards needing to make good decisions about resource allocations, the demand for HSURC's research evidence will grow. When good researchers meet enthusiastic Traders, exciting things could happen.

Winner Number 8: health system planners and administrators

The absolute number of administrative staff will likely decline in our proposed system, but managers will have substantially more power to make changes. New job opportunities for people with management and planning skills will open up at the regional level as well.

Administrators of health care delivery organizations—primary care centres, hospitals, and long-term-care facilities—will have much more freedom to make operational decisions. With the province clarifying health outcome expectations, the delivery system will be challenged, but also free to design services and hire staff that produce good results. Their role as good Traders will be reinforced, not thwarted.

John Harwood is the executive director of the Sault Ste. Marie Group Health Centre, an out-patient service offering primary and secondary care. He already works in a system based on capitation. His centre is one of Ontario's ninety HSOs (health service organizations) and it serves more than 33,000 regular patients from the area. But he complains that the Ministry of Health interferes too often with the centre's day-to-day operational decisions. "We only have one oncologist," he explained, "and he's putting in ridiculous hours trying to look after all our cancer patients and handle a huge volume of outside referrals from fee-for-service doctors in the community." Harwood already has another oncologist lined up for hire, but "the Ministry is balking at approving it. My hands are tied and I'm worried about how long it will be before my lone oncologist gives up on us."

Under our proposal, the number of medical specialists at the secondary level will be determined by the number of referrals from primary care centres. There will be no need for complicated bureaucratic planning processes. The market demand generated by the primary care centres will decide the number of doctors who could make a living in any community. Primary care centres will be free to cross regional borders to purchase secondary care. If the centre's patients can get better service for elective surgery in the region next door, then the centre's own region has more of an incentive to improve its service levels.

Hospital executives with a strong track record in worker-sensitive total quality management (TQM) and continuous quality improvement (CQI) will also emerge as winners in the new system. Many Canadian hospitals are already pursuing TQM, hoping this will give them a competitive edge. But right now only a handful of CEOs have extensive experience with it. Those who do are leaders who know how to flatten and democratize the traditional hierarchical culture of the hospital and how to make better use of data to analyse problems and test solutions. They are beacons of experience for others to learn from and emulate.

To get a quick view of the future for administrators, consider what has already occurred in Prince Albert, Saskatchewan. There, a district health board now controls pooled funding for all health services, except those for physicians and drugs.*

Stan Rice is a champion beef farmer who used to be the pharmacist at the Saskatoon Community Clinic and, later on, the administrator of the Prince Albert Community Clinic. Today, he's the executive director of the Prince Albert District Health Board, serving a region of 47,000 people. Like many other small Canadian cities, Prince Albert has one Catholic and one non-denominational hospital, with a combined capacity of 140 beds. Each hospital had pretty much duplicated all the services delivered by the other, until the provincial government set up the district health board in June 1992. By November 1993, the two hospitals had rationalized all clinical departments except internal medicine. Now reconfigured, the Catholic hospital provides long-term care, internal medicine, and ambulatory care. The public hospital delivers all the other acute-care hospital services.

In the first year following this consolidation, the Prince Albert Health Board saved $1.1 million out of a $32 million acute-care hospital budget. The number of home care services ballooned by 30 percent. The acute care hospitals had twenty-six long-term-care patients waiting for alternative placement when the district board was established. The following year, only one patient was waiting for relocation.

The board also acted to close a small hospital about thirty minutes outside Prince Albert and open a community health

---

* Although the pooled funding available to the board does not cover resources for physician care or for drugs, many doctors are coming forward expressing an interest in alternatives to fee-for-service payment.

centre on the same site, and to set up a single-entry system for assessing long-term-care clients.

Unlike administrators in other provinces, Stan Rice doesn't have to worry about the future of his hospital or his agency. He spends all his time trying to improve the overall health of Prince Albert, and budget flexibility enables him to use whatever services will work best.

Winner No. 9: provincial Ministers of Health

There's nothing more gratifying to a politician than being acknowledged as a good leader. In this respect, Saskatchewan's Health Minister, Louise Simard, has been outstanding. Since her appointment by Premier Roy Romanow in 1991, she has moved quickly to:

- regionalize health system management and service delivery, and
- provide the thirty new district health boards with pooled funding.

None of this was easy. It took courage to wipe out existing boards and replace them with a consolidated structure for governing the entire system. But Ms. Simard didn't blink or back down. Instead, she participated directly in a careful political strategy to win support. In dozens and dozens of community meetings, she talked up the ideas for her reform, bringing people a positive vision of a better system.

And unlike some other health ministers, who are using slash-and-burn tactics to cut both hospitals and community care, Ms. Simard has taken the long view by putting in place two of the key mechanisms for shifting the way resources are allocated. In 1992-93, Saskatchewan's hospital budget *decreased* by over 2 percent, while the home care budget *increased* by over 10 percent. Simard has also announced that the system will move to capitation funding in 1995.* The Ministry of Health has been working with McMaster University researcher Dr. Stephen

---

* Current district budgets reflect historical funding levels, combining previously separate budgets for all services (except drugs and doctors) into one unified pool.

Birch to develop a funding formula that will base capitation funding for their districts on community needs.

Ms. Simard has also been quick to recognize and correct mistakes. The province now has a labour adjustment strategy—a key element that was lacking when her reforms were first implemented.* In fact, throughout the reform process, Saskatchewan's Health Minister (above all others in the country) has shown extraordinary fortitude and a willingness to exert prowess—key Guardian characteristics.

New Brunswick's Health Minister, Dr. Russell King, consolidated the province's fifty-one hospital boards into eight regional boards, but he did so very suddenly, without key stakeholder input. Although a more democratic process is preferable, sometimes governments do need to make changes suddenly. Occasionally, surprise tactics can succeed. In a similar fashion, former British Columbia Health Minister Elizabeth Cull showed considerable fortitude in closing the Shaughnessy Hospital. The announcement itself was somewhat unexpected, even though rumours had been circulating for years of the hospital's likely demise. Cull, since promoted to Finance Minister, was clear that the decision was irrevocable and saw to it that the implementation avoided patient and staff disruption.

Other Ministers of Health could benefit from Ms. Simard's example: move public opinion as much as you can, then change the rules of the game, creating new interests to carry the reforms forward with new momentum. Nothing adds more to a politician's job satisfaction than being able to point to a successfully implemented policy and know that he or she helped make it happen.

Winner No. 10: public servants in Ministries of Health

New roles for provincial health ministries will make work for its public servants much more rewarding than it is today. Currently, they too often lack clear objectives, are subject to unrealistic demands, and spend almost all their time helping to put out political fires. To complicate matters, in the past five years or so, provincial governments have been asked to manage their

---

* However, Saskatchewan's health care unions still feel it should be more labour-friendly.

health care systems instead of just writing cheques. But this new responsibility didn't come with new resources. Nor is there much hope in the current period of economic restraint that health ministries will convince finance departments that they need more staff to do this new job.

But the new system gives provincial ministries a strong and clear job description based on "steering," one that leaves the "rowing" to others.[16] Re-establishing the primacy of their Guardian responsibilities will go a long way towards changing the culture within health ministries, making them happier and more productive workplaces. The structure of their organization will change, too, as ministries develop ways to respond to system concerns within a region and as they assume responsibility for evaluating the system's performance.

Already, Saskatchewan has begun to move in this direction by setting up a District Development Branch and a Health Reform Directorate. Ministry officials know that the battleground over resources has shifted to the regions, and the constant pull to fight fires to address local problems will follow.

Relieved of these major distractions, government officials will be able to tackle their real job. We predict that once they get the chance to really steer the system, once they are able to concentrate on guarding it and the public's health, working life in Ministries of Health will be transformed. Public service jobs will be more gratifying and less frustrating.

Winner Number 11: central agencies of government

Central agencies of government—those that oversee other departments, including the premier's office, policy and priorities committees of cabinet, cabinet office, the Finance Ministry, and, in many provinces, the treasury board or management board—view provincial responsibility for health care with some trepidation. They know the system has a strong tendency towards continuous expansion, and they worry about meeting new demands for care and service as new technologies emerge and as the population grows and ages.

That's why provincial treasurers will heave a sigh of relief when changes to the basic rules for funding and organizing health care make the system more efficient and effective. Setting an overall budget for health and devolving much of the decision-making to the regions and primary care centres will create a more stable and predictable fiscal climate.

Provincial premiers, too, will discover that health reform can be a political plus. In the summer of 1993, Prince Edward Island Premier Catherine Callbeck introduced legislation to set up locally elected regional authorities to replace the existing boards of hospitals and community service agencies, without substantial outcries.[17] Saskatchewan's Premier, Roy Romanow, stood behind his Health Minister as she proceeded to regionalize the system. He withstood a lot of criticism for cutting off fifty-two hospitals from acute-care funding. And, as the system began to produce savings, he didn't grab all the money—he allowed some of it to be reallocated to improve district services. In consequence, he's managed to retain much of his popularity. A much more responsive and efficient health care system will be in place before Mr. Romanow has to face another election. Other Premiers should take note. Health reform done properly can be a political winner.

Winner Number 12: the human services sector

Canada spends more per capita on health care than any other country with a publicly financed health care system. However, we are not so generous with our other social programs. Our record on childhood poverty is a disgrace compared to any other developed country but the United States. The current economic recession is being used by some as an excuse to cut our social safety net to ribbons. A more efficient health care system isn't the whole answer to these problems, but it would allow us to reallocate billions of dollars to child care, housing, income maintenance, and other worthwhile social initiatives.[18]

The Art of the Possible

Now that we have identified those who have an interest in supporting reform, what is the next hurdle?

For governments to implement health reform, an appropriate political strategy is essential. To prime the pump, they need to change some key beliefs among the media, the public, and the major players in the health field before taking the first steps to create publicly financed competition at the primary care level.

Once this is in place, new interest groups will be created. These, in turn, will accelerate changes in beliefs about what's possible and necessary, and the stage will be set for further reforms.

For example, the most recent recession allowed provincial governments to negotiate fixed budgets for doctors' billings, something they have been trying to do for a very long time. Almost immediately, provincial medical associations began demanding controls on the numbers of new doctors entering the system—a policy that organized medicine had firmly resisted for fifteen years.

Two key strategies can help change beliefs:

- facilitating a coalition for change; and
- organizing opportunities for public debate.

Many patients in our system—including seniors, women, and people with HIV infection, mental illness, and chronic conditions—are very poorly served by the health care system. Hundreds of thousands of its employees are fed up with deteriorating working conditions and their inability to influence decisions. Both groups could work together more effectively if they were organized into a grand coalition for reform.

Two things get in the way of this happening. Many splits among and within these groups have created a culture of "warring clans," making it hard for members from disparate groups to even remember that they have interests in common. A second problem is that repressed interests often get co-opted by the medical profession or administrators and wind up serving their interests instead of those of consumers and workers.[19]

Political leaders looking for support have to help the repressed interests see that they have a collective interest in health reform. Then they need to establish forums so their voices can be heard. If governments really want reform, the best advice we can offer them is to identify and help to mobilize those individuals and groups who stand to gain the most from the changes.

Lessons from Ontario: creating coalitions for change

At present, there is no cohesive coalition for health care reform, and there are few opportunities for public debate and dialogue about the issue. Some governments have even made public debate more difficult by dealing with dominant interest groups behind closed doors. That's what Ontario did when it created its Joint Management Committee (JMC) with doctors and the Joint Policy and Planning Committee with hospitals. But there is an alternative to this kind of exclusive bargaining.

In 1981, the Ontario Medical Association outmanoeuvred the new Health Minister, Larry Grossman, when they signed a very rich deal that increased the doctors' fee schedule by 60 percent over five years.* An ambitious politician, Grossman had his eye on the Premier's job, but he knew that to win caucus approval he had to get the health portfolio under control first.

Grossman knew that changing the rules can help create new interests in the system. In the early 1980s, Ontario's community health centre program was in limbo.** Grossman commissioned Dr. Fraser Mustard (now head of the Canadian Institute for Advanced Research) to chair a task force on primary care. Mustard worked quickly, taking only six months to report back that community health centres made sense. Almost immediately, Grossman announced that the community health centre program was no longer experimental. He also promised to develop new centres and provided $50,000 in funding for a new Association of Ontario Health Centres. Bingo! A new interest group was created.

Through a series of forums known as the "Deerhurst Process" (named after the resort where one of the first meetings was held), Grossman began to discuss other plans for the health system's future with the Ontario Hospital Association, the Registered Nurses' Association of Ontario, and the Ontario Medical Association. While this was going on, his senior policy advisers were meeting with many members of the "repressed" interest groups in the system—mental health advocates, representatives of community health centres, and health care unions—to try to convince

---

* The cost of living during that period only rose 30 percent. Some analysts still joke about the time "Larry wrestled the OMA to the ceiling."

** In fact, Grossman's predecessor as Health Minister, Dennis Timbrell, came close to killing them off altogether. Today, Mr. Timbrell is the president of the Ontario Hospital Association.

these groups to pull together to take on the dominant interests in the system.

Grossman's campaign peaked in April 1983 when he brought together nearly three hundred people from all parts of Ontario's health care system at a large Scarborough hotel for three days. There were only a couple of dozen delegates from organized medicine, and other dominant interest groups were also in a minority. Grossman's people had put together a background document for the conference that outlined the "facts" for health policy reform—including the evidence that health care is, overall, a minor determinant of health and that the health care system could be organized more efficiently. Helping to make these points were a host of internationally renowned speakers, but most of the conference time was devoted to small group sessions at which fifteen delegates got the chance to debate the issues, assisted by a trained facilitator. In these small groups, the dominant interests had to confront a ragtag opposition of consumers and community health advocates, and they usually came out second-best. During and after this meeting, the OMA and other dominant groups began to moderate some of their positions—an example of what Paul Sabatier calls "policy-oriented learning."

Unfortunately, the whole process came to a crashing halt when Grossman was promoted to Treasury. Ministry officials quickly scuttled the forums, and policy debates in health retreated once again into backroom discussions with doctors and hospitals.

All the same, Grossman's approach to health reform is highly relevant to the political challenges facing us today. Smart governments will follow his lead, seeking out and helping to organize allies for reform among the "repressed" interests in the system.

Consolidating a Coherent Consumer Voice

It takes great courage for government leaders to actually help organizations to take them on in policy debates. And yet this kind of support is necessary if we wish to have a truly balanced debate, since the "repressed" interests in our system generally lack resources and access to expert policy advice.

Consumer groups are really the new kids on the block when it comes to health policy. When seniors, disabled people, or groups addressing mental illness, AIDS, or breast cancer enter the fray, they usually arrive with a strong critique of the delivery system. And often their criticisms take aim at the dominant structural interests in the system—doctors and hospitals.

It won't be easy for all these different groups to come together with one coherent voice. Most see their issues in isolation from the more general systemic problems that plague the system. For example, AIDS activists often identify homophobia as the real culprit, while breast cancer support groups often point to sexism. While discrimination does, of course, play a part in some of the difficulties they experience in getting the care they need, these groups also have a lot to gain from a total reform of the system.

Each consumer group naturally wants more attention and more resources for its own issue. Many who focus on a specific disease think a cure is just around the corner, if only society would spend more money looking for one. They don't realize how rare real cures are in health care. Apart from antibiotic drugs and a few surefire surgical treatments, most health care services only help to *control* serious illnesses, not *cure* them. In most cases, cures will remain elusive, no matter how much money we spend trying to find them.

And there's another issue for professional policy analysts weighing the recommendations from consumer coalitions—are they cost-effective? When the Seniors' Alliance in Ontario came together in a consumer group, they were committed to improving the long-term-care system for all seniors. The need to target scarce resources on the frail elderly, for reasons of effectiveness and efficiency, conflicted with the Alliance's desire to see more "wellness" programs for healthy seniors. Many seniors' groups would like to see more "aging-in-place" services, like snow shovelling, yard work, and help with shopping. When targeted at those most at risk of losing their independence, these programs are often a wise investment, but providing them to everyone over sixty-five is a very costly frill, taking resources away from those who really need them.

In 1986, ten consumer groups in Australia developed a plan for consumer input into planning and policy development. With funding from their federal government, the Australian Consumers' Health Forum networks with other consumer and community groups, dispenses grants for research on public participation and social action, and ensures a consumer voice in the health policy process.[20] We could follow their example.

The time is ripe for governments in Canada to cultivate a consumer coalition for health reform. Politicians committed to structural change will need their informed support. Governments can help in two ways: with no-strings financial assistance, and by setting up participatory forums for public debate.

Grey power

For over ten years, successive Ontario governments have been trying to reform the province's long-term-care system. Until recently, they have not had much success. The problem was not a lack of information or policy analysis: virtually everyone agreed about what ailed the system—fragmentation, poor coordination, uneven access, unequal funding levels, too much reliance on institutions, too little funding for community care. All the same, there was little consensus about solutions, until consumers came together and insisted on having a voice in developing policy.

In the summer of 1991, Ontario's NDP government released a policy paper concerning reforms to long-term care, inviting all stakeholders, and especially consumers, to respond.[21] Their paper made proposals essentially identical to those made a year earlier by the Liberal government.[22]

That's when Ted Ball, a former adviser to Larry Grossman who by then was working outside government as a private consultant, invited representatives from the three largest consumer organizations in the province* to explore the possibility of working on a joint response. "The first meeting was pretty tense," says Ball, "because there was some bad feeling among and between the groups. But after some venting of ancient history, we quickly settled down to the business at hand. Everyone clearly understood that working together would be much more powerful than working separately."

Very soon, the largest provincial seniors' organization in the province's history was born: the Senior Citizens' Consumer

---

* The founding groups were: the United Senior Citizens of Ontario, the Ontario Coalition of Senior Citizen Organizations, and the Consumers' Association of Canada (Ontario).

Alliance for Long-Term Care Reform in Ontario. Chaired by Jane Leitch, who was also serving as president of the United Senior Citizens of Ontario, the Alliance had four members from each of its three founding organizations. A sophisticated and politically savvy group, these consumers were determined to influence government policy.

Very quickly, their work intensified as they boned up on the research evidence and began identifying weaknesses in the government's proposals. They also set about raising funds to support their activities from government, philanthropic organizations, and some other private sector groups.

Knowing that many other groups would also be preparing submissions, in the fall of 1991, the Alliance put out a booklet of provocative questions about the proposed reforms, including questions they wanted the government itself to answer.[23] They distributed this booklet to six thousand key interest groups— consumers, professional associations, hospitals, district health councils, nursing homes, home care providers, and many more. The questions themselves prompted many of these organizations to start thinking from a consumer's perspective as they debated the issues and prepared their own responses.

The government had planned a major public consultation on its long-term-care reform, which, in the end, heard from more than seventy thousand people throughout the province. But the Alliance was determined to run its own show. The seniors worried that government facilitators might not ask the right questions and that the consumers' voices might be drowned out by professional groups.[24] So in January 1992, the Alliance hosted a policy conference for six hundred delegates, one-third of whom were consumers. Expert speakers addressed key issues and provided a forum for the Alliance to announce that it was going to hold its own public hearings on long term-care reform the following month.

In February and March, a rotating panel of Alliance members sat through sixteen full days of hearings. "We thought at first we could wrap it up in about four or five days," says Sylvia Cheuy, who worked closely as a consultant to the Alliance, "but the requests started flooding in so fast, we had to expand the entire process. I guess you could say we were victims of our own success." In the end, more than 150 groups and individuals participated—consumers, institutions, a host of professional groups, community agencies, and even government officials. In the evenings, the Alliance invited other groups to sponsor policy forums on a variety of related topics, including organized labour, palliative care, and quality assurance. They also sent for On Lok's executive director, Marie-Louise Ansak, to make a presentation so people would be able to envision a better way of providing coordinated services.

In June 1992, the Alliance put on another equally well-attended conference and used the occasion to release its report. Instead of offering yet another critique, this report offered a completely new vision—a realistic plan for addressing the appalling fragmentation in community-based long-term care.[25] Frances Lankin, Ontario's Health Minister at the time, addressed this conference and signalled her strong interest in the Alliance's recommendations. "I actually read it through cover to cover twice over the week-end," she asserted. Privately, she thanked the seniors profusely for delivering what seemed to her a workable alternative to the government's plan.

Throughout the fall and winter, Alliance members attended a series of meetings with the Minister, her staff, the deputy, and government officials. Despite some natural resistance from the public servants who had drafted the original reform scheme, and from certain provider groups who felt threatened by the Alliance's proposals, when the government released its new policy paper in 1993, the Alliance knew the taste of victory.[26] The new plan substantially followed the consumers' key recommendations for changing the rules of the game—pooling resources for long-term care at the regional level, regional planning and resource allocation through district health councils, and new consolidated structures for assessing eligibility and delivering services at the community level.

Since then, the Alliance has kept a sharp eye on how the plan is being implemented. In the fall of 1993, it released yet another paper signalling early problems and reminding the government what it needs to do to keep reforms on track.[27]

Workers Unite

Organized labour obviously has a lot to gain from system reforms that guarantee job security and better working conditions. Sectoral bargaining in both Quebec and British Columbia has protected workers from the massive layoffs and job losses experienced in other provinces.

Health care unions with similar protections could provide another source of organizing skill and policy leadership to support government health reform plans. But unions could also present a forceful and formidable challenge to governments if no provision is made for sectoral bargaining, wage parity, portability of benefits, recognition of seniority, and employment security. Unions, after all, have largely a Guardian role to play in our system. It is sometimes challenging to find ways of fulfilling these responsibilities that do not distract from the overall system's ability to serve patients better. Some are demonstrating that it can be done, however.

For example, Linda Silas-Martin, the energetic president of the New Brunswick Nurses Union, was determined to focus public attention on the pain her nurses felt at being excluded from the health reform process. In the fall of 1992, the union organized a public meeting to debate health reform during its annual meeting. More than six hundred people attended. It was readily apparent that the nurses understood and supported the need for change. At the same time, however, they expressed legitimate concerns about quality of care and workers losing their jobs.

Two local radio personalities moderated a panel of politicians; the opposition health critics and the health minister, Dr. Russell King—to his credit—all participated. It wasn't long before the sparks began to fly. Questions from the audience challenged the minister to explain why some of the newly created regional boards were holding closed meetings, and what he intended to do about all the layoffs that were happening.

Uncomfortable as it may have been for the minister, many important policy issues related to regionalization got a brisk airing at this event. And perhaps some beliefs changed as well. For example, several regional board members in attendance said they would propose open board meetings to their members. And they did—all regional board meetings are now open to the public. Silas-Martin herself earned political capital and went on to negotiate a better deal with government to protect her members. In other words, Sabatier's policy-oriented learning—however painful—can set the stage for a better reform process.

The Canadian Union of Public Employees also helped the system's policy IQ when it hosted a national health care workers' conference in Montreal, in February 1992. All delegates went away with a set of five research papers outlining major issues of concern.[28] The conference itself was organized in workshops around these policy topics and helped to create a more level playing field for workers confronting these issues. Author and health policy consultant Varda Burstyn attended this conference on behalf of the Windsor Essex Steering Committee on health system reconfiguration. She says it really "helped to clarify and to make more generally known not only the common problems faced by workers across the system, but also a set of possible solutions which could be creatively adapted from one set of jurisdictions to another."

Consumers and Health Workers: Hang Together or Hang Separately?

During the debates over public health insurance in the 1960s and early 1980s, consumers and health care workers agreed on a policy position and, in combination, were a very effective counterbalance to the dominant interests who opposed Medicare and the ban on user fees.

But the issues for health care *system* reform are quite different. What are the prospects today for forging a similar grand alliance of support?

First, we have to recognize that sometimes the interests of consumers and workers are virtually identical and sometimes they collide. It's encouraging, however, to find that when both have the chance to air their perspectives, some policy-oriented learning can moderate their respective positions. For example, some parts of organized labour in British Columbia seemed ready to reject many of the concepts put forward by the British Columbia Royal Commission on Health Care and Costs. They even poked fun at the name of the report—*Closer to Home*—until some allies made it clear that most consumers really *did* want their care provided closer to home. This reoriented the

debate considerably, and British Columbia unions went on to battle for a better labour adjustment deal, one that would protect
security for both workers and consumers.

And there's another issue that should provide some glue to hold
workers and consumers together, Varda Burstyn points out: "Both
want to see more of health care's resources flowing into service
delivery rather than administration." Ontario's senior citizen consumer alliance was shocked to discover that between 35 and 40
percent of long-term-care spending in the community went to
administrative overheads.[29] Some of this overhead was for case
management to help consumers wend their way through a ridicu-
lously complex maze of agencies and service providers. "That's
what convinced us, we needed to tackle consolidation of services
at the delivery level first," says president Jane Leitch. "We wanted
to see a system at the ground level that was more efficient, one that
would concentrate most of the funding on care, not management."

Other indications of overlap in the values and interests of
workers and consumers also offer scope for a grand alliance for
health system reform. For example, both, in a sense, are self-
appointed Guardians of the system—determined to protect the
integrity of public finance and quality of care.

Economics professor Richard Plain from the University of
Alberta has been a very outspoken opponent of moves by Premier
Ralph Klein to privatize the system. In a segment on the TV news-
magazine show "W-5," he pleaded for people to understand that
being able to jump ahead of others by paying cash for a privately
operated magnetic resonance imaging (MRI) scan was a serious
policy departure and one that threatened Medicare itself. Plain is
an active member of the Consumers' Association of Canada
(CAC), a group that has had a health committee for a number of
years. The CAC also added a strong and supportive consumer
voice in the fight to pass the Canada Health Act of 1984.

The Canadian Health Coalition, with membership support from
the Canadian Labour Congress, churches, social service organizations, and consumers, has also opposed privatization of our system.* The Coalition had some success, for example, in focusing
media attention on the negative implications of federal funding

---

* Some individual provinces also have similar health coalitions that have
been actively fighting government cutbacks and privatization.

cutbacks and increased patent protection for brand-name drugs. Just before the recent federal election, it was this tiny group that managed to get a signed letter from the Liberals promising a meaningful federal role in providing "stabilty and predictability in the financing of health care."* Unfortunately, the Coalition is perennially strapped for funding and has had trouble maintaining a consistent public profile because of chronic understaffing. Recently, however, Stephen Learey, a former housing activist with a strong background in community development, was hired as the new executive director. Now that this is a full-time position, the Coalition will have a better chance to organize for health reform.

In the meantime, the Canadian Nurses Association (nursing's national professional association) and the Consumers' Association of Canada are two of the seven members of HEAL, the national health action lobby.** HEAL has issued a number of well-researched discussion papers since its formation in 1991 but also has had difficulty in coming up with positive policies. Their main claim to fame is that, along with the Canadian Health Coalition (and the Liberals and the NDP), they helped to make health care an issue in the 1993 federal election.

Nurturing Nursing

In many ways, nurses are the key to health reform. Nurses are losing their jobs by the thousands. Those who still have jobs are watching their quality of working life deteriorate. New nurses are fleeing to Texas just to find full-time work. But these stories have attracted little public or media attention. Contrast that with the flurry of national media attention Ontario's new doctors got

---

* Of course "zero growth" is stable and predictable, although many would be disappointed with this definition.

** The other members of HEAL are the Canadian Medical Association, the Canadian Public Health Association, the Canadian Psychological Association, the Canadian Hospital Association and the Canadian Long-Term Care Association.

when the province simply threatened to put limits on where they could practise.

Major system reform is just what nurses need to get more autonomy and greater job satisfaction. And there are other reasons why nurses should be front and centre in any coalition for health reform:

- *Numbers*: with over a quarter of a million RNs in the country, nursing is the single largest group of workers in the entire system.
- *Contacts*: nurses also have a long tradition as patient advocates, as the profession closest to consumers. A hospital patient may spend only a few minutes with the doctor each day, while nurses are in and out all the time seeing to her needs.*
- *Commitment to quality*: nurses have a long history of pursuing quality-of-care issues. A 1989 survey found that licensing agencies for nurses were more likely than those for doctors, optometrists, dentists, and pharmacists to have written standards of practice.[30]
- *Nurses are also consumers*: the vast majority of nurses are women, and women are also the most intensive users of health services.**

Nursing has made great strides since the 1970s, when nurses were poorly paid, non-unionized, and mainly trained in hospitals, under often brutal and humiliating conditions. Today most nurses train in community colleges, and degree-based university programs are available across the country. Organized labour represents nursing in every province, and the vast majority of hospital nurses are union members. By the early 1990s, wage levels for nursing in some provinces were approaching what firefighters and police officers earn.

---

* Of course, nurses worry they're doing less and less direct patient care all the time because of staff cutbacks and increased paperwork.

** There are a number of factors related to higher health system use by women—one of the most important is their need for reproductive care. In addition, women, more commonly than men, decide when other family members need health care.

All the same, nursing has never attained the stature it really deserves within the system. There was a brief spate of attention in the mid to late 1980s when a perceived nursing shortage was blamed for cardiac surgery waiting lists. Governments set up a series of provincial and national task forces to improve recruitment of nurses and find ways to keep them in the profession. But a few years later, when the recession hit, the "shortage" disappeared. Nurses returned to work; nursing returned to oblivion.

Nurses also constantly take hits and putdowns from organized medicine and from a great many individual doctors, who appear to view them as unqualified inferiors. For example, Dr. Ken Babey of Mount Forest, Ontario, recently called nurse-practitioners an "unfounded idea,"[31] despite dozens of studies showing these specially trained nurses can provide comparable or even better care for many services usually provided by physicians.

Two prominent nursing leaders recently told us about similar experiences they had with their personal physicians during the 1986 Ontario doctors' strike. In each case the doctor used time during the nurses' medical appointments to give them a lecture on politics—essentially haranguing them for opposing extra-billing.

Organized nursing almost never takes the medical profession to task for these kinds of insults. Nurses are shy about confronting doctors, especially in public. It isn't, well ... it isn't like a nurse. Gail Donner, now a professor of nursing at the University of Toronto, trained in Winnipeg in the early 1960s. She remembers being taught to always stand when a doctor entered the room. "It got so I stood up no matter who came in—doctors, other nurses, even patients." When the OMA tore strips off the ONA for its health reform brochure, the union cringed, but in silence. And so the abuse continues, and nursing's misery is next to invisible.

Now more than ever the profession needs powerful leadership, but organized nursing is itself in disarray. In particular, there are continuing tensions between nursing associations and nurses' unions, and between registered nurses and registered practical nurses. Even the provincial professional associations are plagued by numerous issues that divide the ranks.* Most

---

* One of the most divisive issues for nursing is the profession's pursuit of degree-based entry to practice. The majority of RNs now in practice hold diplomas, not degrees. Many diploma RNs resent the implication that their educational background is now considered insufficient.

nursing leaders are senior and well-educated nurses who now work as administrators rather than at the bedside. There's an interesting contrast here between nursing and medicine. Physicians who become administrators often maintain part-time practices and usually identify themselves as part of the physician brotherhood. Nurse administrators almost never continue clinical practice once promoted and usually identify with other managers rather than fellow nurses.

So what are the chances now for nurses to assume a central role in a new coalition for health reform? Pretty good, we think. In fact, the kinds of reforms we propose might just be the ticket to unite the profession and rejuvenate its flagging leadership. A rallying cry from nurses could also be a magnet for attracting supporters outside the profession and might spark the creation of a new health system reform coalition. Here are just a few examples of what organized nursing could do to set the process in motion.

- Provincial nursing leaders could challenge provincial medical leaders to public debates about health care reform. The media would love to cover these events and it would be a great opportunity to present their respective viewpoints.
- In Ontario, Nova Scotia, Alberta, and other provinces, nurses could lead coalitions to disband the joint management committees and replace them with a series of provincial forums to discuss health reform issues in public.
- Canadian nursing organizations could lobby for a "1-800-4A-NURSE" program, which could be implemented in every province to give advice to patients about how and when to use the health care system.

Effective nursing leadership will identify and debate in public the hidden turf wars between medicine and nursing instead of papering over these differences. These nursing leaders will not shy away from pointing out that physicians have full employment, and often provide unnecessary services, while nurses are losing their jobs. They will expose the costly encroachment of medicine into traditional nursing areas as well: lifestyle counselling has become a growth area for many doctors. They will restore the status of the nurse-practitioner as a more cost-effective alternative to physicians. The public will learn that our failure to employ human resources cost-effectively has been a flagrant and costly error.

Organized Medicine or Reorganized Medicine?

Provided they are "doctor-friendly," some health system reforms are even getting a boost from organized medicine. The Canadian Medical Association, for example, has recently taken giant steps in the right direction. Under the leadership of secretary-general Leo-Paul Landry, and with help from a talented staff, the CMA has made a strong effort to play a broker role within the profession. It has been active on policy issues like decentralization and the quality of medical care and has convened groups of medical organizations to discuss these and other common issues. Dr. Ronald Wensel, vice-president of medicine for the University of Alberta Hospitals in Edmonton, chairs the CMA's committee on quality of care. He says doctors have three options given the financial squeeze our system is feeling: "They can ignore the problem and hope it goes away, head for the barricades and develop a bunker mentality in an effort to protect their turf, or occupy the driver's seat by dealing with quality-related issues."[32]

Things are less rosy, however, at the provincial level, where the leadership of medical associations is more mixed. Some—like the British Columbia Medical Association (BCMA)—sound as if they need to be rescued from Jurassic Park. In 1992, the BCMA's board passed a resolution calling for an end to Medicare, claiming it was unaffordable and denied "free citizens the right ... to purchase services in a free-competitive market."[33] Where more policy-aware leaders do emerge, they face a constant barrage of criticism from members of the ultra-right—a perpetual goading that hampers the associations from being more effective policy brokers for health care system reform.*

---

* Of course, being the dominant structural interest in health care, doctors haven't lost any of their traditional powers. And as long as they can say yea or nay to policy options behind closed doors, they won't need to broker in public.

At this point, neither the CMA nor the provincial medical associations have enough manoeuvring room. All the same, medicine does produce some very progressive physicians, and many of these doctors might be eager to participate in a more balanced policy debate. Some could, in fact, become vital allies in a coalition for more enlightened policy change, providing a counterweight to the more self-serving interests in medicine.

Consider Dr. Gary Gibson, a family physician from Cambridge, Ontario, and professor of family medicine at the University of Western Ontario. Dr. Gibson believes that doctors should be leading the way in cutting health care costs. "The scientific evidence that much of what we're doing is wasteful and/or useless is in our medical journals but is largely ignored," he wrote in an opinion piece published by the *Globe and Mail*.[34] "Where is our leadership?" he asked. In response, Dr. Gibson received numerous letters and phone calls from "family physicians, specialists, professors, deans, economists, patients, bureaucrats, politicians, and some past and present leaders of the profession [who] all said, in effect, 'Right on. Let's get on with it.' " [35]

A Grand Alliance for Health Reform

The politics of health care are challenging. Hospitals and doctors—the dominant interests in the system—are concentrated and powerful. Other health care workers and consumers—the "repressed" interests—are disorganized and weak. The question is, can we transform them into a challenging interest group, one that can give the more powerful dominant interests a run for their money? To make this happen, governments interested in health reform will need to rebalance the distribution of power by furnishing the "repressed" interests with help in getting together, with forums for public debate and—most important—with resources.

Mastering the art of the possible takes courage, strategy, and perseverance. We can learn a lot from the debates over public health insurance about how to do it well. The issues may be different because this time we're talking about restructuring health care delivery, but the strategy is virtually identical.

The country is also very fortunate to have Saskatchewan's and Quebec's examples to draw on. If the health reforms being incubated there actually succeed in improving quality and containing costs—and we think it highly likely—other provinces will be under tremendous pressure to follow suit. And they'll have to get their supporters lined up quickly.

Of course, most of the action on health system reform will take place within provinces, within regions, and at the community level. And so, to this point, we've focused on political strategies for achieving reforms at the provincial level. But Ottawa also has an important role to play in making Medicare work—including a role in supporting health care system reform. After all, at least part of the present difficulties provinces face were "made in Ottawa."

A New Federal Role in Health Reform

You'll remember from Chapters 1 and 2 why federal involvement in health and health care policy is so vital to Medicare's integrity and continued viability. Canadian jurisprudence, the Canada Health Act, and a host of federal and provincial reports all justify a federal presence in health and health care policy and offer some guidance about what the most appropriate role might be at the national level.

Here are some suggestions we think Ottawa should follow in order to become a better Guardian of the public's health and the public's health care system:

- Canada needs an overall strategy for health—one based on clear goals for improving the health status of Canadians. The federal government should take the overall responsibility for creating the social, economic, and physical environments that would support achieving these goals.
- Ottawa should transfer enough targeted cash to the provinces so that they can provide reasonably equal access to health and social services. These cash transfers should grow at the same rate as the country's economy (measured by the gross national product). The federal government should retain the right to withhold portions of these cash transfers from any province in breach of national standards for health insurance.

- During the election campaign, Jean Chrétien promised
to hold a national health forum, now promised for the
spring of 1994. The time is ripe for such an event. We'd
suggest that this forum be used to plan a National Council on Health which would have two key responsibilities:
    1. It would provide expert advice to the Conference of
    Deputy Ministers of Health.
    2. It would become a permanent policy forum for
    national debates about Canada's health policy—acti-
    vating professional and consumer participation. As
    British health policy analyst Rudolf Klein notes, we
    need to construct permanent structures that will
    improve our capacity to discuss key health policy
    questions.[36] It's time to take health policy out of the
    backrooms and into the open.

The Media is the Messenger

The media component of a comprehensive communications strategy is of paramount importance. It can make or break reform.

Returning to Jane Jacobs's model of Guardians and Traders,
we should point out here that members of the news media—like
those who work in government or serve on boards—are essentially Guardians. They too must shun trade—it's highly unethical for a reporter to accept any kind of reward for doing a
favourable story; no quid pro quo is permitted to journalists of
integrity. Newshounds esteem loyalty when they insist on protecting their sources. Newspaper publishers and broadcasters
are also famous for dispensing largesse—raising funds for various charitable causes and often matching dollar-for-dollar the
donations they collect.

But it is in their role as protectors of the public that the media
fulfil the essential role of the Guardian. Reporters love it when
they get to take vengeance on the cheaters in our society by holding them up to public scrutiny. Their work often exposes greed,
fraud, and other types of misbehaviour that might never come to
light without their vigilance. To get a good story, reporters sometimes have to deceive for the sake of the task—never revealing
their angle when doing interviews, for example. Editorials give

the media the chance to exert prowess by pronouncing yea or nay on key issues.

The media are often Guardians of other Guardians.[37] That's the role they play when their editorials lambaste governments for overzealous or wrongheaded public policy. Many government initiatives fail because reporters and journalists (and, by extension, the public) ultimately reject them as harmful. But the converse is also true—promising policies can get a real boost from media support.

Historically, the quality of media coverage of health issues in Canada has been rather mixed.[38] There have been, and still are, numerous examples of what Jonathan Lomas calls "orchestrated media outrage." Health care providers understandably object to any policy that might reduce their income. What, after all, could be more human? Their reaction to funding cutbacks—usually a howl of protest that the system needs more resources—is entirely predictable, however badly it corresponds to what the system really needs. These kinds of stories have always been newsworthy, and the media give them lots of play, even today.

But lately we've observed a decided improvement in health care reporting. In general, we're finding more balance in the coverage and more thoughtful analysis. Journalists and broadcasters—especially those with health beat experience—seem much less likely nowadays to fall victim to one-sided arguments. Opposing points of view are getting more print space and air time. For example, stories about surgical waiting lists have always been good copy—tales of woe and doctors asking for more money—but a recent story in the *Toronto Star* by health reporter Lisa Priest identified the key role of management in trimming waiting times.[39]

This is helping the public to advance further and further in its understanding of health policy. Rod Mickleburgh, a veteran reporter who covers health policy for the *Globe and Mail*, agrees that health coverage is now more even-handed: "It's partly because the players in the system are moderating their views too. For example, doctors today are far less likely to blindly defend fee-for-service payment the way they used to; they're much more open to the alternatives. The same goes for hospital administrators; they're much less strident in their attacks on funders, and far more willing to look at their overall role in the system."

Still, Mickleburgh worries about the future of Medicare as the public leans towards simple solutions to complex problems: "User fees are terribly seductive at a time when the public views government spending as out of control. It's incredibly hard for journalists to explain that we could lose Medicare altogether if we don't draw the line. The difficulty rests with pitting a subtle but correct argument against one that's wrong but easy to understand."

In fact, this is the nub of the problem. Mastering health policy imposes one of the steepest learning curves imaginable. We know of no other policy area more complex than health and its relationship to health care. And we know of no system more difficult to comprehend than the intricate inner workings of health care financing and health care delivery. To the rookie reporter, all this complexity can be overwhelming.

Doing a good job covering the scientific aspects of health care also poses unique difficulties. Technocrats and scientists are often quite uncomfortable talking with the press. The jargon they use can be impenetrable. "And they always insist on qualifying their research findings. By the time they've finished explaining this exception and that limitation, you're not sure what you can report in a few sentences and still be accurate," says Michael Moralis, former health care reporter for several small Ontario dailies, as well as for *Hospital News*.

For journalists without a background in evaluation, it's easy to go astray. Take just one example. For years, health researchers have been demonstrating that treatment rates often vary greatly from one area to another, from one hospital to another, or even from one doctor to another.[40] But while variation studies *are* a red flag that something may be wrong, they cannot tell us *what* it is that's wrong. In fact, variations can only be explained after further investigation is done to pinpoint the causes.

That's what went wrong when journalists reported on a study of breast cancer treatment variation put out by the Institute of Clinical Evaluative Sciences in Toronto. Like many other variation studies, this one found huge county-to-county differences in the rates of breast-conserving surgery for cancer patients. The far north showed the most dramatic disparity. More than three-quarters of breast cancer patients in Cochrane, Ontario, were treated with lumpectomy, compared to fewer than one-tenth of patients in Kenora.

While this clearly indicated that something is wrong in the system, some journalists jumped way ahead of the evidence and concluded that greedy and misinformed surgeons were denying women the chance to choose lumpectomies and radiation and were subjecting them to unnecessary radical mastectomies.[41] While this interpretation might be valid, the study certainly couldn't demonstrate it. Also, there could be other, equally valid explanations for the variation. Consider just one: perhaps the women in Kenora had breast cancers that were too far advanced for lumpectomy. If this were the real reason behind the variation, blaming surgeons would be totally unjust. It would be more appropriate to point the finger at an inadequate primary care system and haphazard screening. The point is that without additional research to explain the variation, and without consensus about what constitutes appropriate care, it is impossible to determine which rate is right.

All of these points and more came out in subsequent news stories, opinion pieces, columns, and letters to the editor. A real public debate ensued, and it helped raise public awareness on a topic that rarely gets an airing outside the back rooms of medical academe. Some scientists clearly wish it had remained there.[42] But the genie is out of the bottle now, and we predict that he won't go back. For example, we expect that research on the extremely high variability of hysterectomies will trigger similar howls of outrage and a strong demand for more investigation to explain and resolve the underlying problem. Public interest in regional variations, appropriateness rates, and other telling signs of our system's performance will mushroom. The editorial pages of our newspapers and the public affairs shows on radio and television will continue to be key forums for active policy debates. Contrary opinions will wage battle in the open. Policy-oriented learning will flourish. And the media will be at the centre of it all. For nowhere is the debate more public than when it reaches you at the breakfast table or in your living room.

History Repeats Itself?

Baseball great Yogi Berra once said, "It's déjà vu all over again!" Yogi could have been commenting on Canadian health care policy. Something wonderful is happening in Saskatchewan again.[43] The country watches with awe. Pretty soon all Canadians are singing from the same song book. That's the story of public health insurance in this country. The question is, can we "play it again, Sam" with health care system reform?

It didn't take much time for public health insurance to catch on, and for thirty years it hasn't really been much of a partisan issue for our politicians. Conservatives, Liberals, and New Democrats all came to learn that public finance is simply a more equitable and affordable way to provide health care coverage. All the same, the whole idea was considered pretty radical when Saskatchewan began the process.

Our proposals for reforming the system may strike some of you as similarly radical. But consider the alternatives. We can hack the system to pieces, cutting programs here, slicing eligibility there, until Medicare becomes little more than a fond memory. Or, we can give our system the "strong medicine" it really needs and avoid all this unnecessary surgery.

We're absolutely convinced that it's not too late to save Medicare. Thanks to public health insurance, there's more than enough money to provide even more comprehensive care—but not if we remain bound to current rules for organizing and paying for it.

We have to act now. Remember, the sooner we take our medicine, the sooner we'll all start feeling better.

Notes

CHAPTER 1

1. M.M. Rachlis, C. Kushner, "Under the Knife," *Report on Business Magazine*, October 1992.
2. One of the authors (C.K.) debated this proposal with Mr. Walker on Newsworld's "Coast to Coast," 30 March 1993.
3. Sandro Contenta, "Putting a human face on Alberta's Ralphonomics," *Toronto Star*, 2 February 1994.
4. Editorial, "Opting out has its price," *Vancouver Sun*, 27 August 1992.
5. *Toronto Star*, 12 September 1993.
6. "Canadian Cancer Statistics 1993," Statistics Canada, Health and Welfare Canada, National Cancer Institute. Ottawa, 1993.
7. T. Whelan et al., "Adjuvant radiotherapy for early breast cancer: patterns of practice in Ontario," *Canadian Medical Association Journal*, 149 (1993): 1273–77. The British Columbia Cancer Control Agency does have clinical guidelines. Other provincial cancer agencies are considering developing their own.
8. *Globe and Mail*, 10 November 1993.
9. Personal communication with Dr. William Meakin, senior policy adviser to the Ontario Cancer Treatment and Research Foundation.
10. Part of the problem here is a worldwide shortage of radiotherapy technicians.
11. See, for example, B. Aarsteinsen, "Cancer therapy backlog likely for years to come," *Toronto Star*, 12 September 1993.
12. M. Simpson et al., "Doctor patient communication: the Toronto consensus statement," *British Medical Journal*, 303 (1991): 1385–87; L.F. Degner, J.M. Farber, T.F. Hack, *Communication between Cancer Patients and Health Care Professionals: An Annotated Bibliography* (Toronto: Canadian Cancer Society, 1989); K. Jenkins, "Doctors don't realize CA patients often left in dark," *The Medical Post*, 13 October 1987; "Consensus statement from the workshop on the teaching and assessment of communication skills in Canadian medical schools," *Canadian Medical Association Journal*, 147 (1992): 1149–50.
13. For a summary of recent provincial inquiries, see: S.L. Mhatre, R.B. Deber, "From equal access to health care to equitable access to health: A review of Canadian provincial health commissions and reports," *International Journal of Health Services*, 22 (1992): 645–68.
14. For more on values and health care, see: R. Priester et al., "A values framework for health system reform," *Health Affairs*, 11(1) (1992): 84–107.
15. Some might argue that section 36 refers solely to the formal program of equalization payments. However, only subsection (2) refers specifically to equalization payments. Because subsection (1) does not, it could be interpreted to allow for a series of global objectives to be achieved by the equalization program *and other federal programs as necessary*, using the legal principle of *"inclusio unius est exclusio alterius."*

16. The preamble to the act says (in part):
"Whereas the Parliament of Canada recognizes:

"...that Canadians can achieve further improvements in their well-being through combining individual lifestyles that emphasize fitness, prevention and health promotion with collective action against the social, environmental and occupational causes of disease, and that they desire a system of health services that will promote such physical, and mental health and such protection against disease;

"- that future improvements in health will require the cooperative partnership of governments, health professionals, voluntary organizations and individual Canadians;

"- that continued access to quality health care without financial or other barriers will be critical to maintaining and improving the health and well-being of Canadians.

"AND WHEREAS the Parliament of Canada wishes to encourage the development of health services throughout Canada by assisting the provinces in meeting the costs thereof."

Section 3 of the act says:

"It is hereby declared that the primary objective of Canadian health care policy is to protect, promote and restore the physical and mental well-being of residents of Canada and to facilitate reasonable access to health services without financial or other barriers."

17. Gallup, September 1993.

18. Ibid.

19. The Constitution of 1867 refers to the provincial legislatures having the exclusive right to make laws in relation to: "The Establishment, Maintenance, and Management of Hospitals, Asylums, Charities, and Eleemosynary Institutions in and for the Province, other than Marine Hospitals."

20. There were other bodies with more limited powers of regulation in Ontario going back to 1792. See: E. Macnab, *A Legal History of the Health Professions in Ontario. (A study for the Committee on the Healing Arts)* (Toronto: Queen's Printer for Ontario, 1970).

21. Y. Parent, C. Strohmenger, *Demographic and Health Indicators: Presentation and Interpretation (Table 28)* (Ottawa: Statistics Canada,1985).

22. T. McKeown, *The Role of Medicine: Dream, Mirage, or Nemesis* (Princeton, NJ: Princeton University Press, 1979); R. Reves, "Declining fertility in England and Wales as a major cause of the twentieth century decline in mortality: The role of changing family size and age structure in infectious disease mortality in infancy," *American Journal of Epidemiology*, 122 (1985): 112–26.

23. R.G. Evans, G.L. Stoddart, "Producing health, consuming health care," *Social Science and Medicine*, 31 (1990): 1347–64.

24. V.W. Sidel, R. Sidel, *A Healthy State: An International Perspective on the Crisis in United States Medical Care* (New York: Pantheon Books, 1983), 153.

25. Some of these beliefs have been derived from previous work by Professor Jonathan Lomas of McMaster University.

26. The World Health Organization, Health and Welfare Canada, the Canadian Public Health Association, *Ottawa Charter for Health Promotion* (Ottawa: 1986).

27. The Healthy Public Policy Committee of the Premier's Council on Health Strategy, *Nurturing Health: A Framework on the Determinants of Health* (Toronto: Premier's Council on Health Strategy, 1991).

28. *Report of the Commission of Enquiry on Health and Social Services* (Chair, M. Jean Rochon) (Quebec: Government of Quebec,1988).

29. Ibid.

30. S. Veen et al., "Impairments, disabilities, and handicaps of very preterm and very-low-birthweight infants at five years of age," *Lancet*, 338 (1991): 33–36; P. Wysong,

"Preemies' learning handicaps may not show up until school," *Medical Post*, 23 April 1991.

31. United States General Accounting Office, *Breast Cancer 1971–91: Prevention, Treatment, and Research* (Washington: 1991); J.C. Bailor, "Cancer in Canada: Recent trends in mortality," Proceedings of the OCTRF Cansai Epidemiology Seminar, *Chronic Diseases in Canada*, 13(6, supplement) (1992): S2–S8.

32. The Healthy Public Policy Committee of the Premier's Council on Health Strategy, *Nurturing Health: A Framework on the Determinants of Health* (Toronto: Premier's Council on Health Strategy, 1991); M.C. Wolfson et al., "Career earnings and death: A longitudinal analysis of older Canadian men," *Canadian Institute for Advanced Research* (Population Health Program Working Paper No. 12) (Toronto, 1991).

33. L. Payer, *Medicine and Culture* (Markham, Ontario: Penguin Books, 1989).

34. A. Leon et al., "Leisure time physical activity levels and risk of coronary heart disease and death," *Journal of the American Medical Association*, 258 (1987): 2388–95; R. Paffenbarger et al., "Physical activity levels, all cause mortality and longevity of college alumni," *New England Journal of Medicine*, 314 (1986): 605–13.

35. E.H.W. Kluge, C. Lucock, *New Human Reproductive Technologies: A Preliminary Perspective of the Canadian Medical Association* (Ottawa: The Canadian Medical Association, 1991).

36. *Proceed with Care. The Final Report of the Royal Commission on New Reproductive Technologies* (Ottawa: 1993).

37. N.J. Vetter, D.A. Jones, C.R. Victor, "Effect of health visitors working with elderly patients in general practice: a randomised controlled trial," *British Medical Journal*, 288 (1984): 369–72; C. Hendricksen, E. Lund, E. Stromgard, "Consequences of assessment and intervention among elderly people: A three-year randomized, controlled trial," *British Medical Journal*, 289 (1984): 1522–24; M.S.J. Pathy et al., "Randomised trial of case finding and surveillance of elderly people at home," *Lancet*, 340 (1992): 890–93.

38. For example, see: Jane Jacobs, *The Death and Life of Great American Cities* (Toronto: Vintage Books, 1961).

39. S.M. Lipset, *Continental Divide: The Values and Institutions of the United States and Canada* (New York: Rutledge, 1990).

40. Jane Jacobs, "Two ways to live: Jane Jacobs speaks to David Warren," *The Idler*, 38 (Summer 1993): 7.

41. G.L. Stoddart et al., "Why not user charges? The real issues," The Ontario Premier's Council on Health, Well-Being and Social Justice. Toronto, 1993; R.G. Evans, M.L. Barer, G.L. Stoddart, "The truth about user fees," *Policy Options*, October 1993: 4–9.

42. Leo Charbonneau, "User fees inevitable, Quebec treasury says," *Medical Post*, 16 February 1993; "Klein to seek Medicare user fees," *Globe and Mail*, 13 January 1993.

43. R.G. Evans, *Strained Mercy: The Economics of Canadian Health Care* (Toronto: Butterworths, 1984).

44. S. Woolhandler, D. Himmelstein, "The deteriorating administrative efficiency of the U.S. health care system," *New England Journal of Medicine*, 324 (1991): 1253–58.

45. Of course, there is still private insurance for drugs, dental care, and other items that might not be covered by the provinces' plans, and 28 percent of our health care spending is from private sources. But there are some similar problems in these markets as there are for physicians' and hospital insurance in the U.S. For a discussion of the market for pharmaceutical insurance, see: *Prescriptions for Health: The Report of the Pharmaceutical Inquiry of Ontario* (Chair, Dr. Frederick H. Lowy), Toronto, 1990.

46. Saskatchewan got the ball rolling when it implemented public hospital insurance in 1947; New Brunswick was the last province to implement public insurance for medical care in 1971.

47. H. Mimoto, P. Cross, "The growth of the federal debt," *Canadian Economic Observer*, Statistics Canada. Ottawa, 1991.

48. M. Mendelson, "Social Policy in Real Time," The Caledon Institute of Social Policy, 1993. Mr. Mendelson, who is the Ontario Deputy Cabinet Secretary, also recently proposed consolidating all federal and provincial debts at the federal level. In return, provinces would have to agree to a constitutional amendment requiring them to balance their budgets.

49. Information provided by OECD (Mr. Edwin Bell). January 13, 1994. The data used are for 1990.

50. Linda McQuaig, *The Wealthy Banker's Wife: The Assault on Equality in Canada* (Toronto: Penguin, 1993).

51. In 1992, Canada was fourteenth out of twenty-four OECD countries in the proportion of Gross Domestic Product collected as tax revenue. *The Economist*, 4 September 1993: 103.

52. *The Idler*, 138 (Summer 1993).

53. As argued in T. Tremayne-Lloyd, L. Stoltz, "The Maintenance of National Standards within the Canadian Health Care System: Legal and Constitutional Options," (Prepared for the Health Action Lobby). Toronto, 1991.

54. [1982] 2 S.C.R. 112, pp. 141–142. As quoted in T. Tremayne-Lloyd, L. Stoltz, "The Maintenance of National Standards within the Canadian Health Care System."

CHAPTER 2

1. For a review of most of these reports, see: Douglas E. Angus, *Review of Significant Health Care Commissions and Task Forces in Canada Since 1983–84* (Ottawa: the Canadian Hospital Association, the Canadian Medical Association, and the Canadian Nurses Association, 1991).

2. Health and Welfare Canada, "National Health Expenditures, 1975–1987." Ottawa, 1990.

3. Coverage varies considerably across the country. For up-to-date information contact the Canadian Life and Health Insurance Association, 1 Queen Street East, Toronto, Ontario, M5C 2X9: telephone 416–777–2221.

4. See, for example, Chapter 3 in C.D. Naylor, *Private Practice, Public Payment: Canadian Medicine and the Politics of Health Insurance 1911-1966* (Kingston: McGill-Queen's University Press, 1986).

5. Eugene Vayda and Raisa Deber, "The Canadian Health Care System: A Developmental Overview," in *Canadian Health Care and the State: A Century of Evolution*, ed: C. David Naylor (Montreal/Kingston: McGill-Queen's University Press, 1992): 126.

6. L.H. Thomas, *The Making of a Socialist: The Recollections of T.C. Douglas* (Edmonton: University of Alberta Press, 1984): 7.

7. Allan E. Blakeney, "The Political Perspective: Planning and Implementing the Canadian System," in *Looking North for Health Care: What we can learn from Canada's health care system*, eds: Arnold Bennett and Orville Adams (New York: Jossey-Bass, 1993): 71–72.

8. L.H. Thomas, *The Making of a Socialist*.

9. Malcolm Taylor, *Health Insurance and Canadian Public Policy: The Seven Decisions that Created the Canadian Health Insurance System* (Montreal: McGill-Queen's University Press, 1978): 170.

10. M. Taylor, *Health Insurance and Canadian Public Policy*.

11. M. Rachlis and C. Kushner, *Second Opinion: What's Wrong with Canada's Health Care System and How to Fix It* (Toronto: HarperCollins Canada, 1989).

12. Eugene Vayda and Raisa Deber, "The Canadian Health Care System: A Developmental Overview," 127.

13. M. Taylor, *Health Insurance and Canadian Public Policy*.

14. M. Taylor, *Health Insurance and Canadian Public Policy*.

15. Most provinces passed complementary legislation, but others simply entered into voluntary agreements with provincial medical associations.

16. For a discussion of these, see The Parliamentary Task Force on Federal-Provincial Fiscal Arrangements (Chair, Mr. Herb Breau), *Fiscal Federalism in Canada*. (Ottawa: House of Commons, 1981).

17. The actual time of the elimination of the EPF cash transfers depends on assumptions for economic growth, inflation, and population growth. The estimate of 2002 uses the federal government's estimates as published in the 1991 budget.

18. Paul Boothe and Barbara Johnston, "Stealing the Emperor's Clothes: Deficit offloading and national standards in health care," *Commentary*, 41 (1993): 1–12.

19. For example, see K. Leveno, F.G. Cunningham, S. Nelson et al., "A prospective comparison of selective and universal electronic fetal monitoring in 34,995 cases," *New England Journal of Medicine*, 315 (1986): 615–619.

20. J. Kennell, M. Klaus, S. Robertson, C. Hinkley, "Continuous emotional support during labor in a U.S. hospital: a randomized controlled trial," *Journal of the American Medical Association*, 265 (1991): 2197–2201.

21. For example, The National Council of Welfare, *Health, Health Care, and Medicare*, 1990.

22. Robert G. Evans, "Health care in the Canadian Community" in *Looking North for Health Care* (New York: Jossey-Bass, 1993): 25.

23. Health and Welfare Canada, *National Health Expenditures in Canada, 1984*.

24. Policy Planning and Information Branch, Health and Welfare Canada, "Health Expenditures in Canada: Fact Sheets," February 1993.

25. Ibid.

26. Robert G. Evans, "Health Care Reform: 'The Issue from Hell,'" *Policy Options*, July-August, 1993. Professor Evans acknowledges that without these two recessions the cost controls imposed on our health care system might have been less vigorously applied.

27. George J. Scheiber, Jean-Pierre Poullier, Leslie M. Greenwald, "U.S. health expenditure performance: An international comparison and data update," *Health Care Financing Review*, 13(4) (1992): 1–88.

28. Figures were calculated from provincial budgets for 1993–94.

29. Bill C–69 (passed in 1990) and Bill C–20 (passed in 1992) singled out the three wealthiest provinces (Alberta, British Columbia, and Ontario) and put a 5 percent growth cap on federal cost-sharing under the Canada Assistance Plan (CAP) for social assistance and related services. Until then, Ottawa had been paying half the costs of these programs. The Ontario government has estimated that in 1992–93, Ottawa's contribution made up less than 30 percent of the costs of these programs and services.

30. Hospital Medical Records Institute, *Comparative Analysis of the HMRI Database*, December 1992: 6–7.

31. Information on the numbers of hospitals beds and budgets was provided by Mr. Paul Gamble, Executive Director, Hospital Council of Metropolitan Toronto. October 1993.

32. "Decision set in stone," *The Lethbridge Herald*, 19 May 1993.

33. On October 4, 1993, the province announced the deferral of a number of construction projects, including St. Michael's. However, the project has not been cancelled outright.

34. The Caldwell Partners, *Governance of Hospitals in Canada: A Power Struggle*, 1992.

35. "Report of the Investigation by Edward Lane, Ralph Coombs and Donald Holmes of St. Michael's Hospital," 30 August 1991.

36. J.E.F. Hastings, F.D. Mott, A. Barclay, D. Hewitt, "Prepaid group practice in Sault Ste. Marie, Ontario: Part I: analysis of utilization records," *Medical Care*, 11 (1973): 91–103; Saskatchewan Department of Health, *Community Clinic Study* (Regina: 1983); W.G. Manning et al., "A controlled trial of the effect of a prepaid group practice on the use of services," *New England Journal of Medicine*, 310 (1984): 1505–1510; J.E. Ware, W.H. Rogers, A.R. Davies, "Comparisons of health outcomes at a health maintenance organisation with those of fee-for-service care," *The Lancet*, Vol. 1 (1986): 1017–22; E.M. Sloss et al., "Effect of a health maintenance organization on physiologic health: results from a randomized trial," *Annals of Internal Medicine*, 106 (1987): 130–38. A.R. Davies et al., "Consumer Acceptance of prepaid and fee-for-service medical care: results from a randomized controlled trial," *Health Services Research*, 21 (1986): 429–52.
37. D.J. Roch, Robert G. Evans, David Pascoe, "Manitoba and Medicare," *Manitoba Health* (March 1985): 21.
38. Alice Baumgart, "The Nursing Workforce in Canada" in *Canadian Nursing Faces the Future*, eds: Alice Baumgart, Jenniece Larsen (Toronto: C.V. Masby Co., 1988).
39. According to a 1991 report by the Ontario Medical Association ("An Evaluation of the G467 Billing Code in the Province of Ontario"), 3 percent of the doctors billing for this service in 1986–87 accounted for almost 43 percent of the total service volume. Further data taken from notes attached to the terms of reference for a Ministry of Health Review of Physiotherapy Services, 1992.

CHAPTER 3

1. *Ontario Medicine*, 6 April 1992.
2. "Stelco fined $20,000 over worker's death," *Toronto Star*, 17 October 1990.
3. "Rail crash couple remain in hospital," *Toronto Sun*, 17 February 1993.
4. "Stop the carnage on rail crossings Ottawa warned," *Toronto Star*, 23 February 1990.
5. Gary Oakes, "Leniency cost life of woman judge says," *Toronto Star*, 16 September 1989.
6. R.G. Evans, G.L. Stoddart, "Producing health, consuming health care," *Social Science and Medicine*, 31 (1990): 1347–63.
7. Lynn Payer, *Medicine and Culture* (New York: Penguin Books, 1988); Sylvia Tesh, *Hidden Arguments: Political Ideology and Disease Prevention Policy* (New Brunswick, NJ: Rutgers University Press, 1990).
8. King James I, "Counterblaste to Tobacco" (1608), quoted in Peter Taylor, *Smoke Ring: The Politics of Tobacco* (London: The Bodley Head, 1984).
9. M.M. Rachlis, "Overview of the magnitude of the tobacco problem". Presentation to the First National Conference on Tobacco or Health in Ottawa on October 21, 1993.
10. Ibid.
11. B.C. Ministry of Health, Office of Health Promotion and the Social Planning and Research Council of B.C., *Examples and Outcomes of Healthy Public Policy, 1993*.
12. *Toronto Star*, 28 August 1993.
13. A.B. Miller, "Planning Cancer Control Strategies," *Chronic Diseases in Canada*, 13 (supplement) (1992): S1-S40.
14. K.E. Warner, L.M. Goldenhar, C.G. McLaughlin, "Cigarette advertising and magazine coverage of the hazards of smoking," *New England Journal of Medicine*, 326 (1992): 305–309.
15. As quoted in Kenneth E. Warner *Selling Smoke: Cigarette Advertising and Public Health* (Washington: American Public Health Association, 1986).
16. C. Godfrey, A. Maynard, "Economic aspects of tobacco use and taxation policy," *British Medical Journal*, 297 (1988): 339–343. D.E. Peterson, S.L. Zeger, P.L. Remington, et al. "The effect of state cigarette tax increases on cigarette sales 1955 to

1988," *American Journal of Public Health*, 82 (1992): 94-96. R.C. Allen, *The health and economic impact of tobacco tax rollbacks*, Harvard University mimeo, 1994.

17. R.W. Pollay, A.M. Lavack, "The targeting of youths by cigarette marketers: Archival evidence on trial," *Advances in Consumer Research*, 20 (1992): 266–271.

18. P.M. Fisher, M.P. Schwartz, J.W. Richards, et al. "Brand logo recognition by children aged 3 to 6 years: Mickey Mouse and Old Joe the Camel, *Journal of the American Medical Association*, 266 (1991): 3145–3148.

19. J.R. DiFranza, J.W. Richards, P.M. Paulman, et al. "RJR Nabisco's cartoon camel promotes Camel cigarettes to children," *Journal of the American Medical Association*, 266 (1991): 3149–3153.

20. Jack Micay, "Grim reaper posed to reap a windfall," *Toronto Star*, 2 February 1994.

21. Ibid.

22. Lysiane Gagnon, "The solution to smuggling is to levy an export tax on tobacco products," *The Globe and Mail*, 5 February 1994.

23. K. Milton, "Diet and primate evolution," *Scientific American* (August 1993): 86–93.

24. G. Rose, "Sick individuals and sick populations," *International Journal of Epidemiology,* 14 (1985): 32–38.

25. L. Lytle, "Latest supermodels are also super-thin, health experts warn," *Toronto Star*, 24 April 1993.

26. "The body game," *People Magazine*, 11 January 1993.

27. P. Mustajoki, "Could mannequins menstruate?" *British Medical Journal*, 305 (1992): 1575–76.

28. Jared Diamond, *The Third Chimpanzee: The Evolution and Future of the Human Animal* (New York: HarperCollins, 1992).

29. M.C. Moore-Ede, C.A. Cziesler, G.S. Richardson, "Circadian timekeeping in health and disease," *New England Journal of Medicine*, 309 (1983): 469–76.

30. Canadian Centre for Occupational Health and Safety, *Rotational Shiftwork: A Summary of the Adverse Effects and Improvement Strategies* (Hamilton: 1987); "Rotating shift work, sleep, and accidents related to sleepiness in hospital nurses," *American Journal of Public Health*, 82 (1992): 1011–14.

31. C.A. Czeisler, M.C. Moore-Ede, R.M. Coleman, "Rotating shift work schedules that disrupt sleep are improved by applying circadian principles," *Science*, 217 (1982): 460–62; K. Orth-Gomer, "Intervention on coronary risk factors by adapting a shift work schedule to biologic rhythmicity," *Psychosomatic Medicine*, 45 (1983): 407–15.

32. N. Belloc, L. Breslow, "Relationship of physical health status and health practices," *Preventive Medicine*, 1 (1972): 409–21; N. Belloc, "Relationship of health practices and mortality," *Preventive Medicine*, 2 (1973): 67–81; J.P. Hirdes, W.F. Forbes, "The importance of social relationships, socioeconomic status and health practices with respect to mortality among healthy Ontario males," *Journal of Clinical Epidemiology,* 45 (1992): 175–82.

33. Standing Committee on Justice and the Solicitor General (Chair, Dr. Bob Horner), *Crime Prevention in Canada: Toward a National Strategy* (Canada: House of Commons, February 1993).

34. S. Fine, "Justice committee targets poverty: Changing social causes of rising crime seen as wiser strategy than filling jails," *Globe and Mail*, 27 February 1993.

35. M.B. Jones, D.R. Offord, "Reduction in antisocial behaviour in poor children by nonschool skill development," *Journal of Child Psychology and Psychiatry*, 30 (1989): 737–50.

36. S.J. Suomi, "Early stress and adult emotional reactivity in rhesus monkeys," *The Childhood Environment and Adult Disease* (Ciba Foundation Symposium 156) (Chichester: Wiley, 1991): 171–88; S.J. Suomi, "Primate separation models of affective

disorders," in *Neurobiology of Learning, Emotion and Affect,* ed. John Madden IV (New York: Raven Press Ltd., 1991).

37. M. Wolfson et al., "Career earnings and death: A longitudinal analysis of older Canadian men," *The Gerontologist* (1993).

38. M.G. Marmot et al., "Health inequalities among British civil servants: the White-hall II study," *Lancet,* 337 (1991): 1387–93; M.G. Marmot et al., "Employment grade and coronary heart disease in British civil servants," *Journal of Epidemiology and Community Health,* 32 (1978): 244–49; M.G. Marmot, M.J. Shipley, G. Rose, "Inequalities in death—specific explanations of a general pattern?" *Lancet,* Vol. 1 (1984): 1003–6.

39. R.G. Wilkinson, "Income distribution and life expectancy," *British Medical Journal,* 304 (1992): 165–68; R.G. Wilkinson, "National mortality rates: the impact of inequality," *American Journal of Public Health,* 82 (1992): 1082–84.

40. R.G. Wilkinson, "Income Distribution and Life Expectancy."

41. T.M. Smeeding, "Why the U.S. antipoverty system doesn't work very well," *Challenge,* (January-February 1992): 30–35.

42. K. Liu et al., "International infant mortality rankings: A look behind the numbers," *Health Care Financing Review,* 13(4) (1992):105–18.

43. T.M. Smeeding, "Why the U.S. antipoverty system doesn't work very well."

44. Ibid.

45. *Globe and Mail,* 24 November 1993.

46. *Globe and Mail,* 25 November 1993.

47. Margaret Philip, "Child poverty rising in Canada," *Globe and Mail,* 25 November 1993.

48. A. Antonovsky, "Can attitudes contribute to health?" *Advances,* 8(4) (1992): 33–49; A. Langius, H. Bjorvell, A. Antonovsky, "The sense of coherence concept and its relation to personality traits in Swedish samples," *Scandinavian Journal of Caring Science,* 6(3) (1992): 165–70.

49. Differences in size and structure are very important for establishing sex roles and family structure. For example, male and female chimpanzees are almost the same size and mutually polygamous. Male and female gibbons are nearly identical in size and live monogamously. Male gorillas are twice the size of females and live in small groups with a dominant male who has a harem of three to six females. In the most extreme mammalian example, the male elephant seal is nearly seven times the size of the female and dominant males have average harems of 50 females. Jared Diamond, *The Third Chimpanzee: The Evolution and Future of the Human Animal* (New York: HarperCollins, 1992).

50. R. Haliechuk, "Don't prosecute all wife assaults, judge suggests," *Toronto Star,* 16 January 1990.

51. E. Stark, A.H. Flitcraft, "Women and children at risk," *International Journal of Health Services,* 18 (1988): 97–118; Ontario Medical Association, "Reports on Wife Assault," Toronto, 1991.

52. As reported on CBC Radio's "As It Happens," 1 February 1994.

53. P.G. Jaffe, J.K. Thompson, M.J. Paquin, "Immediate family crisis intervention as preventative mental health: the family consultant service," *Professional Psychology,* (November 1978): 551–60.

54. J. Hurowitz, "Toward a social policy for health," *New England Journal of Medicine,* 329 (1993): 130–33.

55. K. Dunn, "Health care focuses on sickness instead of what keeps us fit," *Montreal Gazette,* 23 April 1993.

56. Ibid.

57. Most of this history is taken from George A. Rosen, *A History of Public Health* (New York: MD Publications, Inc., 1976).

58. Ibid., 197.

59. Ibid.

60. John Snow, *Snow on Cholera* (London: Oxford University Press, 1936).

61. R. Sheppard, "An apology for the excesses of the eighties," *Globe and Mail*, 13 September 1993.

62. Canadian Press, "Tory paper calls safety not barrier to jobs, *Globe and Mail*, 24 September 1993.

63. S. McCarthy, "UI changes necessary business group says," *Toronto Star*, 9 February 1993.

64. P. Wallich, "Are economy watchers chasing a mirage?" *Scientific American* (June 1993): 141.

65. R. Evans, *Strained Mercy: The Economics of Canadian Health Care* (Toronto: Butterworths, 1984).

66. *Challenge* (Newsletter of the Canadian Healthy Communities Network) 4(1) (1993): 2.

67. *Toronto Star*, 24 November 1993.

68. Ontario Prevention Clearing House, "Newsletter," 3:5 (January 1993).

69. H.M. Stevenson, M. Burke, "Bureaucratic logic in new social movement clothing: The limits of health promotion research," *Canadian Journal of Public Health* (1992, supplement): S47–53.

70. G. Rosen, *A History of Public Health*, 86.

CHAPTER 4

1. Hon. Frances Lankin, speech to the National Physicians Conference, Ottawa, 22 June 1992.

2. Caesarian Birth Planning Committee, *Appropriate Use of Caesarean Section: Recommendations for a Quality Assurance Program* (Toronto: Government of Ontario, Queen's Printer, March 1991).

3. After episiotomy, anterior rupture of the membranes, repair of obstetrical laceration, and circumcision. Hospital Medical Records Institute, "Comparative Analysis of the HMRI Database," (December 1992): 41.

4. Ibid.

5. K.J. Carlson, D.H. Nichols, I. Schiff, "Indications for hysterectomy," *New England Journal of Medicine*, 328 (1993): 856–60.

6. Elizabeth Douglas, "Many hysterectomies really 'mutilation,'" *Medical Post*, 18 January 1994.

7. Hospital Medical Records Institute, "Comparative Analysis of the HMRI Database" (December 1992): 41.

8. Personal communication with Dr. Marsha Cohen.

9. Marsha Cohen, "Hysterectomy rates in Ontario," in *The Ontario Practice Atlas* (Toronto: The Institute for Clinical Evaluative Sciences, 1994).

10. Personal communication with Dr. Marsha Cohen.

11. T.A. Brennan et al., "Incidence of adverse events and negligence in hospitalized patients: Results of the Harvard Medical Malpractice Study I," *New England Journal of Medicine*, 324 (1991): 370–76; L.L. Leape et al., "The nature of adverse events in hospitalized patients: Results of the Harvard Medical Practice Study II," *New England Journal of Medicine*, 324 (1991): 377–84.

12. R. Mickleburgh, "Doctors worried about negligence," *Globe and Mail*, 8 March 1991.

13. T.A. Brennan et al., "Incidence of adverse events and negligence in hospitalized patients: Results of the Harvard Medical Malpractice Study I".

14. Assuming New York State population in 1984 of 17.7 million, Canadian popula-tion in 1994 of 28 million, a rate of death due to negligence of 0.00039, and a rate of permanent disability of 0.000099 (from page 373 of the Harvard study).

15. Task Force on the Use and Provision of Medical Services (Chair, Mr. Graham Scott), *1989–1990 Annual Report*: 11.

16. A selection of this literature includes: D.M. Vickery et al., "Effect of self-care educa-tion program on medical visits," *Journal of the American Medical Association*, 250 (1983): 2952–56; C.R. Roberts et al., "Reducing physician visits for colds through con-sumer education," *Journal of the American Medical Association*, 250 (1983): 1986–89; A. Stergachis, "Use of a controlled trial to evaluate the impact of self-care on health services utilization," *Journal of Ambulatory Care Management*, 9 (1986): 16–22.

17. *Hospital News* (June 1992): 4.

18. John Wennberg, "On the status of the scientific basis of clinical medicine and the need for better science policy to promote the evaluative clinical sciences," a presenta-tion to the International Conference on Quality Assurance and Effectiveness in Health Care, Toronto, 9 November 1989.

19. Working group on Quality Assurance and Effectiveness in Health Care, *Report to the Conference of Deputy Ministers of Health* (Ottawa: Health and Welfare Canada and Statistics Canada, 1990).

20. Anne-Marie Ugnat, David C. Naylor, "Small Area Variations in the Use of Coro-nary Surgery in Ontario, 1981–1989," Institute for Clinical Evaluative Studies, Working Paper Series No. 2, March 1993.

21. E. Chen, C.D. Naylor, "Variation in hospital length of stay for acute myocardial infarction in Ontario, Canada, during fiscal 1990: A population-based analysis," Institute for Clinical Evaluative Studies, Working Paper Series No. 3, March 1993.

22. C. Brender et al., "Surgical treatment for benign prostatic hyperplasia," *Cancer*, 70 (1992, supplement): 371–73.

23. H. Lepor, G. Rigaud, "The efficacy of transurethral resection of the prostate in men with moderate symptoms of prostatism," *Journal of Urology*, 143 (1990): 533–37; C. Moller-Nielson et al., "Sexual life following 'minimal' and 'total' prostate resection," *Urology International*, 40 (1987): 3–4.

24. John Wennberg, "On the status of the scientific basis of clinical medicine."

25. J.F. Kasper, A.G. Mulley, J.E. Wennberg, "Developing shared decision-making programs to improve the quality of health care," *Quality Review Bulletin*, 18 (1992): 183–90. For more information on the Foundation for Informed Medical Decision Making write to: P.O. Box C-17, Hanover, New Hampshire, USA 03755. Telephone: 603-650-1180.

26. John Wennberg, "On the status of the scientific basis of clinical medicine."

27. S.A. Brown, D.E. Grimes, "A meta-analysis of process of care, clinical outcomes, and cost-effectiveness of nurses in primary care roles: nurse practitioners and mid-wives," prepared for and published by the American Nurses Association, Division of Health Policy, July 1992.

28. Organisation for Economic Cooperation and Development, *Measuring Health Care, 1960–1983* (Paris: OECD, 1985).

29. J. Pickleman, "Controversies in biliary tract surgery," *Canadian Journal of Surgery*, 29 (1986): 429–33. Some members of the Canadian surgical community take issue with this position. See I.J.S. Moore, "Gallstones: Who should be treated and how?" *Family Practice*, 12 April 1993; C. Thomas, "Symptomatic Gallstones signal for surgery," *Ontario Medicine*, 20 March 1989.

30. D.F. Ransohoff et al., "Prophylactic cholecystectomy or expectant management for silent gallstones," *Annals of Internal Medicine*, 99 (1983): 199–204; C.K. McSherry et al., "The natural history of diagnosed gallstone disease in symptomatic and asymptomatic patients," *Annals of Surgery*, 202 (1985): 59–63.

31. "Canadian Consensus Conference on Cholesterol: Final Report," *Canadian Medical Association Journal* 139 (supplement) (1988): 1–8.

32. Canadian Task Force on the Periodic Health Examination, "Periodic health examination, 1993 (update: 2), "Lowering the blood total cholesterol level to prevent coronary heart disease," *Canadian Medical Association Journal*, 148 (1993): 521–38

33. Task Force on the Use and Provision of Medical Service, 1989–90. Annual Report, Toronto, 1990.

34. G. Barley, "College vs OMA: Gloves doffed in guidelines scrap," *Ontario Medicine*, 19 February 1990.

35. C. Fooks, M. Rachlis, C. Kushner, "Concepts of Quality of Care: National survey of five self-regulating health professions in Canada," *Quality Assurance in Health Care*, 2 (1990): 89–109.

36. B. Lown, "Sudden cardiac death: the major challenge confronting contemporary cardiology," *American Journal of Cardiology*, 43 (1979): 313–28.

37. The Cardiac Arrythmia Suppression Trial (CAST) investigators, "Preliminary report: effect of encainide and flecainide on mortality in a randomized trial of arrythmia suppression after myocardial infarction," *New England Journal of Medicine*, 321 (1989): 406–12.

38. G. Barley, "Heart drug study sets alarm bells ringing," *Ontario Medicine*, 4 September 1989.

39. J.B. McKinlay, S.M. McKinlay, "From promising report to standard procedure: Seven stages in the career of a medical innovation," *Millbank Memorial Fund Quarterly*, 59 (1981): 374–411.

40. Patients in the control group for this study—which would be considered highly unethical by today's standards—were actually anaesthetized and given a skin incision in the sham operation. L.A. Cobb et al., "An evaluation of internal mammary artery ligation by a double-blind technique," *New England Journal of Medicine*, 260 (1959): 1115–18; E.G. Diamond, C.F. Kittle, J.E. Crockett, "Comparison of internal mammary ligation and sham operation for angina pectoris," *American Journal of Cardiology*, 5 (1960): 484–86.

41. A.B. Miller, "Planning cancer control strategies," *Chronic Diseases in Canada*, 13 (supplement) (1992): S23–S25.

42. A.B. Miller et al., "Canadian Breast Cancer Screening Study 1: Breast cancer detection and death rates among women aged 40–49 years," *Canadian Medical Association Journal*, 147(10) (1992): 1459–76; A.B. Miller et al., "Canadian Breast Cancer Screening Study 2: Breast cancer detection and death rates among women aged 50–59 years," *Canadian Medical Association Journal*, 147(10) (1992): 1477–88.

43. B. Goldman, "When considering attacks against the National Breast Screening Study, consider the sources," *Canadian Medical Association Journal*, 148 (1993): 427–28; C. Gray, "U.S. resistance to Canadian mammogram study not only about data," *Canadian Medical Association Journal*, 148 (1993): 622–23.

44. "American doctors concur with Canadian study: mammograms of no benefit to women under 50," *Medical Post*, 23 March 1993.

45. L. Nystrom et al., "Breast cancer screening with mammography: overview of Swedish randomised trials," *Lancet*, 341 (1993): 973–78; V. Beral, "Breast cancer: mammographic screening," *Lancet*, 341 (1993): 1509–10; "Analyses cast more doubt on value of mammograms," *Globe and Mail*, 26 February 1993.

46. Diana Swift, "American Cancer Institute revises guidelines," *Medical Post*, 2 November 1993.

47. A.L. Cochrane, W.W. Holland, "Validation of screening procedures," *British Medical Bulletin*, 27 (1971): 3–8.

48. Several screening trials for lung cancer have shown that screening does not increase life expectancy: J.C. Baillar III, "Screening for lung cancer – where are we now?" *American*

Review of Respiratory Disease, 130 (1984): 541–42; R. Fontana et al., "Lung cancer screening: The Mayo program," *Journal of Occupational Medicine*, 28 (1986): 746–50.

49. D.L. Sackett et al., *Clinical Epidemiology: A Basic Science for Clinical Medicine* (2nd edition) (Toronto: Little, Brown and Co., 1991): 162.

50. Ibid; D. Cadman et al., "Assessing the effectiveness of community screening programs," *Journal of the American Medical Association*, 251 (1984): 1580.

51. Health and Welfare Canada, *National Health Expenditures in Canada 1975–1987*. Ottawa, 1990.

52. J. Abelson, "NHRPD budget trends," Centre for Health Economics and Policy Analysis. Hamilton, 1993.

53. *The Report of the British Columbia Royal Commission on Health Care and Costs* (Victoria, 1991): B-21.

54. *The Report of the New Brunswick Commission on Selected Health Care Programs* (Fredericton, 1989): 80.

55. C. Fooks, M. Rachlis, C. Kushner, "Concepts of Quality of Care: National survey of five self-regulating health professions in Canada," *Quality Assurance in Health Care*, 2 (1990): 89–109.

56. *The Regulated Health Professions Act*, 1993.

57. R.G. McAuley et al., "Five-year results of the peer assessment program of the College of Physicians and Surgeons of Ontario," *Canadian Medical Association Journal*, 143 (1990): 1193–99.

58. *Globe and Mail*, 17 December 1990.

59. Ibid.

60. "Some hospitals have utilization review committees with involvement of the medical staff, and some have regular utilization review rounds, however, the coordination role of the utilization review committees, even where they exist, is limited." *Report of the New Brunswick Commission on Selected Health Care Programs* (Fredericton, 1989): 80.

61. P. Norman, S. Kostovcik, A. Lanning, "Elective repeat caesarian sections: How many could be vaginal births?" *Canadian Medical Association Journal*, 149 (1993): 431–34.

62. Ibid.

63. J.M. Eisenberg, *Doctors' Decisions and the Cost of Medical Care: The Reasons for Doctors' Practice Patterns and Ways to Change Them* (Ann Arbor, MI: Health Administration Perspectives Press,1986): 137.

64. M.R. Chassin, S.M. McCue, "A randomized trial of medical quality assurance: improving physicians use of pelvimetry," *Journal of the American Medical Association*, 256 (1986): 1012–16; W. Schaffner et al., "Improving antibiotic prescribing in office practice: a controlled trial of three educational methods," *Journal of the American Medical Association*, 250 (1983): 1728–32;

65. J. Avorn, S.B. Soumerai, "Improving drug-therapy decisions through educational outreach: a randomized controlled trial of academically-based detailing," *New England Journal of Medicine*, 308 (1983): 1457–63.

66. *Globe and Mail*, 31 August 1993.

67. R.W. Brooks-Hill, R.A. Buckingham, "Evaluating the effectiveness of a process medical audit in a teaching general hospital," *Canadian Medical Association Journal*, 134 (1986): 350–52; J. Kosecoff et al., "Effects of the National Institutes of Health consensus development program on physician practice," *Journal of the American Medical Association*, 258 (1987): 2708–13; G.M. Anderson, J. Lomas, "Recent trends in Cesarian section rates in Ontario," *Canadian Medical Association Journal*, 141 (1989): 1049–53.

68. D. Berwick, "Continuous improvement as an ideal in health care," *New England Journal of Medicine*, 320 (1989): 53–56; D. Berwick, "Health services research and quality of care: Assignments for the 1990s," *Medical Care*, 27 (1989): 763–71.

69. Alexandra Paul, "Nurses vent rage at cost-cutting health consultant," *Winnipeg Free Press*, 20 April 1993.

70. B.L. Davies et al., *Canadian Medical Association Journal*, 148 (1993): 1737–42. This study cites many randomized trials of electronic fetal monitoring as well as various reviews of the area.

71. Ibid.

72. J. Kennel et al., "Continuous emotional support during labor in a U.S. hospital: a randomized controlled trial," *Journal of the American Medical Association*, 265 (1991): 2197–2201.

73. J. Lomas et al., "Do practice guidelines guide practice? The effect of a consensus statement on the practice of physicians," *New England Journal of Medicine*, 321 (1989): 1306–11.

74. American College of Obstetricians and Gynecologists Committee on Obstetrics, Committee Statement, "Maternal and Fetal Medicine: Guidelines for Vaginal Delivery after a Previous Caesarean Birth," Washington, DC, November 1984.

75. According to a study in Montreal, older obstetricians were less likely to offer their patients an opportunity for a vaginal birth after a previous Caesarean. G. Goldman et al., "Factors influencing the practice of vaginal birth after caesarean section," *American Journal of Public Health*, 83 (1993): 1104–8.

76. J. Lomas et al., "Opinion leaders vs audit and feedback to implement practice guidelines: delivery after previous caesarian section," *Journal of the American Medical Association*, 265 (1991): 2202–7.

77. G. Laffel, D.M. Berwick, "Quality in health care," *Journal of the American Medical Association*, 268 (1992): 407–409.

CHAPTER 5

1. *Globe and Mail*, 19 March 1992.

2. "The Pharmacy Practice 200: An Exclusive IMS Report on the Top 200 Drugs of '92," *Pharmacy Practice*, 8 (December 1992): 27–34.

3. From the Canadian Society of Hospital Pharmacists (Ontario) brief to the Ontario Hospital Association's 1992 Annual Meeting.

4. Joel Lexchin, "Prescribing and drug costs in the province of Ontario," *International Journal of Health Services*, 22(3) (1992): 471–87.

5. *Toronto Star*, 4 May 1993.

6. Ibid.

7. T.R. Frieden, R.J. Mangi, "Inappropriate use of oral ciprofloxacin," *Journal of the American Medical Association*, 264 (1990): 1438–40.

8. "The Pharmacy Practice 200: An Exclusive IMS Report on the Top 200 Drugs of '92."

9. "Ciprofloxacin," *Medical Letter on Drugs and Therapeutics*, 30 (1988): 11–13.

10. T.R. Frieden, R.J. Mangi, "Inappropriate use of oral ciprofloxacin."

11. *Ottawa Citizen*, 5 March 1989.

12. Ibid.

13. J. Lexchin, "Adverse Drug Reactions: Review of the Canadian literature," *Canadian Family Physician*, 37 (1991): 109–18; W.A. Ray, M.R. Griffin, R.I. Shorr, "Adverse drug reactions and the elderly," *Health Affairs*, 9(3) (1990): 114–22.

14. P.A. Dieppe, S.J. Frankel, B. Toth, "Is research into the treatment of osteoarthritis with non-steroidal anti-inflammatory drugs misdirected?" *Lancet*, 341 (1993): 353–54.

15. Ibid.

16. M.C. Allison et al., "Gastrointestinal damage associated with the use of nonsteroidal anti-inflammatory drugs," *New England Journal of Medicine*, 327 (1992): 749–54. Of the NSAID patients, 8.4 percent died as the result of bleeding or perforated peptic ulcer, or perforations in the small-bowel or large bowel, compared to only 3 percent of patients who were not taking this type of medication.

17. "Epidemic-like increase in NSAID-induced ulcer complications," *Canadian Doctor*, February 1989.

18. W.A. Ray et al., "Psychotropic drug use and the risk of hip fracture," *New England Journal of Medicine*, 316 (1987): 363–69; W.A. Ray, M.R. Griffin, W. Downey, "Benzodiazepines of long- and short-elimination half life and the risk of hip fracture," *Journal of the American Medical Association*, 262 (1989): 3303–7.

19. W.A. Ray, M.R. Griffin, and R.I. Sharr, "Adverse Drug Reactions and the Elderly," *Health Affairs*, 9(3) (Fall 1990): 114–22.

20. C. Inake Neutel, "Gender and family income in psychotropic drugs and alcohol use," *Chronic Diseases in Canada*, 13(3) (1992): 42–46.

21. "The Pharmacy Practice 200: An Exclusive IMS Report on the Top 200 Drugs of '92."

22. U.S. Department of Health and Human Services, Public Health Service, Agency for Health Care Policy and Research, "Acute pain management: operative or medical procedures and trauma," Rockville MD, 1992.

23. Joel Katz et al., "Pre-emptive analgesia," *Anaesthesiology*, 77 (1992): 439–46.

24. K.J.S. Anand, P.R. Hickey, "Halothane-morphine compared with high dose sufentanil for anaesthesia and postoperative analgesia in neonatal cardiac surgery," *New England Journal of Medicine*, 326 (1992): 1–9.

25. L.A. Pica et al., "Hypertension follow–up survey, Laval, Quebec, 1988," *Canadian Journal of Public Health*, 84 (1993): 174–76.

26. *Toronto Star*, 28 January 1993.

27. A.P. Williams and Rhonda Cockerill, "Report on the 1989 survey of the prescribing experiences and attitudes toward prescription drugs of Ontario physicians," prepared for the Pharmaceutical Inquiry of Ontario (Lowy Commission), December 1989.

28. For the lower estimate, see Task Force on the Use and Provision of Medical Services, "Quality Assurance and Resource Management—the Medical Services Challenges for the 1990s," November 1990. For the higher figure, see B.K. Cypress, "Drug utilization in general and family practice by characteristics of physicians and office visits," National Ambulatory Medical Care Survey, NCHS advance data, 1983, March 28: 87.

29. D. Drake and M. Uhlman, *Making Medicine, Making Money* (Kansas City: Andrews and McMeel, 1993): 26.

30. *Globe and Mail*, 26 October 1988.

31. D. Drake, M. Uhlman, *Making Medicine, Making Money*: 102.

32. *Toronto Star*, 4 April 1993.

33. Ibid.

34. Ibid.

35. Ibid.

36. J. Avorn, M. Chen, R. Hartley, "Scientific versus commercial sources of influence on the prescribing behavior of physicians," *American Journal of Medicine*, 73 (1982): 4–8.

37. Unpublished data from a study entitled "Journal editors and the news media," conducted by M. Wilkes, U.C.L.A., in Department of Health and Human Services, Office of the Inspector General, "Prescription drug advertisements in medical journals," 1992.

38. Ibid.

39. R. Mickleburgh, "More substance less glitz urged in drug advertising," *Globe and Mail*, 14 January 1993.

40. J.F. Fries et al., "A re-evaluation of aspirin therapy in rheumatoid arthritis," *Archives of Internal Medicine*, 153 (1993): 2465–71.

41. R.E. Araino, S.A. Zelenitsky, "Ketorolac (Toradol): a marketing phenomenon," *Canadian Medical Association Journal*, 148 (1993): 1686–88"

42. Sara Lewis, "Ketorolac in Europe," *Lancet*, 343 (1994): 784.

43. *Globe and Mail*, 14 January 1993.

44. D. Drake and M. Uhlman, *Making Medicine, Making Money.*

45. *Globe and Mail*, 28 December 1991.

46. Nicholas Regush, *Safety Last: The Failure of the Consumer Health Protection System in Canada* (Toronto: Key Porter Books, 1993): 125.

47. D. Drake and M. Uhlman, *Making Medicine Making Money*: 10–11.

48. The Centre for Evaluation of Medicines, *The optimal prescribing bulletin*, Vol. 1, No. 1, St. Joseph's Hospital, Hamilton, 1993.

49. D. Drake and M. Uhlman, *Making Medicine, Making Money*: 11.

50. D. Moulton, "Cooperative drug purchases latest joint initiative of Atlantic premiers," *Medical Post*, 7 December 1993.

51. P.L. Doering et al., "Therapeutic substitution in the health maintenance organization outpatient environment," *Drug Intelligence and Clinical Pharmacy*, 22 (1988): 125–30.

52. Personal communication with Dr. Pete Penna, director of clinical pharmacy services, Group Health Cooperative of Puget Sound, October 1988.

53. "The management of raised blood pressure in New Zealand. A Consensus Development Conference Report to the National Advisory Committee on Core Health and Disability Services," Wellington, NZ, 1992.

54. J. Avorn and S. Sumerai, "Improving drug therapy decisions through a randomized controlled trial of academically-based 'detailing,'" *New England Journal of Medicine*, 308 (1993): 1457–63.

55. The Canadian Medical Association, "Physicians and the pharmaceutical industry," *Canadian Medical Association Journal*, 146 (1992): 388A–388C.

56. Education Council, Residency Training Programme in Internal Medicine, Department of Medicine, McMaster University, "Development of residency program guidelines for interaction with the pharmaceutical industry," *Canadian Medical Association Journal*, 149 (1993): 405–8.

57. G. Guyatt, "Academic medicine and the pharmaceutical industry: a cautionary tale," *Canadian Medical Association Journal*. On press at time of publication.

58. *Medical Post*, 27 February 1990.

59. *Globe and Mail*, 22 December 1988.

60. *Medical Post*, 27 February 1990.

61. *Family Practice*, 15 June 1992.

62. "Drug Company freebies don't sway doctors," *Medical Post*, 7 September 1993.

63. *Toronto Star*, 17 December 1992.

64. *Globe and Mail*, 15 February 1993.

65. The letter is dated 1 December 1992.

66. *Globe and Mail*, 5 February 1993.

67. J. Lexchin, "Effect of generic drug competition on the price of prescription drugs in Ontario," *Canadian Medical Association Journal*, 148(1) (1993): 35–38.

68. *Globe and Mail*, 22 October 1992.

69. H.E. Eastman, letter to the editor, *Globe and Mail*, 12 September 1992. Bill C-91 did allow the PMPRB to adjust Canadian prices according to international prices, but the drug companies got around this regulation by voluntarily taking their products off patent. In most cases it takes five to eight years to bring a generic copy to the marketplace. During this period, the brand-name company is protected from any competition and can maintain high profits. A. Chamberlain, "Drug firms must pay for overcharging," *Toronto Star*, 4 January 1994.

70. Canadian Health Coalition and the Medical Reform Group, "Brief to the Bank, Trade and Commerce Committee of the Senate of Canada on Bill C-91," January 1993: 3.

71. GreenShield Pre-paid Services, Inc., "A report on drug costs," Toronto, Green-Shield, April 1992.

72. *Toronto Star*, 30 November 1992.

73. *Globe and Mail*, 31 March 1993.

74. Notes for remarks by the Honorable Michel Côté, Minister of Consumer and Corporate Affairs, for a press statement, 27 June 1986.

75. D. Spurgeon, "Brand-name drug companies to hold winning hand in GATT talks," *Canadian Medical Association Journal*, 146 (1992): 1429–33.

76. The Canadian Drug Manufacturers Association, "Bill C-91: An Act to Amend the Patent Act; Position Paper," 11 September 1992: 6.

77. "Apotex allowed to sell heart drug, Merck to fight cheaper version," *Toronto Star*, 3 September 1993.

78. Stevie Cameron, "How the drug-makers influence the policy-makers," *Globe and Mail*, 30 November 1992.

79. D. Moulton, "C-91 connection to drug company grant poses problems for N.S. University," *Medical Post*, 9 March 1993.

80. *Medical Post*, 3 November 1992.

81. "There's more than meets the eye in amendments to drug patent legislation," *CMA News*, January 1993.

82. J. Edward, "Science supports the case for brand-name drugs," *Globe and Mail*, 29 December 1992.

83. G. Guyatt, "Higher costs for health care, higher profit for industry," *Globe and Mail*, 14 January 1993.

84. *Globe and Mail*, 18 May 1993.

85. W. Kondro, "Canada: MRC partnership with drug industry," *Lancet*, 341 (1993): 1402.

86. Nicholas Regush, *Safety Last*.

87. *Ottawa Citizen*, 10 October 1987.

88. *Ottawa Citizen*, 16 October 1987.

89. "U.S. drug firms want to abolish provincial rules," *Toronto Star*, 18 February 1993.

CHAPTER 6

1. K. Swedburgh et al., on behalf of the CONSENSUS II Study Group, "Effects of early administration of enalapril on mortality in patients with acute myocardial infarction: Results of the Cooperative North Scandinavian Enalapril Survival Study II (CONSENSUS II)," *New England Journal of Medicine,* 327 (1992): 678–84.

2. "Klein to seek medicare user fees," *Globe and Mail*, 13 January 1993.

3. "User fees inevitable, Quebec treasury says," *Medical Post*, 16 February 1993.

4. G.L. Stoddart et al., "Why not user charges? The real issues," The Ontario Premier's Council on Health, Well-Being and Social Justice. Toronto, 1993; R.G. Evans, M.L. Barer, G.L. Stoddart, "The truth about user fees," *Policy Options*, October 1993: 4–9.

5. R.G. Evans, M.L. Barer, G.L. Stoddart, "The truth about user fees."

6. The charges were $1.50 for each physicians' office visit, $2.00 for each physician's home, emergency, or out-patient visit, $2.50 for each in-patient day during the first thirty days of hospitalization, and $1.50 for each in-patient day from the thirty-first to the ninetieth day of hospitalization. There was an annual ceiling of $180 for each family. Individuals and families receiving government social assistance were exempt from the charges. (All figures are in 1968 dollars.)

7. R.G. Beck, J.M. Horne, "Study of user charges in Saskatchewan 1968–1971," in *User Charges for Health Services: A Report of the Ontario Council of Health* (Toronto: Ontario Council of Health, 1979): 133–62.

8. W.G. Manning et al., "Health insurance and the demand for medical care: evidence from a randomized experiment," *American Economic Review*, 77 (1987): 251–77.

9. For example, compared to first-dollar coverage, the poorest third decreased their use of any health service by 13 percent, with a 25 percent coinsurance rate, compared to an 8 percent decrease for the highest-income third.

10. R.G. Evans, M.L. Barer, G.L. Stoddart, "The truth about user fees."

11. M.C. Fahs, "Physician response to the United Mine Workers' cost-sharing program: The other side of the coin," Health Services Research, 27(1) (1992): 25–45.

12. R.G. Evans, M.L. Barer, G.L. Stoddart, "The truth about user fees."

13. B. Foxman et al., Journal of Chronic Disease, 40 (1987): 429–37. The use of antibiotics was 46 percent lower in the group subject to user charges, but the proportion that was inappropriate remained the same. The authors concluded that the rate of use of antibiotics was proportional to the rate of physician visits and that the decreased use of antibiotics in the user charge group was related to the decreased physician encounters in this group. They recommend that user charges are effective in decreasing the use of antibiotics but not in improving the appropriateness of their prescription.

14. A.L. Siu et al., "Inappropriate use of hospitals in a randomized trial of health insurance plans," New England Journal of Medicine, 315 (1986): 1259–66.

15. The proportion of admissions judged inappropriate was 24 percent in the full coverage group and 22 percent in the user charge group. The proportion of overall hospital days judged inappropriate was 35 percent in the full coverage group and 34 percent in the user charge group.

16. A.L. Siu et al., "Inappropriate use of hospitals in a randomized trial of health insurance plans."

17. As we discuss in Chapter 2, the Canada Health Act refers to services being available according to their "medical necessity." We note that this term has never been operationally defined. However, it is clear that the intent of the terminology in the medicare legislation since Tommy Douglas's original hospital insurance plan in 1947 is that people should have access to services according to their need.

18. R.H. Brook et al., "Does free care improve adults' health? Results from a randomized controlled trial," New England Journal of Medicine, 309 (1983): 1426–34.

19. E.B. Keeler et al., "How free care reduced hypertension in the Health Insurance Experiment," Journal of the American Medical Association, 254 (1985): 1926–31.

20. Ibid. In the RAND HIE, fifty-year-old men with hypertension had a five-year death rate of about 50 per 1,000. This was increased by 10.5 deaths per 1,000 if they were allocated to an insurance plan with user charges.

21. N. Lurie et al., "Termination from Medi-Cal—Does it effect Health?" New England Journal of Medicine, 311 (1984): 480–84; N. Lurie et al., "Termination from Medi-Cal benefits: a follow-up study one year later," New England Journal of Medicine, 314 (1986): 1266–68; M.O. Mundinger, "Health service funding cuts and the declining health of the poor," New England Journal of Medicine, 313 (1985): 44–47.

22. G.J. Scheiber, J.P. Poullier, L.M. Greenwald, "U.S. health care expenditure performance: an international comparison and data update," Health Care Financing Review, 13(4) (1992): 1–88.

23. C.A. Cowan, P.A. McDonnell, "Business, households, and governments: health spending, 1991," Health Care Financing Review, 14(3) (1993): 227–48.

24. G.M. Anderson et al., "Use of coronary artery bypass surgery in the United States and Canada: Influence of age and income," Journal of the American Medical Association, 269 (1993): 1661–66.

25. A study of British civil servants showed that the senior administrators were one-fourth as likely to die of heart disease as those at the lowest levels of the civil service: G. Rose, M.G.T. Marmot, "Social class and coronary heart disease," British Heart Journal, 45 (1981): 13–19. The doctors who participated in the Harvard Physicians' Health Study Research Group had only one-eighth of the cardiovascular disease death rate of the general population. A comparison only with the poor would show this figure

to be even lower: M. Angell, "Privilege and health—what is the connection?" *New England Journal of Medicine*, 329 (1993): 126–27.

26. R. Mickleburgh, "Surgery bypasses wealth," *Globe and Mail*, 7 April 1993.

27. B.J. McNeil, R. Weichselbaum, S.G. Pauker, "Fallacy of the five year survival in lung cancer," *New England Journal of Medicine*, 299 (1978): 1397–1401.

28. N.P. Roos et al., "Mortality and reoperation after open and transurethral resection of the prostate for benign prostatic hyperplasia," *New England Journal of Medicine*, 320 (1989): 1120–24; Paul Cotton, "Case for prostate therapy wanes despite more treatment options," *Journal of the American Medical Association*, 266 (1991): 459–60.

29. M.L. Millenson, "Video gives prostate patients reason to 'pause,'" *The Medical Post*, 22 October 1991; M. Nicholson, "Interactive video series benefits patients and doctors," *The Medical Post*, 19 November 1991. For more information contact the Foundation for Informed Medical Decision Making. P.O. Box C-17, Hanover, New Hampshire, USA 03755.

30. M. Simpson et al., "Doctor patient communication: the Toronto consensus statement," *British Medical Journal*, 303 (1991): 1385–87.

31. L.F. Degner, J.M. Farber, T.F. Hack, *Communication between Cancer Patients and Health Care Professionals: An Annotated Bibliography* (Toronto: Canadian Cancer Society, 1989); K. Jenkins, "Doctors don't realize CA patients often left in dark," *The Medical Post*, 13 October 1987; T. Murray, "Reports from International Consensus Conference on Doctor Patient Communication," *The Medical Post*, 3 December 1991.

32. H.B. Beckman, R.M. Frankel, "The effect of physician behaviour on the collection of data," *Annals of Internal Medicine*, 101 (1984): 692–96.

33. "Consensus statement from the workshop on the teaching and assessment of communication skills in Canadian medical schools," *Canadian Medical Association Journal*, 147 (1992): 1149–50.

34. Simpson et al., "Doctor Patient Communication."

35. Elizabeth MacNab, *A Legal History of Health Professions in Ontario* (Toronto: The Committee on the Healing Arts, Queen's Printer, 1970); Paul Starr, *The Social Transformation of American Medicine* (New York: Basic Books, 1982).

36. Ibid. In fact, the Council of the College of Physicians and Surgeons of Ontario originally included homeopaths and they were not struck off until the twentieth century.

37. S.A. Brown, D.E. Grimes, "A meta-analysis of process of care, clinical outcomes, and cost-effectiveness of nurses in primary care roles: Nurse practitioners and midwives," prepared for and published by the American Nurses Association, Division of Health Policy, July 1992.

38. A. Mitchell et al., "Evaluation of graduating neonatal nurse practitioners," *Pediatrics*, 88 (1991): 789–94.

39. D.E. Everitt, J. Avorn, M.W. Baker, "Clinical decision-making in the evaluation and treatment of insomnia," *The American Journal of Medicine*, 89 (1990): 357–62; J. Avorn, D.E. Everitt, M.W. Baker, "The neglected medical history and therapeutic choices for abdominal pain," *Archives of Internal Medicine*, 151 (1991): 694–98.

40. W.O. Spitzer et al., "The Burlington randomized trial of the nurse practitioner," *New England Journal of Medicine*, 290 (1974): 251–56.

41. R.W. Sutherland, M.J. Fulton, *Health Care in Canada* (Ottawa: The Health Group, 1988).

42. J.E.F. Hastings et al., "Prepaid group practice in Sault Ste Marie, Ontario: Part I: analysis of utilization records," *Medical Care*, 11 (1973): 91–103; H.S. Luft, *Health Maintenance Organizations: Dimensions of Performance* (New York: John Wiley and Sons, 1981): 58–75.

43. W.W. Rosser, J.M. Forster, "Reform of the primary care system in Ontario," unpublished mimeo, August 1993; Ontario Chapter of the Canadian College of Family Physicians, "Position paper on alternate payment mechanisms," July 1992.

NOTES 365

44. W.G. Manning et al. "A controlled trial of the effect of a prepaid group practice on the use of services," *New England Journal of Medicine*, 310 (1984): 1505–10; J.E. Ware et al., *The Lancet*, Vol. 1 (1986): 1017–22.

45. E.M. Sloss et al., "Effect of a health maintenance organization on physiologic health: results from a randomized trial," *Annals of Internal Medicine*, 106 (1987): 130–38; A.R. Davies et al., "Consumer acceptance of prepaid and fee for-service medical care: results from a randomized controlled trial," *Health Services Research*, 21 (1986). 429–52. There were some minor differences in outcomes among sub-groups. Higher-income patients who started the study in poor health had slightly better health outcomes from the HMO while low-income patients who started the study in poor health had slightly poorer outcomes from the HMO. Additionally, the patients allocated to the HMO were somewhat less satisfied with the care they received. This decreased satisfaction seems to have been due to patients equating increasing number of services with better quality. Finally, the study, while expensive and thorough, only investigated one HMO. Technically, the results might not apply to other non-fee-for-service organizations. However, the Group Health Cooperative of Puget Sound is non-profit and is governed by a board made up of recipients and providers of the service. In these characteristics, it resembles many of Canada's hospital boards.

46. L. Bozzoni, "Local community services centres (CLSCs) in Quebec: Description, evaluation, perspectives," *Journal of Public Health Policy*, 9 (1988): 346–75.

47. J.E.F. Hastings et al., "Prepaid group practice in Sault Ste. Marie," Saskatchewan Department of Health, Community Clinic Study, Regina, 1983.

48. M. Renaud et al., "Practice settings and prescribing profiles: The simulation of tension headaches to general practitioners working in different practice settings in the Montreal area," *American Journal of Public Health*, 70 (1980): 1068–73.

49. R.N. Battista, "Adult cancer prevention in primary care: Patterns of practice in Quebec," *American Journal of Public Health*, 73 (1983): 1036–41.

50. R.N. Battista, J.I. Williams, L.A. MacFarlane, "Determinants of primary medical practice in adult cancer prevention," *Medical Care*, 24 (1986): 216–24.

51. R. Allard et al., "Delays in the primary vaccination of children," *Canadian Medical Association Journal*, 133 (1985): 108–10.

52. R. Pineault et al., "Characteristics of physicians practicing in alternative primary care settings: A Quebec study of local community service center physicians," *International Journal of Health Services*, 21 (1991): 49–58.

53. E.J. Topol et al., "A randomized controlled trial of hospital discharge three days after myocardial infarction in the era of reperfusion," *New England Journal of Medicine*, 318 (1988): 1083–88.

54. See a series of articles in the *Journal of the American Medical Association*, 264 (1990).

55. R.B. Saltman, C. von Otter, *Planned Markets and Public Competition* (Buckingham: Open University Press, 1992); A. Webb, G. Wistow, *Planning, Need and Scarcity: Essays on the Personal Social Services* (London: Allen and Unwin, 1986); A. McGuire, "Measuring performance in the health care sector: the whys and the hows," in *The Challenges of Medical Practice Variations,* eds: F. Anderson, G. Mooney (London: MacMillan Press, 1990).

56. In 1975, there were 39,104 doctors for 22.9 million Canadians (1 per 585). By 1989, there were 58,942 doctors for 26.5 million Canadians (1 per 450). The doctors included are non-military doctors with a known address in Canada at the end of the year. Retired and semi-retired doctors are excluded from these totals. (Sources: Health and Welfare Canada, *Health Personnel in Canada 1986* and *Health Personnel in Canada 1989.*)

57. Ontario Council of Health, *Medical Manpower for Ontario* (Toronto: Queen's Printer for Ontario, 1983).

58. N. Hall et al., "Randomized trial of a health promotion program for frail elders," *Canadian Journal on Aging*, 11 (1992): 72–91.

59. D.M. Vickery et al., "Effect of self-care education program on medical visits," *Journal of the American Medical Association*, 250 (1983): 2952–56; C.R. Roberts et al., "Reducing physician visits for colds through consumer education," *Journal of the American Medical Association*, 250 (1983): 1986–89; A. Stergachis, "Use of a controlled trial to evaluate the impact of self-care on health services utilization," *Journal of Ambulatory Care Management*, 9(4) (1986): 16–22.

60. J.M. FitzGerald, D. Swan, M.O. Turner, "The role of asthma education," *Canadian Medical Association*, 147 (1992): 855-56; I. Charlton et al., "Evaluation of peak flow and symptoms only self management plans for control of asthma in general practice," *British Medical Journal*, 301 (1990): 1355–59; L. Tougaard et al., "Economic benefits of teaching patients with chronic obstructive pulmonary disease about their illness," *Lancet*, 339 (1992): 1517–20.

61. C. Hendriksen, E. Lund, E. Stromgard, "Consequences of assessment and intervention among elderly people: a three year randomized controlled trial," *British Medical Journal*, 289 (1984): 1522–24; M.S. John Pathy et al., "Randomized trial of case finding and surveillance of elderly people at home," *British Medical Journal*, 340 (1992): 890–93; N.J. Vetter, D.A. Jones, C.R. Victor, "Effect of health visitors working with elderly patients in general practice: a randomised controlled trial," *British Medical Journal*, 288 (1984): 369–72.

62. J. Wasson, C. Gaudette, F. Whaley, "Telephone care as a substitute for routine clinic follow-up," *Journal of the American Medical Association*, 267 (1992): 1788–93.

63. For those who initially rated their health as fair or poor, there were twelve deaths in the traditional care group and four in the telephone group (P = 0.06). Conventional statistical significance usually requires P-values of .05 or less. The P-value indicates the probability that the observed results could have occurred by chance alone. In other words, we could be 94 percent certain that the mortality results are a true bill.

64. J. Tudor Hart, "The inverse care law," *Lancet*, Vol. 1 (1971): 405–12.

65. Press release from meeting of Health Ministers, 28 January 1992.

66. Michelle Noble, "Disincentives on the table," *Ontario Medicine*, 8 March 1993; Matt Borsellino, "Young MDs wary of OMA manpower plan," *Medical Post*, 9 March 1993.

67. Fran Lowry, "Will Ontario's moratorium have a snowball effect?" *Canadian Medical Association Journal*, 149 (1993): 1005–10.

68. Abraham Flexner, *Medical Education in the United States and Canada*, Carnegie Foundation for the Advancement of Teaching, Bulletin No. 4. (New York: 1910).

69. The Community Health Centre Project (Chair, Dr. John Hastings) (Ottawa: Health and Welfare Canada, 1972): The Ontario Task Force to Review Primary Health Care (Chair, Dr. Fraser Mustard), (Toronto: Ontario Ministry of Health, 1981).

70. M. Komaromy et al., "Sexual harassment in medical training," *New England Journal of Medicine*, 328 (1993): 322–26; M.M. Farley, P. Kozarsky, "Sexual harassment in medical training," *New England Journal of Medicine*, 329 (1993): 661; Susan Thorne, "Several medical schools have begun to tackle sexual harassment issue," *Canadian Medical Association Journal*, 147 (1992): 1567–71.

71. R. Moscarello, K.J. Margittai, M. Rossi, "Differences in abuse reported by female and male Canadian medical students," *Canadian Medical Association Journal*, 150 (1994): 357–363. Pippa Wysong, "Female med students suffering widespread abuse," *Medical Post*, 16 February 1993.

72. J.A. Richman et al., "Mental health consequences and correlates of reported medical student abuse," *Journal of the American Medical Association*, 267 (1992): 692–94.

73. Lisa Priest, "Medical students at U of T report harassment," *Toronto Star*, 1 February 1994.

74. C.P. McKegney, "Medical education: a neglectful and abusive family system," *Family Medicine*, 21 (1989): 452–57.

75. A.M. Hayton, "Doctors to be," *Lancet*, 340 (1992): 1546.

76. O. Lechky, "U of T not the only Ontario medical school heavily involved in curriculum renewal," *Canadian Medical Association Journal*, 147 (1992): 1233, 1235–37; J. Shin, R.B. Haynes, M.E. Johnston, "Effect of problem based, self-directed undergraduate education on life long learning," *Canadian Medical Association Journal*, 148 (1993): 969–76.

77. M. Roemer, "Bed supply and hospital utilization: a natural experiment," *Hospitals*, 35 (1961): 36–42.

78. The Diabetes Control and Complications Trial Research Group, "The effect of intensive treatment of diabetes on the development and progression of long-term complications in insulin-dependent diabetes mellitus," *New England Journal of Medicine*, 329 (1993): 977–86.

79. S. Birch et al., "A needs-based approach to resource allocation in health care," *Canadian Public Policy*, 19(1) (1993): 68–85; J. Eyles, S. Birch, "A population needs-based approach to health-care resource allocation and planning in Ontario: a link between policy goals and practice," 84 (1993): 112–17; S. Birch, S. Chambers, "To each according to need: a community-based approach to allocating health care resources," *Canadian Medical Association Journal*, 149 (1993): 607–12.

80. N.P. Roos et al., "Assessing the relationship between health care use and the health of the population: seeking levers for policy makers," paper delivered to the Honda Foundation-Discoveries Symposium, Toronto, 16–18 October 1993.

81. Ibid.

CHAPTER 7

1. *Globe and Mail*, 9 November 1990.

2. Dr. Huckell states that Mr. Mueller had a complete obstruction of his left main coronary artery and his right coronary artery.

3. In fact that figure should have been closer to 10 to 15 percent. See: T. Takaro, R. Pifarre, R. Fish, "Left main coronary artery disease," *Progress in Cardiovascular Diseases*, 28 (1985): 229–34.

4. This story has been constructed from interviews with both Mr. Mueller and Dr. Huckell conducted in April 1991, as well as from an official report from the Vancouver General Hospital written by Michelle Perreault on 7 August 1991.

5. *Globe and Mail*, 5 November 1988; *Toronto Star*, 4 November 1988. Some observers (including the authors) are not so sanguine about the long-term effects (especially the indirect effects) of free trade on health care. However, we agree that in the short-term, the free trade agreement has had little impact on insurance for hospitals and physicians.

6. David Vienneau, "The father of medicare raps Reform," *Toronto Star*, 7 October 1993.

7. G.J. Scheiber, J.P. Poullier, "Overview of international comparisons of health care expenditures," *Health Care Financing Review*, 1989 annual supplement:1–87.

8. G.J. Scheiber, J.P. Poullier, L.M. Greenwald, "U.S. health expenditure performance: An international comparison and data update," *Health Care Financing Review*, 13(4) (1992): 1–88.

9. Health Care Expenditure Fact Sheets, Health & Welfare Canada, February 1993.

10. The Health Insurance Association of America, "Statement of HIAA on access and affordability of health care: Presentation to the Committee on Government Operations of the U.S. House of Representatives," 4 June 1991.

11. M.L. Barer, W.P. Welch, L. Antioch, "Canadian/U.S. health care: Reflections on the HIAA's analysis," *Health Affairs*, 10 (1991): 229–36.

12. R.G. Evans et al., "Controlling health expenditures—the Canadian reality," *New England Journal of Medicine*, 320 (1989): 571–77.

13. S. Woolhandler, D.U. Himmelstein, "The deteriorating administrative efficiency of the US health-care system," *New England Journal of Medicine*, 324 (1991): 1253–58.

14. D.A. Redelmeier, V.R. Fuchs, "Hospital expenditures in the United States and Canada," *New England Journal of Medicine*, 328 (1993): 772–78.

15. National Center for Health Statistics, *Health, United States, 1991* (Hyattsville, Maryland: Public Health Service, 1992). The figures used are for care of civilians in non-federal short-stay hospitals.

16. This statistic was calculated for Ontario using the population of 9,426,200 from the vital statistics of the province for 1988 and the days of care in acute-care hospitals, from *Hospital Statistics 1988–89,* published by the Ontario Ministry of Health.

17. Personal communication with Dr. Geoffrey Anderson, Institute for Clinical Evaluative Sciences, Toronto, Ontario, 22 June 1993.

18. J.L. Rouleau et al., "A comparison of management patterns after acute myocardial infarction in Canada and the United States," *New England Journal of Medicine*, 328 (1993): 779–84. The study did find that there was slightly greater incidence of activity-limiting angina in Canadians versus Americans after an average of 42 months of follow-up (33 percent vs. 27 percent).

19. There are many different ways to count doctors, but using data from Health and Welfare's Health Personnel in Canada (1989) and the U.S. Department of Health and Human Services' *Health United States 1991*, Canada had 449 persons per active, civilian physician and the U.S. had 458 persons per active, non-federal physician.

20. United States General Accounting Office, "Canadian Health Insurance: Lessons for the United States," 1991.

21. J. Iglehart, "Canada's health care system faces its problems," *New England Journal of Medicine*, 322 (1990): 562–68.

22. Charlotte Gray, "Checkbooks in hand, U.S. hospitals come to woo Canada's best and brightest," *Canadian Medical Association Journal*, 147 (1992): 483, 486–87.

23. D.U. Himmelstein, S. Woolhandler, S.M. Wolfe, "The vanishing safety net: New data on uninsured Americans," *International Journal of Health Services*, 22 (1992): 381–96.

24. T. Bodenheimer, "Underinsurance in America," *New England Journal of Medicine*, 327 (1992): 274–78.

25. Ibid.

26. These two examples are taken from Consumer Reports' *How to Solve the Health Care Crisis: Affordable Protection for All Americans* (Yonkers, New York: Consumer Report Books, 1992).

27. D. Wilson, "B.C. investor besieged by U.S. pleas for aid," *Globe and Mail*, 28 May 1990.

28. V.R. Fuchs, J.S. Hahn, "How does Canada do it? A comparison of expenditures for physicians' services in the United States and Canada," *New England Journal of Medicine*, 323 (1990): 884–90.

29. National Center for Health Statistics, *Health United States, 1991*, Tables 49 and 50.

30. J.W. Zylke, "Declining childhood immunization rates becoming cause for concern," *Journal of the American Medical Association*, 266 (1991): 1321.

31. National Center for Health Statistics, *Health United States, 1991,* Table 50.

32. Murray Campbell, "Insidious legacy of neglect," *Globe and Mail*, 7 June 1991.

33. For example, R.H. Brook et al., "Diagnosis and treatment of coronary disease: comparison of doctors' attitudes in the U.S.A. and the U.K.," *Lancet*, Vol. i (1988): 750–53; W.A. Knaus et al., "A comparison of intensive care in the U.S.A. and in France," *Lancet*, Vol. ii (1982): 642–46.

34. R.G. Hughes, S.S. Hunt, H.S. Luft, "Effects of surgeon volume and hospital volume on quality of care in hospitals," *Medical Care*, 25 (1987): 489–503.

35. K.C. Goldberg et al., "Racial and community factors influencing coronary artery bypass graft surgery rates for all 1986 medicare patients," *Journal of the American Medical Association*, 267 (1992): 1473–77; M.B. Wenneker, J.S. Weissman, A.M. Epstein, "The association of payer with utilization of cardiac procedures in Massachusetts," *Journal of the American Medical Association*, 264 (1990): 1255–60.

36. G.M. Anderson et al., "Use of coronary artery bypass surgery in the United States and Canada," *Journal of the American Medical Association*, 269 (1993): 1661–66.

37. G.T. Christakis et al., "The changing pattern of coronary artery bypass surgery," *Circulation*, 80 (supplement 1) (1989): 1151–61; C.D. Naylor, "Queuing for coronary surgery during a severe supply-demand mismatch in a Canadian referral centre: A case study of implicit rationing," Institute for Clinical Evaluative Sciences Working paper No. 1, Sunnybrook Hospital, Toronto.

38. M. Rachlis, J. Olak, C.D. Naylor, "The vital risk of delayed coronary surgery: Lessons from the randomized trials," *Iatrogenics*, 1 (1991): 103–11.

39. G. Christakis et al., "The changing pattern of coronary artery bypass surgery."

40. R. Mulgan, R.L. Logan, "The coronary bypass waiting list: a social evaluation," *New Zealand Medical Journal*, 103 (1990): 371–72; G. Dupuis et al., "The hidden costs of delayed bypass surgery," *Clinical Investigational Medicine*, 13 (supplement) (1990): C35(1).

41. R.G. Evans et al., "Controlling health expenditures—the Canadian reality."

42. Tracey Tyler, "11 delays for surgery killed man widow says," *Toronto Star*, 3 January 1989; Kelly Toughill, "Man, 62, died of heart attack waiting for cardiac operation," *Toronto Star*, 15 October 1989; Matt Maychak, "Wait for surgery was fatal for husband, widow says," *Toronto Star*, 10 November 1988.

43. Rod Mickleburgh, "Cronkite report on surgery delays challenged," *Globe and Mail*, 18 June 1991.

44. C.D. Naylor, "A different view of queues in Ontario," *Health Affairs*, 10 (1991): 110–28.

45. V.L. Kaminski, W.J. Sibbald, E.M. Davis, "Investigation of cardiac surgery at St. Michael's Hospital, Toronto, Ontario: Final Report," February 1989.

46. C.D. Naylor et al., "Revascularization Panel, Consensus Methods Group. Assessment of priority for coronary revascularization procedures," *Lancet*, 335 (1990): 1070–73; C.D. Naylor et al., "Assigning priority to patients requiring coronary revascularization: Consensus principles from a panel of cardiologists and cardiac surgeons," *Canadian Journal of Cardiology*, 7 (1991): 207–13.

47. Sandi Farran, "Rogers 'well' after heart surgery," *Toronto Star*, 12 August 1993.

48. B.G. Morgan, "Patient access to magnetic resonance imaging centers in Orange County, California," *New England Journal of Medicine*, 328 (1993): 884–85.

49. Ibid.

50. As quoted in L.L. Roos et al., "Health and Surgical outcomes in Canada and the United States," *Health Affairs*, 11(2) (1992): 56–72.

51. L.L. Roos et al., "Postsurgical mortality in Manitoba and New England," *Journal of the American Medical Association*, 263 (1990): 2453–58.

52. J.L. Rouleau et al., "A comparison of management patterns after acute myocardial infarction in Canada and the United States."

53. P. Braveman et al., "Adverse outcomes and lack of health insurance among newborns in an eight county area of California, 1982–1986," *New England Journal of Medicine*, 321 (1989): 508–13.

54. J.C. Javitt et al., *New England Journal of Medicine*, 325 (1991): 1418–22; A. Sommer et al., *New England Journal of Medicine*, 325 (1991): 1412–17.

55. J.W. Zylke, "Declining childhood immunization rates becoming cause for concern," *Journal of the American Medical Association*, 266 (1991): 1321.

56. E.E. Calle et al., "Demographic predictors of mammography and pap smear screening in U.S. women," *American Journal of Public Health*, 83 (1993): 53–60.

57. J. Hadley, E.P. Steinberg, J. Feder, *Journal of the American Medical Association*, 265 (1991): 374–79.

58. E. Moy, C. Hogan, "Access to needed follow-up services: Variations among different medicare populations," *Archives of Internal Medicine*, 153 (1993): 1815–23.

59. AFL-CIO Department of Employee Benefits, "The Permanent Replacement of Workers Striking over Health Care Benefits in 1990," June 1991.

60. Address by Ontario Premier Bob Rae to the Ontario Home Builders' Association, 12 January 1993. The New Democratic Party premier must have had his tongue well placed in his cheek when he made this comment since he has always advocated a single-payer plan for the U.S.

61. G.J. Scheiber, J.P. Poullier, L.M. Greenwald, "U.S. health expenditure performance: An international comparison and data update," *Health Care Financing Review*, 13(4) (1992): 1–88.

62. M. Drohan. "No easy cure for German health costs," *Globe and Mail*, 14 February 1994; B.L. Kirkman-Liff, "Physician payment and cost-containment strategies in West Germany: suggestions for medicare reform," *Journal of Health Politics, Policy and Law*, 15 (1990): 69–99.

63. V. Navarro, "Why some countries have national health insurance, and others have national health services, and the United States has neither," *International Journal of Health Services*, 19 (1989): 383–404.

64. T.R. Marmor, D. Boyum, "American medical care reform: Are we doomed to fail?" *Daedalus*, 121(4) (1992): 175–94.

65. W.K. Mariner, "Problems with employer-provided health insurance—the employee retirement income security act and health care reform," *New England Journal of Medicine*, 327 (1992): 1682–85.

66. "Common Cause. Why the United States does not have a national health program: The medical industry complex and its PAC contributions to congressional candidates January 1, 1981, through June 30, 1991," *International Journal of Health Services*, 22 (1992): 619–44.

67. In the United States, the Hill-Burton Act of 1946 (The Hospital Survey and Construction Act). In Canada, the National Health Grants Program of 1948.

68. Paul Starr, *The Social Transformation of American Medicine* (New York: Basic Books, 1982): 285.

69. Ibid.

70. "Hence, the decision which Canadians have to make ... is whether they wish to pay $1.020 million ... in 1971 for a programme administered by the insurance industry, or $837 million for a programme administered by government agencies.
"In our opinion it would be ... uneconomic ... to spend an extra $193 million.... We must choose the most frugal method ... which we know from our hospital insurance experience is equally efficient." Royal Commission on Health Services, 1964.

71. See Paul Starr, *The Social Transformation of American Medicine*, for comment by Taft.

72. S.M. Lipset, *Continental Divide: The Values and Institutions of the United States and Canada* (New York: Routledge, 1990).

73. V. Navarro, "Why some countries have national health insurance, and others have national health services, and the United States has neither"; H. Taylor, U.E. Reinhardt, "Does the system fit?" *Health Management Quarterly*, 1991, third quarter: 2–10.

74. J.B. Benear, letter in the *New England Journal of Medicine*, 327 (1992): 1101. Dr. Benear, who is from Tulsa, Oklahoma, writes regarding an article on primary care in Canada: "Perhaps some of the problems in the U.S. system relative to the systems in other nations arise from tremendous differences in societies. I suspect that the characters of Canadian, British, and German society and perhaps even Japanese society are more similar to each other than any of them is to ours."

75. D.M. Fox, "Policy and politics of research," *Journal of Health, Politics, Policy and Law*, 15 (1990): 481–99.
76. H. Taylor, U.E. Reinhardt, "Does the system fit?"
77. Dashiell Hammett, *The Dain Curse* (Toronto: Vintage Books, 1972).
78. Anon., "Notes and Comments," *New Yorker*, 20 April 1992: 29–30.
79. R. Voelker, "Is reform coverage really universal?" *Journal of the American Medical Association*, 270 (1993): 2663 ff.

CHAPTER 8

1. Hon. M. Lalonde, *A New Perspective on the Health of Canadians* (Ottawa: Health and Welfare Canada, 1974).
2. Hon. S.A. Miller, *White Paper on Health Policy* (Winnipeg: Government of Manitoba, 1972): 7.
3. Hon. Jake Epp, *Achieving Health for All: A Framework for Health Promotion* (Ottawa: House of Commons Canada, 1986); *The Report of the Ontario Panel on Health Goals* (Chair, Dr. Robert Spasoff) (Toronto: Government of Ontario, 1987); *Future Directions for Health Care in Saskatchewan—Report of the Saskatchewan Commission on Directions in Health Care* (Chair, Dr. R. G. Murray) (Regina: Government of Saskatchewan, 1990); *The Rainbow Report: Our Vision of Health. Report of the Premier's Commission on Future Health Care for Albertans* (Chair, Mr. Lou Hyndman) (Edmonton: Government of Alberta, 1990); *Report of the British Columbia Royal Commission on Health Care and Costs* (Chair, Mr. Justice Peter Seaton) (Victoria: Government of British Columbia, 1991); *The First Report of the Standing Committee on Health and Welfare, Social Affairs, Seniors and the Status of Women* (Chair, Mr. Bob Porter, MP) (Ottawa: House of Commons Canada, 1991); *Report of Ontario Health Review Panel* (Chair, Dr. John Evans) (Toronto: Government of Ontario, 1987); *Report of the Commission of Inquiry into Health and Social Services* (Chair, Dr. Jean Rochon) (Quebec, 1988); *Report of the Commission on Selected Health Care Programs* (Co-chairs, Mr. E. Neil McKelvey and Sister Bernadette Levesque) (Fredericton, 1989), *The Report of the Nova Scotia Royal Commission on Health Care* (Chair: Ms. Camille Gallant) (Halifax, 1990); *The Report of the P.E.I. Task Force on Health* (Chair: Dr. D.W. Cudmore) (Charlottetown, 1992). Manitoba Health, *Quality Health for Manitobans: The Action Plan* (Winnipeg, 1992). There have been various reports on Newfoundland over the years, including the *Report on the Reduction of Hospital Services*, Lucy Dobbin Consulting Services (St. John's, 1993).
4. *Report of Ontario Health Review Panel* (Chair, Dr. John Evans) (Toronto: Government of Ontario, 1987).
5. C. Lindblom, "The science of muddling through," *Public Administration Review*, 19 (1959): 79-99.
6. Ontario Government, "Managing Health Care Resources: Meeting Ontario's Priorities," supplementary paper to 1992 budget (Toronto: Government of Ontario, 1992).
7. G. Palmer, S.D. Short, *Health care and public policy—an Australian analysis* (Melbourne: McMillan Company of Australia, 1989): 257.
8. R.R. Alford, *Health Care Politics: Ideological and Interest Group Barriers to Reform* (Chicago: University of Chicago Press, 1975).
9. There are some small nursing homes and labs and drug companies. This analysis, however, applies to the larger and more powerful ones.
10. R.R. Alford, *Health Care Politics: Ideological and Interest Group Barriers to Reform*.
11. In fact, much of the monopoly was created through the closure of rival schools. See B. Ehrenreich, D. English, *For Her Own Good: 150 Years of Experts' Advice to Women* (Garden City, New York: Anchor Books, 1979); Paul Starr, *The Social Transformation of American Medicine* (New York: Basic Books, 1982).

12. As quoted in *Report of the Task Force on the Implementation of Midwifery in Ontario* (Chair, Mary Eberts) (Toronto: Government of Ontario, 1987): 197.

13. *Globe and Mail*, 11 May 1989.

14. K. Dunn, "Wonder why complaints about MDs seem to get nowhere?" *Montreal Gazette*, 3 November 1992.

15. There is some evidence that aggressive use of cholesterol-lowering drugs may, in fact, reduce the plaque in coronary arteries. For example, see D.H. Blankenhorn et al., "Beneficial effects of combined colestipol-niacin therapy on coronary atherosclerosis and coronary venous bypass grafts," *Journal of the American Medical Association*, 257 (1987): 32-33; G. Brown et al., "Regression of coronary artery disease as a result of intensive lipid lowering therapy in men with high levels of apolipoprotien B (FATS)," *New England Journal of Medicine*, 323 (1990): 1289.

16. D. Ornish et al., "The lifestyle heart trial," *Lancet*, 326 (1990): 129.

17. Dr. Ornish has funding to attempt replication of his study in six U.S. sites. See "Lifestyle changes still cut risk of heart disease," *The Medical Post*, 23 November 1993.

18. In 1986 Health and Welfare Canada estimated the cost of treating coronary heart disease at $1.04 billion, excluding the costs of physicians' care (likely another $100 to $200 million).

19. Modified from J. Lomas, "Research and the health policy process: A Canadian perspective," in *Proceedings of the Second Annual Conference of the Centre for Health Economics and Policy Analysis*, ed. C. Fooks (Hamilton: McMaster University, 1989).

20. M.G. Taylor, *Health Insurance and Canadian Public Policy* (Montreal: McGill-Queen's University Press, 1978): 371.

21. World Bank, *World Development Report 1992: Development and the Environment, World Development Indicators* (New York: Oxford University Press, 1992).

22. C.H. Weiss, "Ideology, Interests and Information," Chapter 9 in *Ethics, the Social Sciences, and Policy Analysis*, eds: D. Callahan and B. Jennings, (New York: Plenum Press, 1983): 221-45; D.A. Stone, "Facts," Chapter 13 in *Policy Paradox and Political Reason* (New York: HarperCollins, 1988): 249-64.

23. J. Lomas, "Finding audiences, changing beliefs: the structure of research use in Canadian health policy," *Journal of Health Politics, Policy and Law*, 15 (1990): 525-42.

24. P. Sabatier, "Knowledge, policy-oriented learning, and policy change," *Knowledge: Creation, Diffusion, Utilization*, 8 (1987): 649-92.

25. Justice Emmett Hall, *Canada's National-Provincial Health Program for the 1980s* (Ottawa: Health and Welfare Canada, 1980); R. Plain, "Charging the Sick—observations on the economic aspects of medical-social policy reforms," in *Medicare, the Decisive Year*, proceedings of the Canadian Centre for Policy Alternatives (Ottawa: CPA, 1984).

26. E.W. Barootes, "The role of Saskatchewan in government sponsored health care: a retrospective view," *Annals of the Royal College of Physicians and Surgeons of Canada*, 24 (1991): 117-19.

27. T.R. Marmor, J.B. Christianson, *Health Care Policy: A Political Economy Approach* (Beverly Hills: Sage Publishers, 1982).

28. The state of Oregon used a public process to priorize the benefits covered by Medicaid, the state's health insurance program for the poor. It began by assessing community values, and then ranked condition and treatment pairs according to community values and the scientific evidence of cost-effectiveness. The state had established a firm budget for the Medicaid program, and of the 700 treatments priorized, only 565 remained as benefits Medicaid would cover. Lisa Priest, "Canada eyeing Oregon plan," *Toronto Star*, 18 September 1993; J.W. Fiscus, "State legislature finally approves Oregon health plan," *Medical Post*, 24 August 1993.

29. D. Lett, "Care at risk nurses claim," *Winnipeg Free Press*, 20 September 1993; F. Russell, "Government defeats its own arguments on health care," *Winnipeg Free Press*, 10 July 1993.

30. From a speech by Dennis Timbrell, President, Ontario Hospital Association, October 1993.

31 K. Dunn, "Home care exhausting to older women," *Montreal Gazette*, 12 April 1993.

32. L. Charbonneau, "Particular medical activities all the rage," *Medical Post*, 2 November 1993.

33. Personal communication with Michael Decter, 2 February 1994.

34. Personal communication with Employment and Immigration Canada, 21 December 1993.

35. From 47,633 to 15,011 for psychiatric hospitals and from 844 to 5,836 in general hospitals. D. Wasylenki, P. Goering, E. MacNaughton, "Planning mental health services: background and key issues," *Canadian Journal of Psychiatry*, 37 (1992): 199-206.

36. Ibid. In 1994, Alberta announced plans for a similar commission.

37. C.E. Lindblom, "Still muddling, not yet through," *Public Administration Review*, 39 (1979): 517-36.

CHAPTER 9

1. See: Saskatchewan Health Services Utilization and Research Commission, *Long-Term Care in Saskatchewan, Final Report*, (Saskatoon: January 1994).

2. Dr. Robert Kane, an expert in geriatric research from the University of Minnesota's School of Public Health, notes that some of the replication sites had great difficulty signing up participants. This might reflect the need for better marketing of the program to its intended target group, but Dr. Kane also believes there are a number of factors associated with On Lok's successful programming that may be hard to reproduce in other settings. For example, one of the major barriers to getting a program like On Lok up and running is that participants have to agree to use the doctors employed by the program. Also, On Lok operates an affordable apartment project on one of its sites, meaning that for about fifty of its participants, a trip to the day centre is as close as a ride in an elevator. This obviously saves on transportation costs, and the prospect of more affordable housing is likely an added incentive for poorer participants to join the program. Furthermore, Kane points out that the San Francisco program mainly serves a Chinese population, and he wonders if there are some cultural reasons why On Lok's program arrangements work as well as they do. For example, he asks how many American-born elderly people would really want to come into a day centre for social and health-related activities rather than getting most of their needs seen to at home? As for the excellent clinical care participants receive, Dr. Kane notes that a significant number of On Lok's personnel had professional training in China but are unable to work as professionals in the United States.

3. The results of the randomized controlled trial showed that participants in Beth Abraham's Comprehensive Care Management program, versus those in the control groups, used 32 percent fewer hospital days and 75 percent fewer nursing home days. *New York Doctor*, June 1992.

4. Toronto Hospital news release, 2 June 1993.

5. S. Martinusen et al., "Comparison of cefoxitin and ceftizoxime in a hospital therapeutic interchange program," *Canadian Medical Association Journal*, 148 (1993): 1161-69.

6. J. Wasson et al., "Telephone care as a substitute for routine clinic follow-up," *Journal of the American Medical Association*, 267 (1992): 1788-93.

7. L.I. Stein, "The doctor-nurse game," *Archives of General Psychiatry*, 16 (1967): 699-703; L.I. Stein, D.T. Watts, T. Howell, "The doctor-nurse game revisited," *New England Journal of Medicine*, 322 (1990): 546-49.

8. W.A. Knaus et al., "An evaluation of outcome from intensive care in major medical centres," *Annals of Internal Medicine*, 104 (1986): 410-18.

9. D. Osborne, T. Gaebler, *Re-inventing Government: How the Entrepreneurial Spirit is Transforming the Public Sector* (New York: Penguin Books, 1993).

10. There is no uniform understanding of terms like regionalization, decentralization, deconcentration, and devolution.The following represents our working definition of the terms. *Decentralization*: the transfer of authority *or* ministry personnel to regional or community levels. *Deconcentration*: the transfer of ministry personnel to regional or community levels. *Devolution*: the transfer of planning, management, or budgetary authority to regional or community levels. A. Mills et al., *Health System Decentralization: Concepts, Issues and Country Experience* (Geneva: World Health Organization, 1990).

The difficulty in defining terms has resulted in a further ambiguity concerning several key issues involved in regionalization:

1. What are the purposes of regionalization?
2. What roles do the provinces, regions, and communities play?
3. How are the regions and communities funded?

11. The CMA Working Group on Regionalization and Decentralization, *The Language of Health System Reform* (Ottawa: Canadian Medical Association, 1993); A. Mills et al., *Health System Decentralization: Concepts, Issues and Country Experience* (Geneva: World Health Organization, 1990).

12. Consultative Council on Medical and Allied Services, *Interim Report on the Future Provision of Medical and Allied Services* (London: His Majesty's Stationery Office, 1920).

13. Ontario Premier's Council on Health Strategy, *Towards Health Outcomes: Goals 2 and 4, objectives and targets* (Toronto, 1991); Government of New Brunswick, *Toward a Comprehensive Health Strategy: Health 2000 Vision, Principles and Goals* (Fredericton, 1989); Nova Scotia Provincial Health Council, *Toward Achieving Nova Scotia's Health Goals: An Initial Plan of Action for Health Care Reform* (Halifax, December 1992); Quebec Ministry of Health and Social Services, *The Policy on Health and Well-being* (Quebec City, 1992).

14. K. Liu et al., "International infant mortality rankings: A look behind the numbers," *Health Care Financing Review*, 13(2) (1992): 105-18; J.C. Bailor, E.M. Smith, "Progress against cancer?" *New England Journal of Medicine*, 314 (1986): 1226-32; J.C. Bailor, "Cancer in Canada: Recent trends in mortality," *Chronic Diseases in Canada*, 13(6) (supplement) (1992): S2-S8; L. Goldman, E.F. Cook, "The decline in ischemic heart disease mortality rates: An analysis of the comparative effects of medical interventions and changes in lifestyle," *Annals of Internal Medicine*, 101 (1984): 825-36.

15. This taxonomy was first suggested by Professor Stephen Birch and his colleagues at McMaster University.

16. D.D. Rutstein et al., "Measuring the quality of medical care: A clinical method," *New England Journal of Medicine*, 294 (1976): 582-88.

17. Ibid.

18. D.D. Rutstein et al., "Measuring the quality of medical care: Second revision of tables of indexes," *New England Journal of Medicine*, 302 (1980): 1146; J.R.H. Charlton et al., "Geographical variation in mortality from conditions amenable to medical intervention in England and Wales," *Lancet*, Vol. i (1983): 691-96; S. Woolhandler et al., "Medical care and mortality: Racial differences in preventable deaths," *International Journal of Health Services*, 15 (1985): 1-11; K. Poikolainen, J. Eskola, "The effect of health services on mortality: Decline in death rates from amenable and non-amenable causes in Finland," *Lancet*, Vol. i (1986): 199-202; J.R.H. Charlton, R. Velez, "Some international comparisons of mortality amenable to medical intervention," 292 (1986): 295-301; J.P. Mackenbach, M.H. Bouvier-Colle, E. Jougla, " 'Avoidable' mortality and health services: A review of aggregate data studies," *Journal of Epidemiology and Community Health*, 44

(1990): 106-11; J.P. Mackenbach, "Health care expenditures and mortality from amenable conditions in the European Community," *Health Policy*, 19 (1991): 245-55.

19. For example, see C. Gray, "Practice guidelines often ignored," *Ontario Medicine*, 8 November 1993.

20. T.J. Montague et al., "Changes in acute myocardial infarction risk and patterns of practice for patients older and younger than 70 years, 1987-90," *Canadian Journal of Cardiology*, 8 (1992): 596-600.

21. R.B. Saltman, C. von Otter, *Planned Markets and Public Competition: Strategic Reform in Northern Health Systems* (Philadelphia: Open University Press, 1992): 27-29.

22. A. McGuire, "Measuring performance in the health care sector: the whys and the hows," in *The Challenges of Medical Practice Variations*, eds: F. Anderson, G. Mooney (MacMillan Press, 1990).

23. I. Vohlonen, M. Pekurinen, R.B. Saltman, "Re-organizing primary medical care in Finland: the personal doctor program," *Health Policy*, 13 (1989): 65-79.

24. A.L. Siu et al., "A fair approach to comparing quality of care," *Health Affairs*, 10(1) (1991): 62-75; A.L. Siu et al., "Choosing quality of care measures based on expected impact of improved care on health," *Health Services Research*, 27 (1992): 619-50.

25. C. Hertzman, A. Ostry, H. Heacock, *Developing health status indicators from routinely collected data. A report for the British Columbia Royal Commission on Health Care and Costs* (Vancouver, 1991). There are some statistical limitations to interpreting the study because of low numbers of certain events. However, the Coast Garibaldi health unit rate had statistically significantly higher death rates and the Vancouver unit had statistically significantly lower rates than the provincial average.

26. Hospital Medical Records Institute, "Hospital utilization reporting project—Final project report," Toronto, 5 November 1992.

27. In the development of our model we are indebted to R.B. Saltman, C. von Otter, *Planned Markets and Public Competition: Strategic Reform in Northern Health Systems* (Philadelphia: Open University Press, 1992).

A slightly different version of public competition was suggested in the mid-1980s by some Canadians. See G.L. Stoddart, J.R. Seldon, "Publicly financed competition in Canadian health care delivery: A proposed alternative to increased regulation?" in *Proceedings of the Second Canadian Conference on Health Economics: A Silver Anniversary Appraisal*, ed. J.A. Boan (Regina: University of Regina, 1983): 121-43; J.M. Muldoon, G.L. Stoddart, "The potential contribution of a competitive approach to controlling health care expenditures for a hypothetical community: A simulation model," in *Proceedings of the Third Canadian Conference on Health Economics*, ed. J.M. Horne (Winnipeg: University of Manitoba, 1987).

28. Personal communication with Terry Kaufman, executive director, CLSC Notre Dame De Grâce.

29. M. Rachlis, C. Kushner, *Second Opinion: What's Wrong with Canada's Health Care System and How to Fix It* (Toronto: HarperCollins, 1989): 277–280.

30. S. Birch et al., "A needs-based approach to resource allocation in health care," *Canadian Public Policy*, 19(1) (1993): 68-85; J. Eyles, S. Birch, "A population needs-based approach to health-care resource allocation and planning in Ontario: a link between policy goals and practice," *Canadian Journal of Public Health*, 84 (1993): 112-17; S. Birch, S. Chambers, "To each according to need: a community-based approach to allocating health care resources," *Canadian Medical Association Journal*, 149 (1993): 607-12.

31. N.P. Roos et al., "Assessing the relationship between health care use and the health of the population: seeking levers for policy makers," paper delivered to the Honda Foundation Discoveries Symposium, Toronto, 16-18 October 1993.

32. Ibid.

33. B. Jarman, "Underprivileged areas: validation and distribution of scores," *British Medical Journal*, 289 (1984): 1587-92. See also "Is the Jarman score better than

social class at assessing the need for prevention and primary care?" *Family Practice*, 5 (1988): 105-10.

34. J. Abelson, J. Lomas, "Do health service organizations and community health centres have higher disease prevention and health promotion levels than fee-for-service practices?" *Canadian Medical Association Journal*, 142 (1990): 575-81.

35. B. Hutchison et al., "Effect of a financial incentive to reduce hospital utilization in capitated primary care practice," working paper 94-1, Centre for Health Economics and Policy Analysis, McMaster University, Hamilton.

36. Ontario Ministry of Health, "New Beginnings: Draft Discussion Paper on the Review of the HSO Program," February 1991; Jeff Brooke, "HSOs—the future of health care," *Medical Post*, 9 March 1993.

37. See A. Hirschman, *Exit, Voice, and Loyalty* (Cambridge, MA: Harvard University Press, 1970).

38. Some good principles for policy-oriented boards can be found in Dr. John Carver's book, *Boards that Make a Difference: A New Design for Leadership in Nonprofit and Pubic Organizations* (San Francisco: Josey-Bass Publishers, 1990).

39. John Stuart Mill, *Representative Government* (1861).

CHAPTER 10

1. N. Hall et al., "Randomized trial of a health promotion program for frail elders," *Canadian Journal on Aging*, 11 (1992): 72-91; C. Hendriksen, E. Lund, E. Stromgard, "Consequences of assessment and intervention among elderly people: a three year randomized controlled trial," *British Medical Journal*, 289 (1984): 1522-24; N.J. Vetter, D.A. Jones, C.R. Victor, "Effect of health visitors working with elderly patients in general practice: a randomised controlled trial," *British Medical Journal*, 288 (1984): 369-72; M.S. John Pathy et al., "Randomized trial of case finding and surveillance of elderly people at home," *Lancet*, 340 (1992): 890-93; J. Wasson, C. Gaudette, F. Whaley, "Telephone care as a substitute for routine clinic follow-up," *Journal of the American Medical Association*, 267 (1992): 1788-93.

2. College of Family Physicians of Canada, "Position Paper on Alternate Payment Mechanisms," July 1992.

3. "Well-controlled" was considered to be a diastolic reading of <90mm Hg and "fair control" was considered to be 90–99 mmHg. The mean blood pressure of the hypertensive patients fell from 186/110 to 146/84.

4. J.T. Hart et al., "Twenty five years of case finding and audit in a socially deprived community," *British Medical Journal*, 302 (1991): 1509-13.

5. S.L. Kark, *The practice of community-oriented primary care* (New York: Appleton-Century-Crofts, 1989).

6. D.M. Pringle, "Nursing practice in the home: the Role of the Victorian Order of Nurses," in *Canadian Nursing Faces the Future*, eds A.J. Baumgart, J. Larsen (Toronto: C.V. Mosby Co., 1988).

7. The data are from the United States medicare program but are probably fairly applicable to Canada. See J.D. Lubitz, G.F. Riley, "Trends in payments in the last year of life," *New England Journal of Medicine*, 328 (1993): 1092-96. E.J. Emanuel, L.L. Emanuel, "The economics of dying: The illusion of cost savings at the end of life," *New England Journal of Medicine*, 330 (1994): 540-44. Emanuel and Emanuel claim that about 6 percent of total health care costs could be saved by better use of patient choice about health care. However, their methods are somewhat conservative and the difference could easily be 10 percent of overall health care expenditures.

8. D.W. Malloy, G.H. Guyatt, "A comprehensive health care directive in a home for the aged," *Canadian Medical Association Journal*, 145 (1991): 307-11; D.W. Malloy et al., "Two years experience with a comprehensive health care directive in a home

for the aged," *Annals of the Royal College of Physicians and Surgeons of Canada,* 25 (1992): 433-36.

9. L.I. Stein, "The doctor-nurse game," *Archives of General Psychiatry,* 16 (1967): 699-703.

10. L.I. Stein, D.T. Watts, T. Howell, "The doctor-nurse game revisited," 322 (1990): 546-49.

11. S.J. Weiss, H P Davis, "Validity and reliability of the collaborative practice scales," *Nursing Research,* 34 (1985): 299-305.

12. Statistics Canada information for 1992. For community (public) health—6,425 full-time, 2,775 part-time, 660 not stated. For home care—4,311 full-time, 2,381 part-time, 209 not stated. For physicians' offices/family practice—2,541 full-time, 2,898 part-time, 157 not stated.

13. B. Ehrenreich, D. English, *For Her Own Good: 150 Years of Experts' Advice to Women* (Garden City, New York: Anchor Books, 1979).

14. T.L. Halbert et al., "Population-based health promotion: A new agenda for public health nurses," *Canadian Journal of Public Health,* 84 (1993): 243-45.

15. For a recent "horror story" of poor discharge planning, see H. Henderson, "Did health system contribute to Rose's painful death?" *Toronto Star,* 5 February 1994.

16. Remarks of Mary Jean Gallagher on the Windsor-Essex County's "Win/Win in Health," 27 January 1994.

17. J. Lomas, "Finding Audiences, Changing Beliefs: the structure of research use in Canadian health policy," *Journal of Health Politics, Policy and Law,* 15 (1990): 3.

18. D. Ornish et al., "The Lifestyle Heart Trial," *Lancet,* 326 (1990): 129-33.

19. Ibid.

20. H. Yki-Jarvihen, "Pathogenesis of non-insulin dependent diabetes mellitus," *Lancet,* 343 (1994): 91-95.

21. P. Manga et al., *The Effectiveness and Cost-effectiveness of Chiropractic Management of Low Back Pain* (Toronto: Kenilworth Publishers, 1993); P.G. Shekelle et al., "Spinal manipulation for low-back pain," *Annals of Internal Medicine,* 117(7) (1992): 590-98.

22. N. Frasure-Smith, R. Prince, "The ischemic heart disease life stress monitoring program: Impact on mortality," *Psychosomatic Medicine,* 47 (1985): 431-45; N. Frasure-Smith, R. Prince, "Long-term follow-up of the ischemic heart disease life stress monitoring program," *Psychosomatic Medicine,* 51 (1989): 485-513; N. Frasure-Smith, "In hospital symptoms of psychological stress as predictors of long-term outcome after acute myocardial infarction in men," *The American Journal of Cardiology,* 67 (1991): 121-27.

CHAPTER 11

1. Manitoba Health, Education, and Social Policy Subcommittee of Cabinet, *White Paper on Health Policy,* 1972.

2. M.M. Rachlis, C. Kushner, *Second Opinion: What's Wrong with Canada's Health Care System and How to Fix It* (Toronto: HarperCollins, 1989): 326.

3. *Preserving Universal Medicare, A Government of Canada Position Paper,* 1983.

4. Monique Bégin, *Medicare: Canada's Right to Health* (Montreal: Optimum Publishing International, 1984): 195.

5. *Ontario Medicine,* 23 November 1993.

6. Ibid.

7. The Kaiser-Permanente health maintenance organization (HMO) system in the United States administers routine questionnaires to a random sample of all in-patients and out-patients.

8. Assuming collaborative primary care practices based on family physician-nurse teams serving between 1,000 and 2,000 patients (depending on the needs and location of

patients being seen), the system would need 12,000 to 24,000 new primary care nurses, with increases in home care and other community nursing positions to likely 50,000 full-time positions. There are currently 24,000 full-time and another 20,000 part-time community nurses including public health, home nursing, physicians' offices, etc.

9. *Globe and Mail*, 27 April 1992.

10. Assuming few plumbers would make less than $25 per hour, with a 37.5-hour week and time-and-one-half for overtime. We also understand that most plumbers cannot *choose* to work fifty hours per week and most doctors can.

11. According to the Ontario Health Insurance Plan, in 1992-93 the average gross Medicare billing by family doctors (with billings of at least $30,000) was $188,000. With a 40 percent overhead, the average family doctor would net $113,000. Ontario family doctors with more than five years' experience working in community health centres make $120,000 plus extensive benefits. Some work 37-hour weeks with limited call. Others work 50-plus hours doing obstetrics and taking frequent calls. Doctors working for sessional fees in family planning clinics make over $50 per hour. Doctors in Ontario have historically earned more than those in most other provinces. By contrast, in Quebec, where doctors make less than their counterparts anywhere in North America, CLSC family doctors with more than five years' experience earn about $77,000 for a 35-hour week.

12. *Toronto Star*, 14 September 1992.

13. B.C. Ministry of Health, "A Report on the Health of British Columbians, Provincial Health Officer's Annual Report, 1992."

14. The Commission studied large hospitals and small ones separately, but the results were similar. The reports are: "Barriers to Community Care" and "Preliminary Report on Base, Regional, and Large Community Hospitals in Saskatchewan."

15. *Globe and Mail*, 1 June 1993.

16. D. Osborne, T. Gaebler, *Reinventing Government: How the Entrepreneurial Spirit is Transforming the Public Sector* (New York: Penguin Books, 1992).

17. *Medical Post*, 24 August 1993.

18. M. Rachlis, C. Kushner, *Second Opinion: What's Wrong with Canada's Health Care System and How to Fix It* (Toronto: HarperCollins, 1989).

19. B. Checkoway, M. Doyle, "Community organizing lessons for health care consumers," *Journal of Health, Politics, Policy, and Law*, 5 (1980): 213-26; B. Checkoway, "The empire strikes back: More lessons for health care consumers," *Journal of Health Politics, Policy, and Law*, 7 (1982): 111-27; M. O'Neill, "Community participation in Quebec's health system: A strategy to curtail community empowerment?" *International Journal of Health Services*, 22 (1992): 287-301.

20. Australian National Health Strategy, "Healthy Participation: Achieving greater public participation and accountability in the Australian health care system," Background Paper No. 12 (Canberra, Australia, March 1993).

21. Government of Ontario, *Redirection of Long-Term Care and Support Services in Ontario, Ministry of Health and Ministry of Community and Social Services, and the Office of Seniors Issues* (Toronto: Queens Park, 1991).

22. Government of Ontario, *Strategies for Change, Ministry of Health and Ministry of Community and Social Services* (Toronto: Queen's Park, 1990).

23. Senior Citizens' Alliance for Long-Term Care Reform, Public Hearings Paper, November 1991.

24. Jane Aronson, "Are we really listening? Beyond the official discourse on the needs of old people," *Canadian Social Work Review*, 9(1) (1992): 73-87.

25. Senior Citizens' Consumer Alliance for Long-Term Care Reform, Consumer Report on Long-Term Care Reform—advance copy, June 1992.

26. Government of Ontario, *Partnerships in Long-Term Care: A New Way to Plan, Manage and Deliver Service and Community Support; A Policy Framework, Ministry of Health, Ministry of Community and Social Services, Ministry of Citizenship*, April 1993.

27. Senior Citizens' Alliance on Long-Term Care Reform, Consumer Response to the Ontario Government's Long-Term Care Reform Policies, October 1993.

28. CUPE's policy papers covered the following topics: 1) where the money comes from; 2) the shift to community care; 3) health care restructuring—a union response; 4) Total Quality Management: reorganizing health care work; 5) the Americanization of health care; 6) an uncertain future.

29. Price Waterhouse consultant Neil Stuart derived this estimate from data presented in: Price Waterhouse Management Consultants, "Operational Review of the Ontario Home Care Program," Toronto, 1989.

30. C. Fooks, M. Rachlis, C. Kushner, "Concepts of Quality of Care: National survey of five self-regulating health professions in Canada," *Quality Assurance in Health Care*, 2 (1990): 89-109.

31. M. Quinn, "Nurse practitioners instead of MDs: An uncharted idea ready to fly," *Family Practice*, 15 November 1993.

32. Michael O'Reilly, "Hospitals apply business techniques in attempt to cut cost of delivering care," *Canadian Medical Association Journal*, 149 (1993): 1718. We would like to see organized medicine feeling a sense of ownership for quality issues but we would like to see doctors develop a more collaborative approach with other professions and with administrators.

33. British Columbia Medical Association, *Info/Board*, Report of June 3–4/92 board meeting.

34. Gary Gibson, "Doctors must choose the way to go," *Globe and Mail*, 18 June 1993.

35. Gary Gibson, "The troops are ready. Are the leaders?" *Canadian Medical Association Journal*, 149(6) (1993): 863-64.

36. R. Klein, "Dimensions of rationing: who should do what?" *British Medical Journal*, 307 (1993): 309-11.

37. Jane Jacobs, *Systems of Survival: A Dialogue on the Moral Foundations of Commerce and Politics* (New York: Random House, 1993).

38. M. Rachlis, C. Kushner, *Second Opinion: What's Wrong with Canada's Health Care System* (Toronto: HarperCollins, 1989): Chapter 6.

39. Lisa Priest, *Toronto Star*, 30 January 1994.

40. The Organization for Economic Cooperation and Development, *Measuring Health Care 1960-1983: Expenditures, Costs, and Performance* (Paris: OECD, 1985): 117; E. Vayda, W.R. Mindell, I.M. Rutkow, "A decade of surgery in Canada, England and Wales, and the United States," *The Archives of Surgery*, 117 (1982): 846-53; W.R. Mindell, E. Vayda, B. Cardillo, "Ten-year trends in Canada for selected operations," *Canadian Medical Association Journal*, 127 (1982): 123-27; E. Vayda et al., "Five-year study of surgical rates in Ontario's counties," *Canadian Medical Association Journal*, 131 (1984): 111-15; Working Group on Quality Assurance and Effectiveness in Health Care, *Report to the Conference of Deputy Ministers of Health* (Ottawa: Health and Welfare Canada and Statistics Canada, 1990).

41. For example, Margaret Wente did a column: "The Odds On Winning the Surgical Lottery—Women," 6 November 1993; L. Erichs, "Who's to blame for so many mastectomies?" *Family Practice*, 6 December 1993.

42. Letters to *Ontario Medicine*, 13 December 1993.

43. This does not mean we have no criticisms of the Saskatchewan record. We do. In particular we object to the cuts made to the province's drug benefits program and the failure to make the government's plan for a comprehensive labour adjustment strategy mandatory in every district. Even so, most of what is happening in Saskatchewan is very exciting.

Index